# Complementary and Alternative Medicine

# SOURCEBOOK

*Sixth Edition*

## Health Reference Series

*Sixth Edition*

# Complementary and Alternative Medicine SOURCEBOOK

*Basic Consumer Health Information about Ayurveda, Acupuncture, Aromatherapy, Chiropractic Care, Diet-Based Therapies, Guided Imagery, Herbal and Vitamin Supplements, Homeopathy, Hypnosis, Massage, Meditation, Naturopathy, Pilates, Reflexology, Reiki, Shiatsu, Tai Chi, Traditional Chinese Medicine, Yoga, and Other Complementary and Alternative Medical Therapies*

*Along with Statistics, Tips for Selecting a Practitioner, Treatments for Specific Health Conditions, a Glossary of Related Terms, and a Directory of Resources for Additional Help and Information*

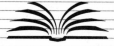

## OMNIGRAPHICS

615 Griswold, Ste. 901, Detroit, MI 48226

Bibliographic Note

Because this page cannot legibly accommodate all the copyright notices, the Bibliographic Note portion of the Preface constitutes an extension of the copyright notice.

\* \* \*

OMNIGRAPHICS

Angela L. Williams, *Managing Editor*

\*\*\*

Copyright © 2018 Omnigraphics

ISBN 978-0-7808-1632-9
E-ISBN 978-0-7808-1633-6

Library of Congress Cataloging-in-Publication Data

Names: Omnigraphics, Inc., issuing body.

Title: Complementary and alternative medicine sourcebook: basic consumer health information about ayurveda, acupuncture, aromatherapy, chiropractic care, diet-based therapies, guided imagery, herbal and vitamin supplements, homeopathy, hypnosis, massage, meditation, naturopathy, pilates, reflexology, reiki, shiatsu, tai chi, traditional chinese medicine, yoga, and other complementary and alternative medical therapies; along with statistics, tips for selecting a practitioner, treatments for specific health conditions, a glossary of related terms, and a directory of resources for additional help and information.

Description: Sixth edition. | Detroit, MI: Omnigraphics, [2018] | Series: Health reference series | Includes bibliographical references and index.

Identifiers: LCCN 2018015924 (print) | LCCN 2018017284 (ebook) | ISBN 9780780816336 (eBook) | ISBN 9780780816329 (hardcover: alk. paper)

Subjects: LCSH: Alternative medicine--Popular works.

Classification: LCC R735 (ebook) | LCC R735.C66 2018 (print) | DDC 610--dc23

LC record available at https://lccn.loc.gov/2018015924

# Table of Contents

## Part II: Alternative Medicine Systems

## Part III: Dietary Supplements

## Part IV: Biologically Based Therapies

## Part V: Mind-Body Medicine

## Part VI: Manipulative and Body-Based Therapies

## Part VII: Energy-Based Therapies

## Part VIII: Alternative Treatments for Specific Diseases and Conditions

## Part IX: Additional Help and Information

# *Preface*

## *About This Book*

Complementary and alternative medicine (CAM) therapies play a key role in the healthcare of many Americans. The National Center for Complementary and Integrative Health (NCCIH) reports that in the United States, approximately 38 percent of adults (about 4 in 10) and approximately 12 percent of children (about 1 in 9) are using some form of CAM. These alternative therapies, alone or in conjunction with mainstream medicines, are often used to treat an increasing variety of diseases and conditions, such as arthritis, anxiety, back pain, cancer, diabetes, heart disease, and sleep problems.

*Complementary and Alternative Medicine Sourcebook, Sixth Edition* provides updated information for people considering these therapies for general well-being or specific health conditions. It discusses how to select a CAM practitioner, talk with a primary healthcare provider about using CAM, evaluate information on the internet, and pay for CAM therapies. It describes whole medical systems, such as Ayurveda, traditional Chinese medicine, Native American medicine, acupuncture, homeopathy, and naturopathy. It also talks about the safe use of dietary supplements, including vitamins, minerals, and herbs. Information on biologically based therapies, mind-body medicine, manipulative and body-based therapies, and energy-based therapies is also included. A glossary of related terms and a directory of additional resources provide additional help and information.

## How to Use This Book

This book is divided into parts and chapters. Parts focus on broad areas of interest. Chapters are devoted to single topics within a part.

*Part I: An Overview of Complementary and Alternative Medicine (CAM)* defines CAM, identifies common therapies, use of CAM in the United States, and answers questions consumers often have about choosing a CAM practitioner and paying for treatments. Statistics on CAM use in specific populations, including women, children. and the elderly, is also included, along with tips on avoiding health fraud and spotting Internet scams.

*Part II: Alternative Medicine Systems* describes whole medical systems practiced in cultures throughout the world that evolved separately from conventional medicine as it is practiced in the United States. These include Ayurvedic medicine and their product caution, traditional Chinese medicine, Native American medicine, acupuncture, acupuncture for cancer, homeopathy and their product caution, and naturopathy.

*Part III: Dietary Supplements* identifies vitamins, minerals, herbs and botanicals, and other food and dietary substances taken to improve health or nutrition. Readers will also find tips on ensuring supplement safety and selecting specific products to support bone and joint health, immune system functioning, mood regulation, probiotics supplements for gastrointestinal health, and weight loss efforts, sports and energy supplements, using dietary supplements wisely, fraudulent in dietary supplements.

*Part IV: Biologically Based Therapies* discusses CAM practices that strive to enhance or improve health using substances found in nature. This part highlights biologically based techniques including apitherapy, aromatherapy and essential oils, and diet-based therapies such as detoxification diets, fasting, popular fad diets, Gerson therapy, and vegetarianism.

*Part V: Mind-Body Medicine describes CAM* techniques that focus on using the mind to improve health or reduce unwanted symptoms, such as biofeedback, deep breathing, guided imagery and hypnosis, meditation, prayer and spirituality, relaxation training, tai chi and qi gong, and yoga. In addition, readers will find information about practices focused on healing via creative expression in art, music, and dance.

*Part VI: Manipulative and Body-Based Therapies* offers information about the Alexander technique aquatic therapy, massage therapy, chiropractic care, craniosacral therapy, Feldenkrais method, and kinesiotherapy, pilates, reflexology, lymphatic drainage, massage therapy, rolfing structural integration, tui na, and other CAM therapies that involve movement or manipulation of one or more parts of the body.

*Part VII: Energy-Based Therapies* discusses CAM therapies that encourage healing through the manipulation of energy fields such as feng shui, shiatsu, reiki, polarity therapy, therapeutic therapy, and magnet therapy.

*Part VIII: Alternative Treatments for Specific Diseases and Conditions* highlights scientific research of CAM therapies for treating arthritis, asthma, cancer, chronic pain, cognitive decline, diabetes, fibromyalgia, headache, hepatitis, low-back pain, menopausal symptoms, seasonal allergies, and sleep disorders. The use of CAM for treating mental health problems, including anxiety and addiction, is also discussed.

*Part IX: Additional Help and Information* provides a glossary of important terms related to complementary and alternative medicine. A directory of organizations that provide information to consumers about complementary and alternative therapies is also included.

## *Bibliographic Note*

This volume contains documents and excerpts from publications issued by the following government agencies: Administration for Children and Families (ACF); Federal Trade Commission (FTC); National Cancer Institute (NCI); National Center for Complementary and Integrative Health (NCCIH); National Endowment for the Arts (NEA); National Heart, Lung, and Blood Institute (NHLBI); National Institute of Environmental Health Sciences (NIEHS); National Institutes of Health (NIH); *NIH News in Health*; Office of Dietary Supplements (ODS); Office on Women's Health (OWH); Substance Abuse and Mental Health Services Administration (SAMHSA); U.S. Bureau of Labor Statistics (BLS); U.S. Department of Agriculture (USDA); U.S. Department of Health and Human Services (HHS); U.S. Department of Veterans Affairs (VA); U.S. Food and Drug Administration (FDA); and U.S. National Library of Medicine (NLM).

It may also contain original material produced by Omnigraphics and reviewed by medical consultants.

## *About the* Health Reference Series

The *Health Reference Series* is designed to provide basic medical information for patients, families, caregivers, and the general public. Each volume takes a particular topic and provides comprehensive coverage. This is especially important for people who may be dealing with a newly diagnosed disease or a chronic disorder in themselves or in a family member. People looking for preventive guidance, information about disease warning signs, medical statistics, and risk factors for health problems will also find answers to their questions in the *Health Reference Series*. The *Series*, however, is not intended to serve as a tool for diagnosing illness, in prescribing treatments, or as a substitute for the physician/patient relationship. All people concerned about medical symptoms or the possibility of disease are encouraged to seek professional care from an appropriate healthcare provider.

## *A Note about Spelling and Style*

*Health Reference Series* editors use *Stedman's Medical Dictionary* as an authority for questions related to the spelling of medical terms and the *Chicago Manual of Style* for questions related to grammatical structures, punctuation, and other editorial concerns. Consistent adherence is not always possible, however, because the individual volumes within the *Series* include many documents from a wide variety of different producers, and the editor's primary goal is to present material from each source as accurately as is possible. This sometimes means that information in different chapters or sections may follow other guidelines and alternate spelling authorities. For example, occasionally a copyright holder may require that eponymous terms be shown in possessive forms (Crohn's disease vs. Crohn disease) or that British spelling norms be retained (leukaemia vs. leukemia).

## *Medical Review*

Omnigraphics contracts with a team of qualified, senior medical professionals who serve as medical consultants for the *Health Reference Series*. As necessary, medical consultants review reprinted and originally written material for currency and accuracy. Citations including the phrase, "Reviewed (month, year)" indicate material reviewed by this team. Medical consultation services are provided to the *Health Reference Series* editors by:

Dr. Vijayalakshmi, MBBS, DGO, MD
Dr. Senthil Selvan, MBBS, DCH, MD
Dr. K. Sivanandham, MBBS, DCH, MS (Research), PhD

## *Our Advisory Board*

We would like to thank the following board members for providing initial guidance on the development of this series:

- Dr. Lynda Baker, Associate Professor of Library and Information Science, Wayne State University, Detroit, MI

- Nancy Bulgarelli, William Beaumont Hospital Library, Royal Oak, MI

- Karen Imarisio, Bloomfield Township Public Library, Bloomfield Township, MI

- Karen Morgan, Mardigian Library, University of Michigan-Dearborn, Dearborn, MI

- Rosemary Orlando, St. Clair Shores Public Library, St. Clair Shores, MI

## Health Reference Series *Update Policy*

The inaugural book in the *Health Reference Series* was the first edition of *Cancer Sourcebook* published in 1989. Since then, the *Series* has been enthusiastically received by librarians and in the medical community. In order to maintain the standard of providing high-quality health information for the layperson the editorial staff at Omnigraphics felt it was necessary to implement a policy of updating volumes when warranted.

Medical researchers have been making tremendous strides, and it is the purpose of the *Health Reference Series* to stay current with the most recent advances. Each decision to update a volume is made on an individual basis. Some of the considerations include how much new information is available and the feedback we receive from people who use the books. If there is a topic you would like to see added to the update list, or an area of medical concern you feel has not been adequately addressed, please write to:

Managing Editor
*Health Reference Series*
Omnigraphics
615 Griswold, Ste. 901
Detroit, MI 48226

# Part One

# An Overview of Complementary and Alternative Medicine (CAM)

# Chapter 1

# *What Is Complementary and Alternative Medicine (CAM)?*

"Complementary and alternative medicine" (CAM) is the term for medical products and practices that are not part of standard medical care.

- **Standard medical care** is medicine that is practiced by health professionals who hold an M.D. (medical doctor) or D.O. (doctor of osteopathy) degree. It is also practiced by other health professionals, such as physical therapists, physician assistants, psychologists, and registered nurses. Standard medicine may also be called biomedicine or allopathic, Western, mainstream, orthodox, or regular medicine. Some standard medical care practitioners are also practitioners of CAM.

- **Complementary medicine** is treatments that are used along with standard medical treatments but are not considered to be standard treatments. One example is using acupuncture to help lessen some side effects of cancer treatment.

This chapter contains text excerpted from the following sources: Text in this chapter begins with text excerpted from "Complementary and Alternative Medicine," National Cancer Institute (NCI), April 10, 2015; Text beginning with the heading "Complementary versus Alternative," is excerpted from "Complementary, Alternative, or Integrative Health: What's in a Name?" National Center for Complementary and Integrative Health (NCCIH), National Institute of Health (NIH), March 2015.

- **Alternative medicines** are treatments that are used instead of standard medical treatments. One example is using a special diet to treat cancer instead of anticancer drugs that are prescribed by an oncologist.

- **Integrative medicine** is a total approach to medical care that combines standard medicine with the CAM practices that have shown to be safe and effective. They treat the patient's mind, body, and spirit.

## Are CAM Approaches Safe?

Some CAM therapies have undergone careful evaluation and have found to be safe and effective. However, there are others that have been found to be ineffective or possibly harmful. Less is known about many CAM therapies, and research has been slower for a number of reasons:

- Time and funding issues
- Problems finding institutions and cancer researchers to work with on the studies
- Regulatory issues

CAM therapies need to be evaluated with the same long and careful research process used to evaluate standard treatments. Standard cancer treatments have generally been studied for safety and effectiveness through an intense scientific process that includes clinical trials with large numbers of patients.

## Natural Does Not Mean Safe

CAM therapies include a wide variety of botanicals and nutritional products, such as dietary supplements, herbal supplements, and vitamins. Many of these "natural" products are considered to be safe because they are present in, or produced by, nature. However, that is not true in all cases. In addition, some may affect how well other medicines work in your body. For example, the herb St. John's wort, which some people use for depression, may cause certain anticancer drugs not to work as well as they should.

Herbal supplements may be harmful when taken by themselves, with other substances, or in large doses. For example, some studies have shown that kava kava, an herb that has been used to help with stress and anxiety, may cause liver damage.

Vitamins can also have unwanted effects in your body. For example, some studies show that high doses of vitamins, even vitamin C, may affect how chemotherapy and radiation work. Too much of any vitamin is not safe, even in a healthy person.

Tell your doctor if you're taking any dietary supplements, no matter how safe you think they are. This is very important. Even though there may be ads or claims that something has been used for years, they do not prove that it's safe or effective.

Supplements do not have to be approved by the federal government before being sold to the public. Also, a prescription is not needed to buy them. Therefore, it's up to consumers to decide what is best for them.

The National Cancer Institute (NCI) and the National Center for Complementary and Integrative Health (NCCIH) are currently sponsoring or cosponsoring various clinical trials that test CAM treatments and therapies in people. Some study the effects of complementary approaches used in addition to conventional treatments, and some compare alternative therapies with conventional treatments.

## Complementary versus Alternative

Many Americans—more than 30 percent of adults and about 12 percent of children—use healthcare approaches developed outside of mainstream Western, or conventional, medicine. When describing these approaches, people often use "alternative" and "complementary" interchangeably, but the two terms refer to different concepts:

- If a nonmainstream practice is used **together with** conventional medicine, it's considered "complementary."

- If a nonmainstream practice is used **in place of** conventional medicine, it's considered "alternative."

True alternative medicine is uncommon. Most people who use nonmainstream approaches use them along with conventional treatments.

## Integrative Medicine

There are many definitions of "integrative" healthcare, but all involve bringing conventional and complementary approaches together in a coordinated way. The use of integrative approaches to health and wellness has grown within care settings across the United States. Researchers are currently exploring the potential benefits of integrative health in a variety of situations, including pain management for military personnel and veterans, relief of symptoms in cancer patients and survivors, and programs to promote healthy behaviors.

## *Integrative Approaches for Pain Management for Military Personnel and Veterans*

Chronic pain is a common problem among active-duty military personnel and veterans. NCCIH, the U.S. Department of Veterans Affairs, and other agencies are sponsoring research to see whether integrative approaches can help. For example, NCCIH-funded studies are testing the effects of adding mindfulness meditation, self-hypnosis, or other complementary approaches to pain management programs for veterans. The goal is to help patients feel and function better and reduce their need for pain medicines that can have serious side effects.

## *Integrative Approaches for Symptom Management in Cancer Patients and Survivors*

Cancer treatment centers with integrative healthcare programs may offer services such as acupuncture and meditation to help manage symptoms and side effects for patients who are receiving conventional cancer treatment. Although research on the potential value of these integrative programs is in its early stages, some studies have had promising results. For example, NCCIH-funded research has suggested that:

- Cancer patients who receive integrative therapies while in the hospital have less pain and anxiety.

- Massage therapy may lead to short-term improvements in pain and mood in patients with advanced cancer.

- Yoga may relieve the persistent fatigue that some women experience after breast cancer treatment.

## *Integrative Approaches and Health-Related Behaviors*

Healthy behaviors, such as eating right, getting enough physical activity, and not smoking, can reduce people's risks of developing serious diseases. Can integrative approaches promote these types of behaviors? Researchers are working to answer this question. Preliminary research suggests that yoga and meditation-based therapies may help smokers quit, and NCCIH-funded studies are testing whether adding mindfulness-based approaches to weight control programs will help people lose weight more successfully.

## So, What Terms Does NCCIH Use?

The NCCIH generally uses the term "complementary health approaches" when discussing practices and products of nonmainstream origin. The NCCIH uses "integrative health" when talking about incorporating complementary approaches into mainstream healthcare.

## Types of Complementary Health Approaches

Most complementary health approaches fall into one of two subgroups—natural products or mind and body practices.

### Natural Products

This group includes a variety of products, such as **herbs** (also known as botanicals), **vitamins** and **minerals**, and **probiotics**. They are widely marketed, readily available to consumers, and often sold as dietary supplements.

According to the 2012 National Health Interview Survey (NHIS), which included a comprehensive survey on the use of complementary health approaches by Americans, 17.7 percent of American adults had used a dietary supplement other than vitamins and minerals in the past year. These products were the most popular complementary health approach in the survey. The most commonly used natural product was fish oil.

Researchers have done large, rigorous studies on a few natural products, but the results often showed that the products didn't work. Research on others is in progress. While there are indications that some may be helpful, more needs to be learned about the effects of these products in the human body and about their safety and potential interactions with medicines and other natural products.

### Mind and Body Practices

Mind and body practices include a large and diverse group of procedures or techniques administered or taught by a trained practitioner or teacher. The 2012 NHIS showed that **yoga, chiropractic and osteopathic manipulation, meditation**, and **massage therapy** are among the most popular mind and body practices used by adults. The popularity of yoga has grown dramatically in recent years, with almost twice as many U.S. adults practicing yoga.

Other mind and body practices include **acupuncture, relaxation techniques** (such as breathing exercises, guided imagery, and

7

progressive muscle relaxation), **tai chi**, **qi gong**, **healing touch**, **hypnotherapy**, and **movement therapies** (such as Feldenkrais method, Alexander technique, Pilates, Rolfing Structural Integration, and Trager psychophysical integration).

The amount of research on mind and body approaches varies widely depending on the practice. For example, researchers have done many studies on yoga, spinal manipulation, and meditation, but there have been fewer studies on some other practices.

### Other Complementary Health Approaches

• The two broad areas discussed above—natural products and mind and body practices—capture most complementary health approaches. However, some approaches may not neatly fit into either of these groups—for example, the practices of **traditional healers**, **Ayurvedic medicine**, **traditional Chinese medicine (TCM)**, **homeopathy**, and **naturopathy**.

# Chapter 2

# *The Use of CAM in the United States*

## *National Health Interview Survey (NHIS) Highlights*

- In 2012, 33.2 percent of U.S. adults used complementary health approaches.

- 11.6 percent of U.S. children age 4–17 used complementary health approaches in 2012. There was no meaningful change from 2007 when 12.0 percent used them.

- In 2012, as in 2007 and 2002, the most commonly used complementary approach was natural products (dietary supplements other than vitamins and minerals). 17.7 percent of adults and 4.9 percent of children age 4–17 used natural products.

- Pain—a condition for which people often use complementary health approaches—is common in U.S. adults. More than half had some pain during the 3 months before the survey.

- U.S. adults who take natural products (dietary supplements other than vitamins and minerals) or who practice yoga were more likely to do so for wellness reasons than for treating a

This chapter includes text excerpted from "Use of Complementary Health Approaches in the U.S.," National Center for Complementary and Integrative Health (NCCIH), September 24, 2017.

specific health condition. In contrast, people who use spinal manipulation more often do so for treatment reasons rather than wellness.

- About 59 million Americans spend money out-of-pocket on complementary health approaches, and their total spending adds up to $30.2 billion a year.

- In 2012, 60 percent of the National Health Interview Survey (NHIS) respondents who used chiropractic care had at least some insurance coverage for it, but rates were much lower for acupuncture (25%) and massage (15%).

## Key Facts about Adults

### Natural Products

- Fish oil was the number one natural product among adults, with 7.8 percent using it in 2012.

- Adult use of fish oil, probiotics or prebiotics, and melatonin increased.

- Adult use of glucosamine/chondroitin, echinacea, and garlic decreased.

- Although dietary supplement users were twice as likely to report wellness rather than treatment as a reason for taking supplements, fewer than 1 in 4 reported reduced stress, better sleep, or feeling better emotionally as a result of using dietary supplements.

### Mind and Body Approaches

- The mind and body approaches most commonly used by adults include yoga, chiropractic or osteopathic manipulation, meditation, and massage therapy.

- The percentage of adults who practice yoga has increased substantially, to 9.5 percent in 2012.

- More than 85 percent of U.S. adults who used yoga perceived reduced stress as a result of practicing yoga.

- Nearly two-thirds of adult yoga users reported that as a result of practicing yoga they were motivated to exercise more regularly, and 4 in 10 reported they were motivated to eat healthier.

- Adult yoga users were more likely to affirm feeling better emotionally than users of dietary supplements or spinal manipulation as a result of using that approach.

- More than 60 percent of U.S. adults using spinal manipulation reported doing so to treat a specific health condition, and more than 50 percent did so for general wellness-related reasons.

### Pain

- About 25 million adults (11.2%) have daily pain—i.e., they reported that they had pain every day in the 3 months before the survey.

- Adults with more severe pain had worse health, used more healthcare, and had more disability than those with less severe pain.

## Key Facts about Children
### Natural Products

- Fish oil was the natural product most commonly used by children, with 1.1 percent using it in 2012.

- Melatonin was the second most natural product used by children in 2012.

### Mind and Body Approaches

- The mind and body approaches most commonly used by children include chiropractic or osteopathic manipulation, yoga, meditation, and massage therapy.

- Yoga has become more popular among children, just as it has among adults. 3.1 percent of U.S. children practiced yoga in 2012.

## Key Facts about Spending and Insurance

- Out-of-pocket spending for complementary health approaches represents 9.2 percent of all out-of-pocket spending on healthcare and 1.1 percent of total healthcare spending.

- In 2012, Americans spent $14.7 billion out-of-pocket on visits to complementary practitioners and $12.8 billion on natural products.

11

- Use rates for chiropractic, acupuncture, and massage among people who had no insurance coverage for these types of care increased, suggesting an increased willingness to pay out-of-pocket.

- In 2012, partial insurance coverage was more common than complete coverage for chiropractic care, acupuncture, and massage.

# Chapter 3

# *CAM Use and Children*

In the past, children were often excluded from research studies due to special protections, and findings from studies of adults were applied to children. Today, the National Institutes of Health (NIH) requires that children be included in all studies unless there are scientific and ethical reasons not to.

## *Patterns in the Use of Complementary Health Approaches for Children*

The National Health Interview Survey (NHIS) included a comprehensive survey on the use of complementary health approaches by almost 45,000 Americans, including more than 10,000 children aged 4–17. The survey found that 11.6 percent of the children had used or been given some form of complementary health product or practice, such as yoga or dietary supplements.

The most frequently used approaches for children were natural products (fish oil, melatonin, and probiotics), and chiropractic or osteopathic manipulation.

For children, complementary health approaches were most often used for back or neck pain, other musculoskeletal conditions, head or chest colds, anxiety or stress, attention deficit hyperactivity disorder (ADHD) or attention deficit disorder (ADD), and insomnia or trouble sleeping.

---

This chapter includes text excerpted from "Children and the Use of Complementary Health Approaches," National Center for Complementary and Integrative Health (NCCIH), March 2017.

Other studies show that children in the United States who use or are given complementary health approaches vary in age and health status. For example:

- Teens are particularly likely to use products that claim to improve sports performance, increase energy levels, or promote weight loss.

- Children with chronic medical conditions, including anxiety, musculoskeletal conditions, and recurrent headaches, are more likely than other children to use complementary health approaches, usually along with conventional care.

## What the Science Says about the Safety and Side Effects of Complementary Health Approaches for Children

- Dietary supplements result in about 23,000 emergency room visits every year. Many of the patients are young adults who come to the emergency room with heart problems from taking weight-loss or energy products. One-fifth of the visits are children, most of whom took a vitamin or mineral when unsupervised. (Child-resistant packaging isn't required for dietary supplements.)

- Some dietary supplements contain contaminants, including drugs, chemicals, or metals.

- Children's small size, developing organs, and immature immune system makes them more vulnerable than adults to having allergic or other adverse reactions to dietary supplements.

- Some products may worsen conditions. For example, since echinacea is a type of ragweed, people sensitive to ragweed may also react to echinacea.

- Do not rely on asthma products sold over-the-counter (OTC) and labeled as homeopathic, the U.S. Food and Drug Administration (FDA) warns. Homeopathic remedies and dietary supplements are not evaluated by the FDA for safety or effectiveness.

- Biofeedback, guided imagery, hypnosis, mindfulness, and yoga are some of the mind and body practices that have the best evidence of being effective for children for various symptoms (such as anxiety and stress) and are low-risk. However, spinal manipulation, a common complementary approach, is associated with rare but serious complications.

14

## More to Consider

- Make sure that you have received an accurate diagnosis from a licensed healthcare provider.

- Educate yourself about the potential risks and benefits of complementary health approaches.

- Ask your healthcare provider about the effectiveness and possible risks of approaches you're considering or already using for yourself.

- Do not replace or delay conventional care or prescribed medications with any health product or practice that hasn't been proven safe and effective.

- If a healthcare provider suggests a complementary approach, do not increase the dose or duration of the treatment beyond what is recommended (more isn't necessarily better).

- If you have any concerns about the effects of a complementary approach, contact your healthcare provider.

- As with all medications and other potentially harmful products, store dietary supplements out of the sight and reach of children.

- The National Center for Complementary and Integrative Health (NCCIH) website offers safety tips on dietary supplements and mind and body practices for children and teens.

- Tell all your healthcare providers about any complementary or integrative health approaches you use. Give them a full picture of what you do to manage your health. This will help ensure coordinated and safe care.

## Selecting a Complementary Health Practitioner

If you're looking for a complementary health practitioner for yourself, be as careful and thorough in your search as you are when looking for conventional care. Be sure to ask about the practitioners:

- Experience in coordinating care with conventional healthcare providers

- Experience in delivering care to children and adolescents

- Education, training, and license

15

# Chapter 4

# *CAM Use in Older Adults*

Many older adults are turning to complementary and integrative health approaches, often as a reflection of a healthy self-empowered approach to well-being. Natural products often sold as dietary supplements are frequently used by many older people for various reasons despite safety concerns or a lack of evidence to support their use. Although there is a widespread public perception that the botanical and traditional agents included in dietary supplements can be viewed as safe, these products can contain pharmacologically active compounds and have the associated dangers.

Mind and body practices, including relaxation techniques and meditative exercise forms such as yoga, tai chi, and qi gong are being widely used by older Americans, both for fitness and relaxation and because of perceived health benefits. A number of systematic reviews point to the potential benefit of mind and body approaches for symptom management, particularly for pain. However, research on these mind and body approaches is still hampered by methodological issues, including a lack of consensus on appropriate controls and lack of intervention standardization. While much of the clinical data is inconclusive, these approaches may help older adults maintain motivation to incorporate physical exercise into their regular activities.

---

This chapter includes text excerpted from "Complementary and Integrative Health for Older Adults," National Center for Complementary and Integrative Health (NCCIH), May 2, 2017.

17

## Complementary and Integrative Health for Older Adults

### Osteoarthritis (OA)

#### Mind and Body Practices for OA

In 2012, the American College of Rheumatology (ACR) issued recommendations for using pharmacologic and nonpharmacologic approaches for osteoarthritis (OA) of the hand, hip, and knee:

- The guidelines conditionally recommend tai chi, along with other nondrug approaches such as manual and thermal therapies, self-management programs, and walking aids, for managing knee OA.

- Acupuncture is also conditionally recommended for those who have chronic moderate-to-severe knee pain and are candidates for total knee replacement but are unwilling or unable to undergo surgical repair.

#### Acupuncture for OA

**The Evidence Base**

- The best evidence on the efficacy of acupuncture for OA consists of a few systematic reviews and one meta-analysis, as well as the 2012 ACR for pharmacologic and nonpharmacologic approaches for OA of the hand, hip, and knee, which conditionally recommend acupuncture for people with chronic moderate-to-severe knee pain and are candidates for total knee replacement but can't or won't undergo the procedure.

**Efficacy**

- A National Center for Complementary and Integrative Health (NCCIH)-funded review of meta-analyses and systematic reviews on acupuncture for chronic back pain, OA, and headache found that acupuncture generally appears better than standard care or waitlist controls for people with OA but may not provide additional benefit for people with OA who are receiving advice and exercise.

- In a systematic review of 10 randomized controlled trials of acupuncture for OA of the knee in 1,456 patients, the authors concluded that these studies provide evidence that acupuncture is an effective treatment for pain and physical dysfunction associated with OA of the knee.

- A 2010 systematic review of 16 trials of 3,498 patients examined the effects of acupuncture in OA in peripheral joints and found that although acupuncture, when compared to a sham treatment, showed statistically significant, short-term improvements in OA pain, the benefits were small and not clinically relevant. In contrast, acupuncture, when compared to a waiting list control, showed statistically significant and clinically relevant benefits in people with peripheral joint OA.

### Safety

- There are few complications associated with acupuncture, but adverse effects such as minor bruising or bleeding can occur; infections can result from the use of nonsterile needles or poor technique from an inexperienced practitioner.

*Massage for OA*

Although there has been much research on massage therapy for pain, there are very few studies that specifically examine the effects of massage therapy on OA symptoms.

### The Evidence Base

- The best evidence on the efficacy of massage therapy for OA comes from small randomized controlled trials. Very few studies have examined massage therapy for OA specifically.

### Efficacy

- Results of a randomized controlled trial of 68 adults with OA of the knee who received standard Swedish massage over 8 weeks demonstrated statistically significant improvements in pain and physical function.

### Safety

- Massage therapy appears to have few risks if it is used appropriately and provided by a trained massage professional.

*Tai Chi for OA*

### The Evidence Base

• The best evidence on the efficacy of tai chi consists of a few small randomized controlled trials, as well as the 2012 ACR guidelines for pharmacologic and nonpharmacologic approaches for OA of the hand, hip, and knee, which conditionally recommend tai chi, along with other nondrug approaches such as self-management programs and walking aids, for managing knee OA.

### Efficacy

• A prospective, single-blind, randomized controlled trial of 40 participants found that tai chi demonstrated significantly greater improvement in pain and physical function, as well as improvement in depression, self-efficacy, and quality of life.

### Safety

• Tai chi is considered to be a safe practice.

### Natural Products for OA

Glucosamine, chondroitin sulfate, or the combination

### The Evidence Base

• The evidence base on the effects of glucosamine and chondroitin sulfate for OA is of sufficient size and quality to permit independent systematic reviews and meta-analyses, and the inclusion of specific recommendations in independent clinical practice guidelines.

### Efficacy

• A Cochrane systematic review of 25 studies found evidence of improvement in pain and function in studies using one manufacturer's preparation of glucosamine, not in studies using preparations from other companies.

• Three reports from the National Institutes of Health (NIH)-funded Glucosamine/Chondroitin Arthritis Intervention Trial (GAIT) compared glucosamine, chondroitin sulfate, the two in combination, celecoxib, and placebo. There were no clinically significant differences in pain or function following 6 months and 2 years of treatment. There was also no evidence that glucosamine, chondroitin, or the combination could prevent the progression of OA, based on joint space width measurements.

- A meta-analysis considered 20 controlled clinical trials comparing chondroitin with placebo or n treatment in 3846 patients with OA of the hip or knee. The investigators concluded that "large-scale, methodologically sound trials indicate that the symptomatic benefit of chondroitin is minimal or nonexistent. Use of chondroitin in routine clinical practice should, therefore, be discouraged."

- A 2010 network meta-analysis analyzed 10 glucosamine and chondroitin trials involving 3,803 patients with knee or hip OA published similar results. The investigators concluded that glucosamine, chondroitin, or a combination did not significantly reduce pain or change joint space compared to placebo.

- A 2014 double-blind randomized placebo-controlled trial compared glucosamine, chondroitin, the combination, or placebo in 605 patients with knee OA. While symptomatic improvement was seen in all four groups over the study period, there were no differences in symptomatic improvement. A very small but statistically significant reduction in joint space narrowing was seen in the glucosamine–chondroitin combination group at 2 years.

**Safety**

Glucosamine and chondroitin appear to be relatively safe and well tolerated when used in suggested doses over a 2-year period. In a few specific situations, however, possible side effects or drug interactions should be considered:

- No serious side effects have been reported in large, well-conducted studies of people taking glucosamine, chondroitin, or both for up to 3 years. However, glucosamine or chondroitin may interact with warfarin.

- Although studies conducted by the U.S. Food and Drug Administration (FDA) show that high doses of glucosamine hydrochloride taken by mouth in rats may promote cartilage regeneration and repair, this dose was also found to cause severe kidney problems in the rats—a serious side effect of the treatment.

## Cognitive Decline and Alzheimer Disease (AD)

*Natural Products for Cognitive Decline and AD*

Although a few trials of natural products for the prevention of cognitive decline or dementia have shown some modest effects, direct evidence is lacking.

### The Evidence Base

- The evidence base on the efficacy of natural products for cognitive function and dementia, including AD, consists of many randomized controlled trials, particularly on omega-3 fatty acids and ginkgo biloba supplementation.

### Efficacy

- **Fish oil/Omega-3s.** Among the nutritional and dietary factors studied to prevent cognitive decline in older adults, the most consistent positive research findings are for omega-3 fatty acids, often measured as how much fish people consumed. However, a 2012 Cochrane review of three randomized controlled trials involving more than 3,500 participants concluded that available evidence shows no benefit of omega-3 supplementation on the cognitive functioning of older people without dementia.

- **Ginkgo.** The Ginkgo Evaluation of Memory (GEM) study, a 6-year trial of the well-characterized ginkgo supplement EGb-761 in more than 3,000 older adults, found that it didn't lower the incidence of dementia, including Alzheimer disease (AD), in older adults. Further analysis of the same data showed that ginkgo did not slow cognitive decline, lower blood pressure, or reduce the incidence of hypertension.

### Safety

- Omega-3 fatty acid supplements usually do not have negative side effects. When side effects do occur, they typically consist of minor gastrointestinal symptoms. Omega-3 supplements may extend bleeding time. People who take anticoagulants or nonsteroidal anti-inflammatory drugs should use caution.

- Side effects of ginkgo supplements may include a headache, nausea, gastrointestinal upset, diarrhea, dizziness, or allergic skin reactions. More severe allergic reactions have occasionally been reported. There are some data to suggest that ginkgo can increase bleeding risk.

## *Sleep Disorders*

### *Mind and Body Practices for Sleep Disorders*

**Relaxation techniques.** Relaxation techniques include progressive relaxation, guided imagery, biofeedback, self-hypnosis, and deep breathing exercises. The goal is similar in all: to consciously produce the body's natural relaxation response, characterized by slower breathing, lower blood pressure, and a feeling of calm and well-being. Relaxation techniques are also used to induce sleep, reduce pain, and calm emotions.

Evidence suggests that using relaxation techniques before bedtime can be helpful components of a successful strategy to improve sleep habits. Other components include maintaining a consistent sleep schedule; avoiding caffeine, alcohol, heavy meals, and strenuous exercise too close to bedtime; and sleeping in a quiet, cool, and dark room.

### The Evidence Base

- The best evidence on the efficacy of relaxation techniques for insomnia consists of independent systematic reviews and meta-analyses, and the inclusion of specific recommendations in independent clinical practice guidelines of the American Academy of Sleep Medicine (AASM).

### Efficacy

- A systematic review of 37 studies found evidence that psychological and behavioral therapies, including relaxation techniques, produced reliable changes in several sleep parameters of participants with primary insomnia or insomnia associated with medical and psychiatric conditions. Relaxation was one of five treatments that met criteria for empirically-supported psychological treatments for insomnia. This review was conducted by a task force commissioned by the AASM in order to update its practice parameters on psychological and behavioral therapies for insomnia.

- The accompanying practice parameter report published by the AASM concluded that several psychological and behavioral interventions, including relaxation training, stimulus control therapy, and cognitive behavioral therapy are effective, and recommended inclusion of at least one in initial treatment strategies for chronic primary and comorbid (secondary) insomnia.

- A meta-analysis of five randomized controlled trials evaluating the efficacy of music-assisted relaxation for sleep quality in adults found that music-assisted relaxation had moderate benefits.

### Safety

- Relaxation techniques are generally considered safe. There have been rare case reports of worsening of symptoms in people with epilepsy or certain psychiatric conditions, or with a history of abuse or trauma.

- Relaxation techniques are generally used as components of a treatment plan, and not as the only approach for potentially serious health conditions.

*Other Mind and Body Practices for Sleep Disorders*

### The Evidence Base

- The best evidence on the efficacy of mindfulness-based stress reduction, yoga, and massage therapy consists of clinical trials reports, mostly from small preliminary studies.

- While there have been many studies of acupuncture for insomnia, the evidence base suffers from trials of poor methodological quality, and high levels of publication bias and heterogeneity in study design.

### Efficacy

- A 2011 randomized trial involving 30 adults with primary chronic insomnia reported initial evidence that mindfulness-based stress reduction was comparable in effectiveness to eszopiclone by a variety of measures. The authors concluded that mindfulness-based stress reduction is a viable treatment for chronic insomnia.

- A 2013 randomized controlled trial evaluated the effect of mindfulness-based stress reduction on sleep quality in 336 Danish women with breast cancer. The investigators reported a small statistically significant improvement in sleep quality just after the intervention, but no long-term effect. An earlier uncontrolled study involving people with different types and stages cancer reported similar findings.

- A small 2012 trial evaluated the effects of yoga, passive stretching, or standard care on insomnia in 44 postmenopausal women in Brazil. The investigators found that participants in the yoga group had significantly lower posttreatment scores for insomnia, compared to the other two groups. They also reported significantly improved posttreatment scores for severity of climacteric symptoms, quality of life, and resistance phase of stress in the yoga group compared to control.

- A small 2011 study compared the effects of Chinese therapeutic massage (Tui na), passive movement, or control (not specified) in 44 postmenopausal women with insomnia in Brazil. The investigators reported evidence of improvements in subjective insomnia scores, as well as scores for anxiety, depression, and quality of life in the group of women treated with massage, compared to those in a passive movement or a control (treatment not specified) group.

- A 2012 Cochrane systematic review considered the evidence from 33 randomized trials of needle acupuncture, electroacupuncture, and acupressure for insomnia. The investigators found evidence that needle acupuncture (but not electroacupuncture) as an adjunct to other treatment might marginally increase the proportion of people with improved sleep quality. Overall they concluded that current evidence is not sufficiently rigorous to support or refute acupuncture for treating insomnia.

### Safety

- Meditation is considered to be safe for healthy people. There have been rare reports that meditation could cause or worsen symptoms in people who have certain psychiatric problems, but this question has not been fully researched. People with physical limitations may not be able to participate in certain meditative practices involving physical movement. Individuals with existing mental or physical health conditions should speak with their healthcare providers prior to starting a meditative practice and make their meditation instructor aware of their condition.

- Overall, clinical trial data suggest yoga, as taught and practiced in these research studies under the guidance of a skilled teacher, has a low rate of minor side effects. However, injuries from yoga, some of them serious, have been reported in the popular press. People with health conditions should work with an experienced teacher who can help modify or avoid some yoga poses to prevent side effects.

- Massage therapy appears to have few risks when performed by a trained practitioner. However, massage therapists should take some precautions with certain health conditions. In some cases, pregnant women should avoid massage therapy. Forceful and deep tissue massage should be avoided by people with conditions such as bleeding disorders or low blood platelet counts, and by people taking anticoagulants. Massage should not be done in any potentially weak area of the skin, such as wounds. Deep or intense pressure should not be used over an area where the patient has a tumor or cancer unless approved by the patient's healthcare provider.

- Acupuncture is generally considered safe when performed by an experienced practitioner using sterile needles. Reports of serious adverse events related to acupuncture are rare but include infections and punctured organs.

### Natural Products for Sleep Disorders

#### Melatonin

Melatonin is a hormone known to shift circadian rhythms. Current evidence suggests that melatonin may be useful in treating several sleep disorders, such as jet lag, delayed sleep phase disorder, and sleep problems related to shift work.

#### The Evidence Base

- The best evidence on the efficacy of melatonin for sleep disorders consists of several systematic reviews and meta-analyses, and the inclusion of recommendations in independent clinical practice guidelines of the AASM.

#### Efficacy

- A practice parameter report issued by the AASM includes the recommendation of melatonin supplements to promote daytime sleep among night shift workers. Studies that support this recommendation found that melatonin administration prior to daytime sleep after night work shifts improved daytime sleep quality and duration, and caused a shift in circadian phase in some but not all participants. It did not enhance alertness at night.

- The AASM guidelines also include the recommendation of melatonin supplements to reduce symptoms of jet lag and improve sleep following travel across multiple time zones. A Cochrane review supporting this recommendation assessed the effectiveness of oral melatonin for alleviating jet lag after air travel across several time zones and concluded that melatonin is remarkably effective in preventing or reducing jet lag, and that occasional short-term use appears to be safe.

- Adults and teens with delayed sleep disorder have trouble falling asleep before 2 a.m. and have trouble waking up in the morning. In a review, the authors suggested that a combination of melatonin supplements, a behavioral approach to delay sleep and wake times, and reduced evening light may even out sleep cycles in people with this disorder.

- A 2014 Cochrane review of three randomized controlled trials involving 209 people with moderate to severe dementia found no evidence that melatonin improved sleep.

- A 2013 meta-analysis of 19 randomized placebo-controlled trials involving 1863 participants with primary sleep disorders found evidence of small but statistically significant improvements in sleep onset latency, total sleep time, and overall sleep quality with melatonin use. These effects do not appear to dissipate with continued melatonin use. The investigators concluded that although the absolute benefit of melatonin compared to placebo is smaller than other pharmacological treatments for insomnia, melatonin may have a role in the treatment of insomnia given its relatively benign side-effect profile compared to these agents.

- A study of 170 participants with insomnia, aged 55 years or older, found that prolonged-release melatonin significantly improved quality of sleep and behavior following wakefulness (BFW), compared with placebo. The authors concluded that the improvements in quality of sleep and BFW were strongly correlated, suggesting a beneficial treatment effect on the restorative value of sleep.

## Safety

- Melatonin supplements appear to be relatively safe for short-term use, although modest adverse effects on mood were seen with melatonin use in elderly people (most of whom had dementia) in one study. The long-term safety of melatonin supplements has not been established.

- Melatonin can have additive effects with alcohol and other sedating medications, and older people should be cautioned about its use.

## *Menopausal Symptoms*

### *Mind and Body Practices for Menopausal Symptoms*

Overall, evidence suggests that some mind and body approaches, such as yoga, tai chi, and meditation-based programs may provide some benefit in reducing common menopausal symptoms.

### The Evidence Base

- The evidence base on the efficacy of mind and body practices for the symptoms of menopause consists of a few reviews of randomized controlled trials.

### Efficacy

- A 2010 review of 21 papers assessed mind and body therapies for menopausal symptoms. The researchers found that yoga, tai chi, and meditation-based programs may be helpful in reducing common menopausal symptoms including the frequency and intensity of hot flashes, sleep and mood disturbances, stress, and muscle and joint pain.

- A 2013 Cochrane review of 16 randomized controlled trials involving 1,155 women found that when acupuncture was compared with sham acupuncture, there was no evidence of a difference in their effect on hot flashes. However, when acupuncture was compared with no treatment, there appeared to be some benefit from acupuncture. Acupuncture was less effective than hormone therapy. The low quality of evidence and lack of control with sham acupuncture for some of the studies led the reviewers to conclude that there is insufficient evidence to determine whether acupuncture is effective for controlling menopausal vasomotor symptoms.

- A study funded by NCCIH found that hypnosis significantly improved various measures of hot flashes in a group of postmenopausal women. Although the mechanism of how clinical hypnosis works is unknown, the women in this same study who practiced hypnosis had significantly greater levels of satisfaction than the control group. An earlier study found that hypnosis appears to reduce perceived hot flashes in breast cancer survivors and may have additional benefits such as improved mood and sleep.

**Safety**

- Meditation is considered to be safe for healthy people. There have been rare reports that meditation could cause or worsen symptoms in people who have certain psychiatric problems, but this question has not been fully researched. People with physical limitations may not be able to participate in certain meditative practices involving physical movement. Individuals with existing mental or physical health conditions should speak with their healthcare providers prior to starting a meditative practice and make their meditation instructor aware of their condition.

- Overall, clinical trial data suggest yoga, as taught and practiced in these research studies under the guidance of a skilled teacher, has a low rate of minor side effects. However, injuries from yoga, some of them serious, have been reported in the popular press. People with health conditions should work with an experienced teacher who can help modify or avoid some yoga poses to prevent side effects.

- Tai chi is considered to be a safe practice.

- There are few complications associated with acupuncture, but adverse effects such as minor bruising or bleeding can occur; infections can result from the use of nonsterile needles or poor technique from an inexperienced practitioner.

*Natural Products for Menopausal Symptoms*

Many natural products have been studied for their effects on menopausal symptoms, but there is little evidence that they are useful. While some herbs and botanicals are often found in over-the-counter (OTC) formulas and combinations, many of these combination products have not been studied. Further, because natural products used for menopausal symptoms can have side effects and can interact with other botanicals or supplements or with medications, research in this area is addressing safety as well as efficacy.

*Black Cohosh (Actaea racemosa, Cimicifuga racemosa)*

### The Evidence Base

- The evidence base on the efficacy of black cohosh for menopausal symptoms consists of many randomized controlled trials and a 2012 Cochrane review.

### Efficacy

- A 2012 Cochrane systematic review on black cohosh for menopausal symptoms concludes that its efficacy has yet to be demonstrated.

- Other research suggests that black cohosh does not act like estrogen, as once was thought.

### Safety

- United States Pharmacopeia experts suggest that women should discontinue use of black cohosh and consult a healthcare practitioner if they have a liver disorder or develop symptoms of liver trouble, such as abdominal pain, dark urine, or jaundice.

- There have been several case reports of hepatitis, as well as liver failure, in women who were taking black cohosh. It is not known if black cohosh was responsible for these problems. Although these cases are very rare and the evidence is not definitive, there is concern about the possible effects of black cohosh on the liver.

## Benign Prostatic Hyperplasia (BPH)

*Natural Products for Benign Prostatic Hyperplasia (BPH)*

- Although several small studies have suggested a modest benefit of saw palmetto for treating symptoms of BPH, a large study evaluating high doses of saw palmetto and a Cochrane review found that saw palmetto was not more effective than placebo for treatment of urinary symptoms related to BPH.

### The Evidence Base

- The evidence base on the efficacy of saw palmetto (Serenoa repens) for benign prostatic hyperplasia consists of several randomized controlled trials and systematic reviews.

### Efficacy

- A 2011 double-blind, placebo-controlled, randomized trial in 369 older men demonstrated that saw palmetto extract administered at up to three times the standard daily dose (320 mg) did not reduce the urinary symptoms associated with BPH more than placebo. In addition, a Cochrane review of nine trials concluded that saw palmetto has not been shown to be more effective than placebo for this use.

### Safety

- Saw palmetto appears to be well tolerated by most users. It may cause mild side effects, including stomach discomfort.

## Age-Related Macular Degeneration (AMD)

### Natural Products for AMD

There is some evidence that natural products such as antioxidant vitamins and minerals may delay the development of advanced age-related macular degeneration (AMD) in people who are at high risk for the disease. However, other studies of vitamin E and beta-carotene supplementation did not show benefit in preventing the onset of AMD.

### The Evidence Base

- The evidence base on the efficacy of dietary supplements on preventing or slowing the progression of AMD consists of a few randomized controlled trials and a few systematic reviews.

### Efficacy

- **Antioxidant vitamins and mineral supplements.** The large NIH-sponsored trial, Age-Related Eye Disease Study (AREDS), which involved 3,640 older adults, found that supplementation with a combination of antioxidant vitamins (vitamins C and E and beta carotene) and zinc helped to prevent AMD from progressing from the intermediate stage to the advanced stage. However, a 2012 Cochrane review of four large, high quality randomized controlled trials involving 62,520 people found evidence that taking vitamin E and beta carotene supplements are unlikely to prevent the onset of AMD.

- **Antioxidants and zinc.** Another 2012 Cochrane review of 13 randomized controlled trials involving 6,150 participants found that supplementation with antioxidants and zinc may be of modest benefit in delaying the progression of AMD.

- **The dietary supplement of vitamins and zinc plus omega-3.** A follow-up study on supplements and AMD, AREDS2, indicated that supplements containing EPA and DHA did not slow the progression of AMD in people who were at high risk of developing the advanced stage of the disease.

- **Ginkgo biloba.** Two small randomized controlled trials have suggested beneficial effects of ginkgo biloba on vision, but a 2013 Cochrane review suggests that larger trials in longer duration are needed to provide a more robust measure of the effect of *ginkgo biloba* on AMD.

### Safety

- Although generally regarded as safe, vitamin supplements may have harmful effects, and clear evidence of benefit is needed before they can be recommended

- Omega-3s appear to be safe for most adults at low-to-moderate doses. The FDA has concluded that omega-3 dietary supplements from fish are "generally recognized as safe." Fish oil supplements may cause minor gastrointestinal upsets, including diarrhea, heartburn, indigestion, and abdominal bloating.

- Side effects of ginkgo supplements may include a headache, nausea, gastrointestinal upset, diarrhea, dizziness, or allergic skin reactions. More severe allergic reactions have occasionally been reported. There are some data to suggest that ginkgo can increase bleeding risk.

## Herpes Zoster (Shingles)

### Mind and Body Practices for Herpes Zoster

There have only been a few studies on the effects of tai chi on cell-mediated immunity to varicella-zoster virus following vaccination, but the results of these studies have shown some benefit. Other interventions such as acupuncture, cupping, neural therapy, and intravenous vitamin C (ascorbic acid) have been studied for their effects on the duration of neuropathic pain and postherpetic neuralgia due to herpes zoster, but these studies have been small.

### Tai Chi

**The Evidence Base**

- The evidence base on the efficacy of tai chi for shingles immunity and health functioning consists of only a few small randomized controlled trials.

**Efficacy**

- A randomized controlled trial in more than 100 healthy older adults found that those people who participated in a 16-week tai chi program had higher levels of cell-mediated immunity to varicella-zoster virus following shingles vaccination than those who received the same vaccine but participated in a health education program instead of tai chi.

**Safety**

- Tai chi is considered to be a safe practice.

# Chapter 5

# *Healthcare Providers and CAM*

## Chapter Contents

# Section 5.1

## *Selecting a CAM Practitioner*

This section contains text excerpted from the following sources: Text
in this section begins with excerpts from "6 Things to Know When
Selecting a Complementary Health Practitioner," National Center
for Complementary and Integrative Health (NCCIH), September 24,
2017; Text under the heading "Finding a Complementary Health
Practitioner" is excerpted from "How to Find a Complementary
Health Practitioner," National Center for Complementary and
Integrative Health (NCCIH), September 24, 2017.

If you're looking for a complementary health practitioner to help
treat a medical problem, it is important to be as careful and thorough
in your search as you are when looking for conventional care.

Here are six tips to help you in your search:

1. If you need names of practitioners in your area, first check
   with your doctor or another healthcare provider. A nearby
   hospital or medical school, professional organizations, state
   regulatory agencies or licensing boards, or even your health
   insurance provider may be helpful. Unfortunately, the
   National Center for Complementary and Integrative Health
   (NCCIH) cannot refer you to practitioners.

2. Find out as much as you can about any potential practitioner,
   including education, training, licensing, and certifications. The
   credentials required for complementary health practitioners
   vary tremendously from state to state and from discipline to
   discipline.

   Once you have found a possible practitioner, here are some
   tips about deciding whether he or she is right for you:

3. Find out whether the practitioner is willing to work together
   with your conventional healthcare providers. For safe,
   coordinated care, it's important for all of the professionals
   involved in your health to communicate and cooperate.

4. Explain all of your health conditions to the practitioner, and
   find out about the practitioner's training and experience in

36

working with people who have your conditions. Choose a practitioner who understands how to work with people with your specific needs, even if general well-being is your goal.

5.  Don't assume that your health insurance will cover the practitioner's services. Contact your health insurance provider and ask. Insurance plans differ greatly in what complementary health approaches they cover, and even if they cover a particular approach, restrictions may apply.

6.  Tell all your healthcare providers about the complementary approaches you use and about all practitioners who are treating you. Keeping your healthcare providers fully informed helps you to stay in control and effectively manage your health.

## Finding a Complementary Health Practitioner

The MedlinePlus Directories page (www.medlineplus.gov/directories.html) from the U.S. National Library of Medicine (NLM) lists organizations for some professions and provides links to directories of libraries and various types of health professionals, services, and facilities.

## Section 5.2

# Tips for Talking with Your Healthcare Providers about CAM

Text in this section begins with excerpts from "4 Tips: Start Talking with Your Health Care Providers about Complementary Health Approaches," National Center for Complementary and Integrative Health (NCCIH), September 24, 2017; Text under the heading "Patient Tips for Discussing CAM with Providers" is excerpted from "Time to Talk about CAM: Health Care Providers and Patients Need to Ask and Tell," National Center for Complementary and Integrative Health (NCCIH), June 4, 2015.

When patients tell their providers about their use of complementary health practices, they can better stay in control and more effectively

37

manage their health. When providers ask their patients, they can ensure that they are fully informed and can help patients make wise healthcare decisions.

Here are four tips to help you and your healthcare providers start talking:

1. **List the complementary health practices you use on your patient history form.** When completing the patient history form, be sure to include everything you use—from acupuncture to zinc. It's important to give healthcare providers a full picture of what you do to manage your health.

2. **At each visit, be sure to tell your providers about what complementary health approaches you are using.** Don't forget to include over-the-counter (OTC) and prescription medicines, as well as dietary and herbal supplements. Make a list in advance and take it with you. Some complementary health approaches can have an effect on conventional medicine, so your provider needs to know.

3. **If you are considering a new complementary health practice, ask questions.** Ask your healthcare providers about its safety, effectiveness, and possible interactions with medications (both prescription and nonprescription).

4. **Don't wait for your providers to ask about any complementary health practice you are using.** Be proactive. Start the conversation.

## Patient Tips for Discussing CAM with Providers

- When completing patient history forms, be sure to include all therapies and treatments you use. Make a list in advance.

- Tell your healthcare providers about all therapies or treatments including over-the-counter and prescription medicines, as well as dietary and herbal supplements.

- Take control. Don't wait for your providers to ask about your CAM use.

- If you are considering a new CAM therapy, ask your healthcare providers about its safety, effectiveness, and possible interactions with medicines (both prescription and over-the-counter).

# Chapter 6

# *Insurance Issues and Paying for CAM Treatment*

## Use of Complementary Health Approaches in the United States

Data from the 2012 National Health Interview Survey (NHIS) show that 33 percent of adults and almost 12 percent of children use complementary health approaches and that the most commonly used approach is natural products (dietary supplements other than vitamins and minerals). Fish oil is the natural product most often used by adults and children. As for mind and body practices, adults and children most often turn to chiropractic or osteopathic manipulation, yoga, meditation, and massage therapy.

### Out-of-Pocket Spending on Complementary Health Approaches

People seem to be willing to pay "out-of-pocket" (not through insurance) for certain complementary health approaches. In fact, out-of-pocket spending on these approaches for Americans age 4 and older

This chapter includes text excerpted from "Paying for Complementary and Integrative Health Approaches," National Center for Complementary and Integrative Health (NCCIH), March 19, 2018.

amounts to an estimated $30.2 billion per year, according to the 2012 NHIS. This includes:

- $14.7 billion out-of-pocket for visits to complementary and integrative health practitioners such as chiropractors, acupuncturists, and massage therapists

- $12.8 billion out-of-pocket on natural products

- About $2.7 billion on self-care approaches (homeopathic medicines and self-help materials, such as books or compact disks (CDs), related to complementary health topics)

This out-of-pocket spending for complementary health approaches represents 9.2 percent of all out-of-pocket spending by Americans on healthcare ($328.8 billion) and 1.1 percent of total healthcare spending ($2.82 trillion).

## *Insurance Coverage of Complementary Health Approaches*

Many Americans use complementary health approaches, but the type of health insurance they have affects their decisions to use these practices. In a study, researchers analyzed 2012 NHIS data on acupuncture, chiropractic, and massage. While use rates for all three approaches rose, the increase was much more pronounced among those who did not have health insurance. For those who had health insurance, coverage for these three approaches was more likely to be partial than full.

If you would like to use a complementary or integrative approach and don't know if your health insurance will cover it, you should contact your health insurance provider to find out.

Some questions to ask your insurance provider include:

- Is this complementary or integrative approach covered by my health condition?

- Does it need to be:
  - Preauthorized or preapproved?
  - Ordered by a prescription?

- Do I need a referral?

- Does coverage require seeing a practitioner in the network?

- Do I have coverage if I go out-of-network?

- Are there any limits and requirements—for example, on the number of visits or the amount you will pay?

- How much do I have to pay out-of-pocket?

Keep records about all contacts you have with your insurance company, including notes on calls and copies of bills, claims, and letters. This may help if you have a claim dispute.

If you're choosing a new health insurance plan, ask the insurance provider about coverage of complementary or integrative health approaches. You should find out if you need a special "rider" or supplement to the standard plan for these approaches to be covered. You should also find out if the insurer offers a discount program in which plan members pay for fees and products out-of-pocket but at a lower rate.

## Asking Practitioners about Payment

If you're planning to see a complementary or integrative practitioner, it's important to understand about payment. Here are some questions to ask:

- **Costs.** What does the first appointment cost? What do follow-up appointments cost? Is there a sliding scale based on income? How many appointments am I likely to need? Are there other costs (e.g., tests, equipment, supplements)?

- **Insurance.** Do you accept my insurance plan? What has been your experience with my plan's coverage for people with my condition? Do I file the claims, or do you take care of that?

## Federal Health Benefits Programs

The federal government helps with some health expenses of people who are eligible for federal health benefit programs, such as programs for veterans, people aged 65 and older (Medicare), and people who cannot afford healthcare (Medicaid, funded jointly with the states).

Information on Medicare and Medicaid is available from the Centers for Medicare & Medicaid Services (CMS). A handbook, *Medicare and You*, explains what services Medicare covers.

# Chapter 7

# *Evaluating Web-Based Health Resources*

## *Are You Reading News or Advertising?*

The Federal Trade Commission (FTC) has warned the public about fake online news sites. The site may look real but is actually an advertisement. The site may use the logos of legitimate news organizations or similar names and web addresses. To get you to sign up for whatever they're selling, they may describe an "investigation" into the effectiveness of the product. But everything is fake: there is no reporter, no news organization, and no investigation. Only the links to a sales site are real. Fake news sites have promoted questionable products, including acai berry for weight loss, work at home opportunities, and debt reduction plans.

You should suspect that a news site may be fake if it:

- Endorses a product. Real news organizations generally don't do this.

- Only quotes people who say good things about the product

- Presents research findings that seem too good to be true. (If something seems too good to be true, it usually is.)

---

This chapter includes text excerpted from "Finding and Evaluating Online Resources," National Center for Complementary and Integrative Health (NCCIH), January 2018.

43

- Contains links to a sales site

- Includes only positive reader comments and you can't add a comment of your own

## How to Protect Yourself from Fake News Sites

If you suspect that a news site is fake, look for a disclaimer somewhere on the page (often in small print) that indicates that the site is an advertisement. Also, don't rely on Internet news reports when making important decisions about your health. If you're considering a health product described in the news, discuss it with your healthcare provider.

## More Questions to Ask When Finding Health Information on Websites

Your search for online health information may start at a known, trusted site, but after following several links, you may find yourself on an unfamiliar site. Can you trust this site? Here are some key questions you need to ask.

### Who Runs and Pays for the Website?

- Any reliable health-related website should make it easy for you to learn who's responsible for the site.

- A web address (such as NCCIH's) that ends in ".gov" means it's a government-sponsored site; ".edu" indicates an educational institution; ".org" usually means a noncommercial organization and ".com" a commercial organization. Some ".org" sites belong to organizations that promote an agenda; their content may be biased.

- Who pays for the site? Does the site sell advertising? Is it sponsored by a company that sells dietary supplements, drugs, or other products or services? Confirm any information you find on a site that sells products with an independent site that doesn't sell products.

### What's the Source of the Information?

- Many health or medical sites post information collected from other websites or sources, which should be identified.

### How Do You Know If the Information Is Accurate?

- The site should describe the evidence (such as articles in medical journals) that the material is based on. Also, opinions or advice should be clearly set apart from information that's "evidence-based" (based on research results).

- Keep in mind that testimonials, anecdotes, unsupported claims, and opinions aren't the same as objective, evidence-based information.

### Is the Information Reviewed by Experts?

- You can be more confident in the quality of medical information on a website if health experts reviewed it. Some websites have an editorial board that reviews content. Others put the names and credentials of reviewers in an acknowledgments section near the end of the page.

### How Current Is the Information?

- Outdated medical information can be misleading or even dangerous. Responsible health websites review and update much of their content on a regular basis, especially fact sheets and lists of frequently asked questions (FAQs). However, content such as news reports or meeting summaries that describe an event usually isn't updated. To find out whether the information is old, look for a date on the page (it's often near the bottom).

### What's the Site's Policy about Linking to Other Sites?

- Some sites don't link to any other sites, some link to any site that asks or pays for a link, and others link only to sites that meet certain criteria. You may be able to find information on the site about its linking policy.

- Unless the site's linking policy is strict, don't assume that the sites that it links to are reliable. You should evaluate the linked sites just as you would any other site that you're visiting for the first time.

### How Does the Site Collect and Handle Personal Information? Is the Site Secure?

- Websites track what pages you're looking at. They may also ask you to "subscribe" or "become a member." Any credible site collecting this kind of information should tell you exactly what it will and won't do with it.

- Many commercial sites sell "aggregate" (collected) data about their users to other companies—information such as what percentage of their users are women over 40. In some cases, they may collect and reuse information that's "personally identifiable," such as your zone improvement plan (ZIP) code, gender, and birth date.

- Read any privacy policy or similar language on the site, and don't sign up for anything you don't fully understand. You can find NCCIH's privacy policy on the NCCIH's website.

- See if the address uniform resource locator (URL) for the site starts with "https://" instead of "HTTP://." Sites that use HTTPS (secure hypertext transfer protocol) are encrypted, less likely to be hacked, and more likely to protect your privacy.

### Can You Communicate with the Owner of the Website?

- You should always be able to contact the site owner if you run across problems or have questions or feedback. If the site hosts online discussion forums or message boards, it should explain the terms of use.

### Is It Safe to Link to Twitter or Facebook through a Website?

- If the site is linked to social networking sites such as Twitter, Facebook, or YouTube, spend some time reading what has been posted to see whether you feel comfortable with the tone before joining in. You may also be able to review past discussions.

# Chapter 8

# *Health Fraud Awareness*

Health fraud is the deceptive sale or advertising of products that claim to be effective against medical conditions or otherwise beneficial to health, but which have not been proven safe and effective for those purposes. In addition to wasting billions of consumers' dollars each year, health scams can lead patients to delay proper treatment and cause serious—and even fatal—injuries.

## *Common Types of Health Fraud*

**Cancer fraud.** Among the many long-running cancer, scams are the Hoxsey Cancer Treatment, an herbal regimen that has no proven benefit. Another scam involves products called black salves. These are offered with the false promise of drawing cancer out from the skin, but they are potentially corrosive to tissues.

Cancer requires individualized treatment by a specialized physician. No single device, remedy, or treatment can treat all types of cancer. Patients looking to try an experimental cancer treatment should enroll in a legitimate clinical study.

**Human immunodeficiency virus (HIV)/acquired immunodeficiency syndrome (AIDS) fraud.** There are legitimate treatments that can help people with the human immunodeficiency virus (HIV).

---

This chapter includes text excerpted from "For Consumers—FDA 101: Health Fraud Awareness," U.S. Food and Drug Administration (FDA), May 12, 2009. Reviewed May 2018.

While early treatment of HIV can delay progression to AIDS, there is currently no cure for the disease.

Relying on unproven products and treatments can be dangerous and cause delays in seeking legitimate medical treatments that have been proven in clinical trials to improve quality of life. Safe, reliable testing to determine whether you have HIV can be done by a medical professional.

To date, there is one U.S. Food and Drug Administration (FDA)-approved testing system that allows individuals to test themselves at home. It is an HIV collection system that tests only for HIV-1, which is the cause of the majority of the world's HIV infections.

The test, sold either as The Home Access HIV-1 Test System or The Home Access Express HIV-1 Test System, allows blood samples to be sent to a laboratory for testing with an FDA approved the HIV-1 test.

**Arthritis fraud.** The Federal Trade Commission (FTC) says consumers spend about $2 billion annually on unproven arthritis remedies that are not backed by adequate science.

**Fraudulent "diagnostic" tests.** Doctors often use in vitro diagnostic (IVD) tests—in tandem with a physical examination and a medical history—to get a picture of a patient's overall health. These tests involve blood, urine, or other specimen samples taken from the body. They help diagnose or measure many conditions, including pregnancy, hepatitis, fertility, HIV, cholesterol, and blood sugar.

It's rare that the use of only one of these tests can provide a meaningful diagnosis. You can buy IVD tests in stores, through the mail, or online. Many of these tests are regulated by the FDA and sold legally. However, many others are marketed illegally and do not meet the FDA's regulatory requirements. These tests may not work or may be harmful.

To find out whether the FDA has cleared or approved an IVD test for a particular purpose, call the FDA at 888-463-6332, or your local FDA district office.

**Bogus dietary supplements.** The array of dietary supplements— including vitamins and minerals, amino acids, enzymes, herbs, animal extracts, and others—has grown tremendously.

Although the benefits of some of these have been documented, the advantages of others are unproven. For example, claims that a supplement allows you to eat all you want and lose weight effortlessly are false.

Claims to treat diseases cause products to be considered drugs. Firms wanting to make such claims legally must follow the FDA's premarket new drug approval process to show that the products are safe and effective.

**Weight loss fraud.** Since 2003, the FDA has worked with national and international partners to take hundreds of compliance actions against companies pushing bogus and misleading weight loss schemes.

The FDA has enhanced efforts to stop sales and importation of—and to warn consumers about—weight loss products that contain dangerous prescription drug ingredients that are not listed on the label.

**Sexual enhancement product fraud.** The FDA has warned consumers about numerous illegal drugs promoted and sold online for treating erectile dysfunction and for enhancing sexual performance.

Although they are marketed as "dietary supplements," these products are really illegal drugs that contain potentially harmful ingredients that are not listed on the label.

**Diabetes fraud.** The FDA has taken numerous compliance actions against sales of fraudulent diabetes "treatments" promoted with bogus claims such as:

- "Drop your blood sugar 50 points in 30 days"
- "Eliminate insulin resistance"
- "Prevent the development of type 2 diabetes"
- "Reduce or eliminate the need for diabetes drugs or insulin"

**Influenza (flu) scams.** Federal agencies have come across contaminated, counterfeit, and subpotent influenza products. The FDA, with U.S. Customs and Border Protection (CBP), has intercepted products claimed to be generic versions of the influenza drug Tamiflu, but which actually contained vitamin C and other substances not shown to be effective in treating or preventing influenza.

## Don't Be a Victim

It's ultimately up to the buyer to beware of potential health fraud. Know of the potential for health fraud and learn about the common techniques and gimmicks that fraudulent marketers use to gain your attention and trust. For instance, testimonials from people who say they have used the product may sound convincing, but these can easily be made up. These "testimonials" are not a substitute for scientific proof.

Also, never diagnose or treat yourself with questionable products. Always check with your healthcare professional before using new medical products.

Be wary of these red flags:

- Claims that a product is a quick, effective cure-all or a diagnostic tool for a wide variety of ailments

- Suggestions that a product can treat or cure diseases

- Promotions using words such as "scientific breakthrough," "miraculous cure," "secret ingredient," and "ancient remedy"

- Text with impressive-sounding terms such as: "hunger stimulation point" and "thermogenesis" for a weight loss product

- Undocumented case histories by consumers or doctors claiming amazing results

- Limited availability and advance payment requirements

- Promises of no-risk, money-back guarantees

- Promises of an "easy" fix

- Claims that the product is "natural" or "nontoxic" (which doesn't necessarily mean safe)

Don't be fooled by professional-looking websites. Avoid websites that fail to list the company's name, physical address, phone number, or other contact information.

# Chapter 9

# *Use Caution: Buying Medical Products Online*

Millions of consumers are using digital media to get health information, applications to monitor health conditions, and social media to find people who share similar health-related concerns and experiences. Some of this information will be up-to-date and trustworthy; some will not. How can you tell the good from the bad?

## *Tweeting, Posting, and Downloading Health Information*

The use of social media for health communication is on the rise—both as a resource for consumers and as an outreach tool for healthcare providers. Facebook, YouTube, Twitter, and other forms of social media provide an opportunity for consumers to share information about personal health experiences and seek information from others. Mobile apps provide a convenient way for users to track health-related information and activities; including when and what medications to take, blood sugar levels, and blood pressure, for example.

This chapter contains text excerpted from the following sources: Text in this chapter begins with excerpts from "Drugs—Health Information on the Web," U.S. Food and Drug Administration (FDA), December 16, 2016; Text under the heading "Buy Prescription Drugs from Licensed U.S. Pharmacies Only" is excerpted from "Consumer Information—Buying Health Products and Services Online," Federal Trade Commission (FTC), September 2011. Reviewed May 2018.

According to the Albert Einstein College of Medicine, social networks can benefit patients and caregivers in providing, among other things:

- Support

- Specialized knowledge from peers

- Improved outcomes

However, like websites, not all social media outlets are safe and reliable. Many of the steps that should be taken to evaluate the safety and reliability of a website should also be used when using social media. For example: Is a product being offered for sale? Is the discussion about a new "miracle" treatment? Or is the source of the discussion or information unclear? Users also must be careful of medical misinformation—information that is outdated or based on word of mouth. Personal blogs and Twitter sites that discuss health matters are seldom if ever, regulated.

## Buy Prescription Drugs from Licensed U.S. Pharmacies Only

What looks like an online pharmacy could be a front for a scammer or identity thief. The sites may use official looking seals and logos, guarantee satisfaction or your money back, and "look" legitimate. All that can be faked.

You could end up with products that are fake, expired, or mislabeled, or products that contain dangerous ingredients. Or you may pay for a prescription and never get your order—or your money back.

So how can you tell if you're dealing with a legitimate U.S. pharmacy? To see if a pharmacy is licensed in the United States, check with the board of pharmacy in the state where it's based. The National Association of Boards of Pharmacy (NABP) has information on each state's board. NABP also has a list of online pharmacies that meet its standards and are accredited through its Verified Internet Pharmacy Practice Sites (VIPPS) program. Reputable pharmacy websites should:

- Require a prescription

- Have a licensed pharmacist to answer your questions

- Provide a physical business address and phone number

## *Talk to Your Doctor or Health Professional*

As you look for answers to your health questions, you might come across websites or ads for pills or other products that make big promises. They may say their product will cure a serious condition like arthritis, diabetes, Alzheimer disease (AD), multiple sclerosis (MS), cancer, human immunodeficiency virus (HIV) acquired immunodeficiency syndrome (AIDS), or a range of conditions. Or the ad might be for a weight-loss pill that says you can lose weight without exercising or changing how you eat. The reality is that most of these "miracle" products are useless, and at best, a waste of money. Others are flat-out dangerous.

Don't trust a website just because it looks professional or has success stories from "real people." And don't put much faith in products advertised as "scientific breakthroughs" or "ancient remedies," or ads that use scientific sounding words like "thermogenesis" or safe-sounding words like "natural." Scammers can be creative. The stories may be made up, or the people may be actors or models paid to praise the product.

Ask your doctor about any product before you try it. Your doctor can tell you about the risks of a product, whether there are reputable studies to support the claims, and its effect on any medicine you're taking or treatments you're getting.

# Part Two

# Alternative Medicine Systems

# Chapter 10

# *Understanding Whole Medical Systems*

Whole medical systems involve complete systems of theory and practice that have evolved independently from or parallel to allopathic (conventional) medicine. Many are traditional systems of medicine that are practiced by individual cultures throughout the world. Major Eastern whole medical systems include traditional Chinese medicine (TCM) and Ayurvedic medicine, one of India's traditional systems of medicine. Major Western whole medical systems include homeopathy and naturopathy. Other systems have been developed by Native American, African, Middle Eastern, Tibetan, and Central and South American cultures.

## *Traditional Chinese Medicine (TCM)*

TCM is a complete system of healing that dates back to 200 B.C. in written form. Korea, Japan, and Vietnam have all developed their own unique versions of traditional medicine based on practices originating in China. In the TCM view, the body is a delicate balance of two opposing and inseparable forces: yin and yang. Yin represents the cold, slow, or passive principle, while yang represents the hot, excited, or active

Text in this chapter begins with excerpts from "Whole Medical Systems: An Overview," National Center for Complementary and Integrative Health (NCCIH), October 2004. Reviewed May 2018; Text under the heading "Native American Medicine" is excerpted from "Healing Ways," U.S. National Library of Medicine (NLM), September 26, 2011. Reviewed May 2018.

principle. Among the major assumptions in TCM are that health is achieved by maintaining the body in a "balanced state" and that disease is due to an internal imbalance of yin and yang. This imbalance leads to blockage in the flow of qi (or vital energy) and of blood along pathways known as meridians. TCM practitioners typically use herbs, acupuncture, and massage to help unblock qi and blood in patients in an attempt to bring the body back into harmony and wellness.

Treatments in TCM are typically tailored to the subtle patterns of disharmony in each patient and are based on an individualized diagnosis. The diagnostic tools differ from those of conventional medicine. There are three main therapeutic modalities:

1. Acupuncture and moxibustion (moxibustion is the application of heat from the burning of the herb moxa at the acupuncture point)

2. Chinese *Materia Medica* (the catalog of natural products used in TCM)

3. Massage and manipulation

Although TCM proposes that natural products cataloged in Chinese *Materia Medica* or acupuncture can be used alone to treat virtually any illness, quite often they are used together and sometimes in combination with other modalities (e.g., massage, moxibustion, diet changes, or exercise).

## *Acupuncture*

A report from a Consensus Development Conference on Acupuncture held at the National Institutes of Health (NIH) states that acupuncture is being "widely" practiced—by thousands of acupuncturists, physicians, dentists, and other practitioners—for relief or prevention of pain and for various other health conditions. In terms of the evidence at that time, acupuncture was considered to have potential clinical value for nausea/vomiting and dental pain, and limited evidence suggested its potential in the treatment of other pain disorders, paralysis and numbness, movement disorders, depression, insomnia, breathlessness, and asthma.

Preclinical studies have documented acupuncture's effects, but they have not been able to fully explain how acupuncture works within the framework of the Western system of medicine.

It is proposed that acupuncture produces its effects by the conduction of electromagnetic signals at a greater-than-normal rate, thus aiding the activity of pain-killing biochemicals, such as endorphins and immune system cells at specific sites in the body. In addition, studies have shown that acupuncture may alter brain chemistry by changing the release of neurotransmitters and neurohormones and affecting the parts of the central nervous system related to sensation and involuntary body functions, such as immune reactions and processes whereby a person's blood pressure, blood flow, and body temperature are regulated.

## *Ayurvedic Medicine*

Ayurveda, which literally means "the science of life," is a natural healing system developed in India. Ayurvedic texts claim that the sages who developed India's original systems of meditation and yoga developed the foundations of this medical system. It is a comprehensive system of medicine that places equal emphasis on the body, mind, and spirit, and strives to restore the innate harmony of the individual. Some of the primary Ayurvedic treatments include diet, exercise, meditation, herbs, massage, exposure to sunlight, and controlled breathing. In India, Ayurvedic treatments have been developed for various diseases (e.g., diabetes, cardiovascular conditions, and neurological disorders). However, a survey of the Indian medical literature indicates that the quality of the published clinical trials generally falls short of contemporary methodological standards with regard to criteria for randomization, sample size, and adequate controls.

## *Homeopathy*

Homeopathy is a complete system of medical theory and practice. Its founder, German physician Samuel Christian Hahnemann (1755–1843), hypothesized that one can select therapies on the basis of how closely symptoms produced by a remedy match the symptoms of the patient's disease. He called this the "principle of similars." Hahnemann proceeded to give repeated doses of many common remedies to healthy volunteers and carefully record the symptoms they produced. This procedure is called a "proving" or, in modern homeopathy, a "human pathogenic trial." As a result of this experience, Hahnemann developed his treatments for sick patients by matching the symptoms produced by a drug to symptoms in sick patients. Hahnemann emphasized from the beginning carefully examining all aspects of a person's health status, including emotional and mental states, and tiny idiosyncratic characteristics.

## Naturopathy

Naturopathy is a system of healing, originating from Europe, that views disease as a manifestation of alterations in the processes by which the body naturally heals itself. It emphasizes health restoration as well as disease treatment. The term "naturopathy" literally translates as "nature disease." Naturopathy, or naturopathic medicine, is practiced throughout Europe, Australia, New Zealand, Canada, and the United States. There are six principles that form the basis of naturopathic practice in North America (not all are unique to naturopathy):

1.  The healing power of nature

2.  Identification and treatment of the cause of disease

3.  The concept of "first do no harm"

4.  The doctor as teacher

5.  Treatment of the whole person

6.  Prevention

The core modalities supporting these principles include diet modification and nutritional supplements, herbal medicine, acupuncture and Chinese medicine, hydrotherapy, massage and joint manipulation, and lifestyle counseling. Treatment protocols combine what the practitioner deems to be the most suitable therapies for the individual patient.

## Native American Medicine

Native concepts of health and illness have sustained diverse peoples since ancient times.

Many traditional healers believe that every person has responsibility for his or her proper behavior and health, and that healing is often done by the patient. Healers, therefore, serve as facilitators and counselors, often using stories, humor, music, tobacco, smudging, medicinal plants, and herbs, and related ceremonies to bring their healing energies into the healing space.

# Chapter 11

# *Acupuncture*

## *Chapter Contents*

# Section 11.1

# *What Is Acupuncture?*

Text beginning with the heading "What Is Acupuncture?" is excerpted from "Acupuncture: In Depth," National Center for Complementary and Integrative Health (NCCIH), January 2016; Text under the heading "Acupuncture May Be Helpful For Chronic Pain: A Meta-Analysis" is excerpted from "Acupuncture May Be Helpful for Chronic Pain: A Meta-Analysis," National Center for Complementary and Integrative Health (NCCIH), September 10, 2012. Reviewed May 2018.

Acupuncture is a technique in which practitioners stimulate specific points on the body—most often by inserting thin needles through the skin. It is one of the practices used in traditional Chinese medicine (TCM).

## *What the Science Says about the Effectiveness of Acupuncture*

Results from a number of studies suggest that acupuncture may help ease types of pain that are often chronic such as low-back pain, neck pain, and osteoarthritis/knee pain. It also may help reduce the frequency of tension headaches and prevent migraine headaches. Therefore, acupuncture appears to be a reasonable option for people with chronic pain to consider. However, clinical practice guidelines are inconsistent in recommendations about acupuncture.

The effects of acupuncture on the brain and body and how best to measure them are only beginning to be understood. Evidence suggests that many factors—like expectation and belief—that are unrelated to acupuncture needling may play important roles in the beneficial effects of acupuncture on pain.

### *For Low-Back Pain*

- An analysis of data on participants in acupuncture studies looked at back and neck pain together and found that actual acupuncture was more helpful than either no acupuncture or simulated acupuncture.

- A review by the Agency for Healthcare Research and Quality (AHRQ) found that acupuncture relieved low-back pain immediately after treatment but not over longer periods of time.

- A systematic review of studies on acupuncture for low-back pain found strong evidence that combining acupuncture with usual care helps more than usual care alone. The same review also found strong evidence that there is no difference between the effects of actual and simulated acupuncture in people with low-back pain.

- Clinical practice guidelines issued by the American Pain Society (APS) and the American College of Physicians (ACP) recommends acupuncture as one of several nondrug approaches physicians should consider when patients with chronic low-back pain do not respond to self-care (practices that people can do by themselves, such as remaining active, applying heat, and taking pain-relieving medications).

### For Neck Pain

- An analysis found that actual acupuncture was more helpful for neck pain than simulated acupuncture, but the analysis was based on a small amount of evidence (only three studies with small study populations).

- A large German study with more than 14,000 participants evaluated adding acupuncture to usual care for neck pain. The researchers found that participants reported greater pain relief than those who didn't receive it; the researchers didn't test actual acupuncture against simulated acupuncture.

### For Osteoarthritis/Knee Pain

- An Australian clinical study involving 282 men and women showed that needle and laser acupuncture were modestly better at relieving knee pain from OA than no treatment, but not better than simulated (sham) laser acupuncture. Participants received 8–12 actual and simulated acupuncture treatments over 12 weeks. These results are generally consistent with previous studies, which showed that acupuncture is consistently better than no treatment but not necessarily better than simulated acupuncture at relieving OA pain.

- A major analysis of data on participants in acupuncture studies found that actual acupuncture was more helpful for OA pain than simulated acupuncture or no acupuncture.

- A systematic review of studies of acupuncture for knee or hip OA concluded that actual acupuncture was more helpful for OA pain than either simulated acupuncture or no acupuncture. However, the difference between actual and simulated acupuncture was very small, while the difference between acupuncture and no acupuncture was large.

### For Headache

- An analysis of data on individual participants in acupuncture studies looked at migraine and tension headaches. The analysis showed that actual acupuncture was more effective than either no acupuncture or simulated acupuncture in reducing headache frequency or severity.

- A systematic review of studies concluded that actual acupuncture, compared with simulated acupuncture or pain-relieving drugs, helped people with tension-type headaches. It suggested that actual acupuncture has a very slight advantage over simulated acupuncture in reducing tension-type headache intensity and the number of headache days per month.

- A systematic review found that adding acupuncture to basic care for migraines helped to reduce migraine frequency. However, in studies that compared actual acupuncture with simulated acupuncture, researchers found that the differences between the two treatments may have been due to chance.

### For Other Conditions

- Results of a systematic review that combined data from 11 clinical trials with more than 1,200 participants suggested that acupuncture (and acupuncture point stimulation) may help with certain symptoms associated with cancer treatments.

- There is not enough evidence to determine if acupuncture can help people with depression.

- Acupuncture has been promoted as a smoking cessation treatment since the 1970s, but research has not shown that it helps people quit the habit.

### What Is Simulated Acupuncture?

In some clinical trials, researchers test a product or practice against an inactive product or technique (called a placebo) to see if the response is due to the test protocol or to something else. Many acupuncture trials rely on a technique called simulated acupuncture, which may use blunt-tipped retractable needles that touch the skin but do not penetrate (in real acupuncture, needles penetrate the skin). Researchers also may simulate acupuncture in other ways. However, in some instances, researchers have observed that simulated acupuncture resulted in some degree of pain relief.

## What the Science Says about Safety and Side Effects of Acupuncture

- Relatively few complications from using acupuncture have been reported. Still, complications have resulted from use of nonsterile needles and improper delivery of treatments.

- When not delivered properly, acupuncture can cause serious adverse effects, including infections, punctured organs, collapsed lungs, and injury to the central nervous system.

- The U.S. Food and Drug Administration (FDA) regulates acupuncture needles as medical devices for use by licensed practitioners and requires that needles be manufactured and labeled according to certain standards. For example, the FDA requires that needles be sterile, nontoxic, and labeled for single use by qualified practitioners only.

## Acupuncture May Be Helpful for Chronic Pain: A Meta-Analysis

A National Center for Complementary and Integrative Health (NCCIH)-funded study, employing individual patient data meta-analyses and published in the *Archives of Internal Medicine*, provides the most rigorous evidence to date that acupuncture may be helpful for chronic pain. In addition, results from the study provide robust evidence that the effects of acupuncture on pain are attributable to two components. The larger component includes factors such as the patient's belief that treatment will be effective, as well as placebo and other context effects. A smaller acupuncture-specific component involves such issues as the locations of specific needling points or depth of needling.

Although millions of Americans use acupuncture each year, often for chronic pain, there has been considerable controversy surrounding its value as a therapy and whether it is anything more than an elaborate placebo. Research exploring a number of possible mechanisms for acupuncture's pain-relieving effects is ongoing.

Researchers from the Acupuncture Trialists' Collaboration, a group that was established to synthesize data from high-quality randomized trials on acupuncture for chronic pain, conducted an analysis of individual patient data from 29 high-quality randomized controlled trials, including a total of 17,922 people. These trials investigated the use of acupuncture for back and neck pain, OA, shoulder pain, or a chronic headache.

For all pain types studied, the researchers found modest but statistically significant differences between acupuncture versus simulated acupuncture approaches (i.e., specific effects), and larger differences between acupuncture versus no-acupuncture controls (i.e., nonspecific effects). (In traditional acupuncture, needles are inserted at specific points on the body. Simulated acupuncture includes a variety of approaches which mimic this procedure; some approaches do not pierce the skin or use specific points on the body.) The sizes of the effects were generally similar across all pain conditions studied.

The authors noted that these findings suggest that the total effects of acupuncture, as experienced by patients in clinical practice, are clinically relevant. They also noted that their study provides the most robust evidence to date that acupuncture is more than just placebo and a reasonable referral option for patients with chronic pain.

# Section 11.2

# *Acupuncture for Cancer*

This section includes text excerpted from
"Acupuncture (PDQ®)–Patient Version," National
Cancer Institute (NCI), March 30, 2018.

Acupuncture applies needles, heat, pressure, and other treatments to places on the skin, called acupuncture points (or acupoints), to control symptoms such as pain or nausea and vomiting. Acupuncture is part of traditional Chinese medicine (TCM). TCM uses acupuncture, diet, herbal therapy, meditation, exercise, and massage to restore health.

Acupuncture is based on the belief that qi (vital energy) flows through the body along paths, called meridians. Qi is said to affect a person's spiritual, emotional, mental, and physical condition.

## How Is Acupuncture Given?

Most acupuncture methods use needles. Disposable, stainless steel needles that are slightly thicker than a human hair are inserted into the skin at acupoints. The acupuncture practitioner chooses the correct acupoints for the problem being treated. The inserted needles may be twirled, moved up and down at different speeds and depths, heated, or charged with a weak electric current.

Acupuncture methods include the following:

- Auricular acupuncture: Acupuncture needles are placed at acupoints on the outer ear that match up with certain parts of the body.

- Electroacupuncture

- Trigger point acupuncture

- Laser acupuncture

- Acupuncture point injection

- Microwave acupuncture

- Acupressure

- Moxibustion

- Cupping

## What Do Patients Feel during Acupuncture?

Patients may have a needling feeling during acupuncture, known as de qi sensation, making them feel heaviness, numbness, or tingling.

## Have Any Laboratory or Animal Studies Been Done Using Acupuncture?

In laboratory studies, tumor samples are used to test a new treatment and find out if it is likely to have any anticancer effects. In animal studies, tests are done to see if a drug, procedure, or treatment is safe and effective in animals. Laboratory and animal studies are done before a treatment is tested in people.

Laboratory and animal studies have tested the effects of acupuncture.

## Have Any Studies Been Done in People?

In 1997, the National Institutes of Health (NIH) began looking at how well acupuncture worked as a complementary therapy for cancer-related symptoms and side effects of cancer treatments. Studies of acupuncture in cancer care also have been done in China and other countries.

### *Nausea and Vomiting Caused by Chemotherapy, Surgery, and Radiation Therapy*

- The strongest evidence for acupuncture has come from clinical trials on the use of acupuncture to relieve nausea and vomiting.

- A 2013 review that included 41 randomized controlled trials found that acupuncture helped treat nausea and vomiting caused by chemotherapy.

- Another review from 11 randomized clinical trials, found that fewer chemotherapy patients in the acupuncture groups had acute vomiting compared to the control group.

- A comparison of studies suggests that the specific acupuncture point used may make a difference in how well acupuncture works to relieve nausea caused by chemotherapy.

- Patients who received either true acupuncture or sham acupuncture were compared to patients who received only standard care to prevent nausea and vomiting from radiation therapy. The study found that patients in both the true and sham acupuncture groups had less nausea and vomiting than those in the standard care group.

### *Pain*

Acupuncture has been studied to help relieve pain in cancer patients. The results are mixed due to small sample sizes and design problems.

#### *Cancer Pain*

- In one review, acupuncture reduced cancer pain in some patients with various cancers, although the studies were small. Another review concluded acupuncture with pain medicine worked better than the pain medicine alone. This review was limited by poor quality of clinical trials.

*Postoperative Pain*

- In several randomized clinical trials on pain after surgery, acupuncture reduced the pain, but sample sizes were small and additional treatments were unknown. Some studies reported that when acupuncture was used with standard care, pain relief was better.

*Muscle and Joint Pain from Aromatase Inhibitors*

- Aromatase inhibitors, a type of hormone therapy for postmenopausal women who have hormone-dependent breast cancer, may cause muscle and joint pain.

- Four randomized controlled trials compared the effects of real and sham acupuncture in reducing pain. All four trials showed no side effects from either real acupuncture or sham acupuncture. One trial showed real acupuncture was better than sham acupuncture in relieving joint and muscle pain, but the other three trials did not. In one of the studies, patients receiving real acupuncture had more pain relief than a control group of patients who were waiting to receive treatment later.

- Observational studies have also reported both real acupuncture and sham acupuncture may relieve pain more than standard care.

- A review of 17,922 patients reported that real acupuncture relieved pain better than sham acupuncture.

- An ongoing randomized clinical trial of 228 patients is comparing real acupuncture, sham acupuncture, and standard care in breast cancer survivors with muscle and joint pain from aromatase inhibitors.

*Peripheral Neuropathy*

- Several small studies have been done on the use of acupuncture in treating peripheral neuropathy caused by chemotherapy or other anticancer drugs. Most of these studies found acupuncture decreased pain and improved nerve function. A randomized controlled trial, however, found that acupuncture did not work better than a placebo.

## Hot Flashes

Hormone therapy may cause hot flashes in women with breast cancer and men with prostate cancer. Studies of the use of acupuncture to relieve hot flashes have shown mixed results.

- Six randomized clinical trials studied the use of acupuncture to prevent hot flashes in breast cancer survivors. These trials found that acupuncture was safe and decreased hot flashes. It was not clear whether real acupuncture worked better than sham acupuncture.

- A 2015 randomized trial of electroacupuncture in breast cancer survivors with hot flashes had four groups for treatment: electroacupuncture, sham acupuncture, gabapentin, and placebo. The trial looked at how well sham acupuncture worked compared to the placebo and compared hot flash relief in all groups. The study found that sham acupuncture worked better than gabapentin or the placebo, and both electroacupuncture and sham acupuncture gave better relief than gabapentin.

- A 2016 randomized trial compared acupuncture plus self-care (as described in an information booklet provided to all patients) to self-care alone in breast cancer survivors. The study found that adding acupuncture reduced hot flashes after 12 weeks of treatment and at the 3- and 6-month follow-up visits. The study also found that acupuncture improved the patients' quality of life.

- A 2016 review of 12 randomized trials in breast cancer survivors with hot flashes included 6 studies that compared real acupuncture with sham acupuncture. Of these, only 2 studies found that real acupuncture had a benefit compared with the sham treatment. The other studies found that acupuncture was no better than hormone therapy, venlafaxine, or relaxation therapy in relieving hot flashes.

- Some studies have reported that acupuncture may relieve hot flashes in prostate cancer patients on androgen-deprivation therapy.

## Fatigue

Fatigue is a common symptom in patients with cancer and a frequent side effect of chemotherapy and radiation therapy.

- Several randomized clinical trials have studied the use of acupuncture in reducing cancer-related fatigue. These trials found that acupuncture improved fatigue when compared to standard care alone. It is not clear whether real acupuncture works better than sham acupuncture.

### Dry Mouth (Xerostomia)

Several clinical trials have studied the effect of acupuncture in the treatment and prevention of xerostomia (dry mouth) caused by radiation therapy in patients with nasopharyngeal carcinoma and head and neck cancer.

- In studies that compared acupuncture with standard care for preventing dry mouth in patients being treated with radiation therapy, patients treated with acupuncture during radiation therapy had fewer symptoms and better saliva flow.

- Two randomized controlled trials compared real and sham acupuncture for the prevention and treatment of dry mouth. These trials found that both real and sham acupuncture increased the flow of saliva.

- A study on the long-term effects of acupuncture on dry mouth found that patients had better saliva flow at 6 months compared to before treatment. Patients who received additional acupuncture had more saliva flow at 3 years compared to patients who did not continue acupuncture treatment.

Other trials are ongoing.

### Lymphedema

There have been a number of case reports and studies that show acupuncture is safe and may decrease swelling and relieve symptoms in patients with lymphedema in the arms and legs. In one randomized clinical trial, acupuncture was found to keep lymphedema from getting worse but did not decrease swelling or symptoms.

### Ileus

After cancer surgery, some patients develop ileus. Randomized clinical trials that studied acupuncture for ileus had mixed results.

### Sleep Problems

A study that compared acupuncture with fluoxetine found that acupuncture worked better in relieving depression and improving sleep. Another study found that acupuncture improved sleep slightly better than standard care.

### The Immune System

Studies that suggest acupuncture may improve the immune system are limited.

### Other Symptoms of Cancer and Side Effects of Cancer Treatment

Other clinical trials in cancer patients have studied the effects of acupuncture on cancer symptoms and side effects caused by cancer treatment, including weight loss, cough, coughing up blood, fever, anxiety, depression, proctitis, speech problems, blocked esophagus, and hiccups. Studies have shown that treatment with acupuncture either relieves symptoms or keeps them from getting worse.

## Have Any Side Effects or Risks Been Reported from Acupuncture?

There have been few complications reported. Problems are caused by using needles that are not sterile and from placing the needle in the wrong place, movement of the patient, or a defect in the needle.
Problems include the following:

- Feeling soreness and pain during treatment
- Feeling tired, lightheaded, or sleepy
- Getting an infection
- A strict clean needle method must be used when acupuncture treatment is given to cancer patients because chemotherapy and radiation therapy weaken the body's immune system.

## Is Acupuncture Approved by the U.S. Food and Drug Administration (FDA)?

The FDA approved acupuncture needles for use by licensed practitioners in 1996. The FDA requires that sterile needles be used and labeled for single use by qualified practitioners only.

More than 40 states and the District of Columbia (D.C.) have laws about acupuncture practice.

# Chapter 12

# *Ayurvedic Medicine*

## *Chapter Contents*

# Section 12.1

# *Understanding Ayurvedic Medicine*

This section includes text excerpted from "Ayurvedic
Medicine: In Depth," National Center for Complementary and
Integrative Health (NCCIH), January 2015.

Ayurvedic medicine (also called Ayurveda) is one of the world's oldest medical systems. It originated in India more than 3,000 years ago and remains one of the country's traditional healthcare systems. Its concepts about health and disease promote the use of herbal compounds, special diets, and other unique health practices. India's government and other institutes throughout the world support clinical and laboratory research on Ayurvedic medicine, within the context of the Eastern belief system. But Ayurvedic medicine isn't widely studied as part of conventional (Western) medicine.

## *Is Ayurvedic Medicine Safe?*

Ayurvedic medicine uses a variety of products and practices. Some of these products—which may contain herbs, minerals, or metals—may be harmful, particularly if used improperly or without the direction of a trained practitioner. For example, some herbs can cause side effects or interact with conventional medicines. Also, ingesting some metals, such as lead, can be poisonous.

## *Is Ayurvedic Medicine Effective?*

Studies have examined Ayurvedic medicine, including herbal products, for specific conditions. However, there aren't enough well-controlled clinical trials and systematic research reviews—the gold standard for Western medical research—to prove that the approaches are beneficial.

## *Keep in Mind*

Tell all your healthcare providers about any complementary and integrative health approaches you use. Give them a full picture of what you do to manage your health. This will help ensure coordinated and safe care.

## What Is Ayurveda?

The term "Ayurveda" combines the Sanskrit words *ayur* (life) and *veda* (science or knowledge). Ayurvedic medicine, as practiced in India, is one of the oldest systems of medicine in the world. Many Ayurvedic practices predate written records and were handed down by word of mouth. Three ancient books known as the Great Trilogy was written in Sanskrit more than 2,000 years ago and are considered the main texts on Ayurvedic medicine—*Caraka Samhita, Sushruta Samhita,* and *Astanga Hridaya.*

Key concepts of Ayurvedic medicine include universal interconnectedness (among people, their health, and the universe), the body's constitution *(prakriti)*, and life forces *(dosha)*, which are often compared to the biologic humors of the ancient Greek system. Using these concepts, Ayurvedic physicians prescribe individualized treatments, including compounds of herbs or proprietary ingredients, and diet, exercise, and lifestyle recommendations.

The majority of India's population uses Ayurvedic medicine exclusively or combined with conventional Western medicine, and it's practiced in varying forms in Southeast Asia.

## What the Science Says about the Safety and Side Effects of Ayurvedic Medicine

Ayurvedic medicine uses a variety of products and practices. Ayurvedic products are made either of herbs only or a combination of herbs, metals, minerals, or other materials in an Ayurvedic practice called *rasa shastra.* Some of these products may be harmful if used improperly or without the direction of a trained practitioner.

### Toxicity

Ayurvedic products have the potential to be toxic. Many materials used in them haven't been studied for safety in controlled clinical trials. In the United States, Ayurvedic products are regulated as dietary supplements. As such, they aren't required to meet the same safety and effectiveness standards as conventional medicines.

A National Center for Complementary and Integrative Health (NCCIH)-funded study examined the content of 193 Ayurvedic products purchased over the Internet and manufactured in either the United States or India. The researchers found that 21 percent of the products contained levels of lead, mercury, and/or arsenic that exceeded the standards for acceptable daily intake.

Other approaches used in Ayurvedic medicine, such as massage, special diets, and cleansing techniques may have side effects as well. To help ensure coordinated and safe care, it's important to tell all your healthcare providers about any Ayurvedic products and practices or other complementary and integrative health approaches you use.

## *What the Science Says about the Effectiveness of Ayurvedic Medicine Research*

Most clinical trials of Ayurvedic approaches have been small, had problems with research designs, or lacked appropriate control groups, potentially affecting research results.

- Researchers have studied Ayurvedic approaches for schizophrenia and for diabetes; however, scientific evidence for its effectiveness for these diseases is inconclusive.

- A preliminary clinical trial funded in part by the NCCIH found that conventional and Ayurvedic treatments for rheumatoid arthritis had similar effectiveness. The conventional drug tested was methotrexate and the Ayurvedic treatment included 40 herbal compounds.

- Ayurvedic practitioners use turmeric for inflammatory conditions, among other disorders. Evidence from clinical trials show that turmeric may help with certain digestive disorders and arthritis, but the research is limited.

- Varieties of boswellia (*Boswellia serrata, Boswellia carterii,* also known as frankincense) produce a resin that has shown anti-inflammatory and immune system effects in laboratory studies. A preliminary clinical trial found that osteoarthritis patients receiving a compound derived from *B. serrata* gum resin had greater decreases in pain compared to patients receiving a placebo.

# Section 12.2

## *Use Caution with Ayurvedic Products*

This section includes text excerpted from "Use
Caution with Ayurvedic Products," U.S. Food and Drug
Administration (FDA), December 15, 2017.

Ayurvedic medicine is a traditional system of healing arts that originated in India. It involves using products such as spices, herbs, vitamins, proteins, minerals, and metals (e.g., mercury, lead, iron, zinc). Some preparations combine herbs with minerals and metals. These products are commonly sold on the Internet or in stores and are represented as "Indian" or "South Asian."

"Consumers should know that Ayurvedic products are generally not reviewed or approved by the U.S. Food and Drug Administration (FDA)," says Mike Levy, Director of the Division of New Drugs and Labeling Compliance in the Office of Compliance, part of the FDA's Center for Drug Evaluation and Research (CDER).

Most Ayurvedic products are marketed either for drug uses not approved by the FDA or as dietary supplements. As such, consumers should understand that these products have not been approved by the FDA before marketing.

"The bottom line," Levy says, "is that consumers need to be on guard when purchasing any product using the Internet, especially medical products." This is an area that is challenging to regulate.

### *Concerns about Heavy Metals*

The presence of metals in some Ayurvedic products makes them potentially harmful. A study published in the *Journal of the American Medical Association (JAMA)*, demonstrated that one-fifth of U.S.-manufactured and Indian-manufactured Ayurvedic products bought on the Internet contained detectable lead, mercury, or arsenic.

Researchers found 25 websites selling Ayurvedic products. After identifying 673 products, they randomly selected 230 for purchase. Of those, they received and analyzed 193 products. Nearly 21 percent were found to contain detectable levels of lead, mercury, or arsenic.

All metal-containing products exceeded one or more standards for acceptable daily metal intake. The researchers concluded that several Indian-manufactured products could result in lead and/or mercury ingestions 100 to 100,000 times greater than acceptable limits.

This study followed a previous study published in JAMA found that one out of five Ayurvedic "herbal medicine products" produced in South Asia and available in South Asian grocery stores in Boston contained potentially harmful levels of lead, mercury, and/or arsenic.

## A Priority for FDA

"This issue has been and will continue to be a priority for FDA," Levy says. The agency has had an import alert on certain Ayurvedic products in place since 2007. This import alert allows FDA personnel to prevent these products from entering the United States.

"Through this import alert, the agency is able to stop commercial import shipments of these products," Levy says, "but individual Internet purchases are harder to monitor."

The FDA is re-evaluating its existing import alert and considering possible enforcement actions related to Ayurvedic products manufactured in the United States.

## Advice for Consumers

- **Be aware that Ayurvedic products do not undergo FDA review.** In accordance with current law, FDA does not evaluate these products before they are marketed. This means their safety, quality, and effectiveness cannot be assured by FDA. Certain populations, including children, are particularly at risk for the toxic effects of heavy metals.

- **Use caution when buying medical products on the Internet.** FDA urges consumers to beware of unregulated Internet drug sellers. Many of their products could pose direct or serious indirect health issues or could contain toxic substances.

- **Tell your healthcare professional about all alternative products.** Some herbs, minerals, and metals can interact with each other and with conventional medications.

# Chapter 13

# *Homeopathy*

## *Chapter Contents*

# Section 13.1

# *Introduction to Homeopathy*

This section includes text excerpted from "Homeopathy,"
National Center for Complementary and Integrative
Health (NCCIH), April 2015.

Homeopathy, also known as homeopathic medicine, is an alternative medical system that was developed in Germany more than 200 years ago.

The alternative medical system of homeopathy was developed in Germany at the end of the 18th century. Supporters of homeopathy point to two unconventional theories: "like cures like"—the notion that a disease can be cured by a substance that produces similar symptoms in healthy people; and "law of minimum dose"—the notion that the lower the dose of the medication, the greater its effectiveness. Many homeopathic remedies are so diluted that no molecules of the original substance remain.

Homeopathic remedies are derived from substances that come from plants, minerals, or animals, such as red onion, arnica (mountain herb), crushed whole bees, white arsenic, poison ivy, belladonna (deadly nightshade), and stinging nettle. Homeopathic remedies are often formulated as sugar pellets to be placed under the tongue; they may also be in other forms, such as ointments, gels, drops, creams, and tablets. Treatments are "individualized" or tailored to each person—it is not uncommon for different people with the same condition to receive different treatments.

## *Regulation of Homeopathic Treatments*

Homeopathic remedies are regulated as drugs under the Federal Food, Drug and Cosmetic Act (FD&C Act). However, under current Agency policy, the U.S. Food and Drug Administration (FDA) does not evaluate the remedies for safety or effectiveness.

The FDA allows homeopathic remedies that meet certain conditions to be marketed without agency preapproval. For example, homeopathic remedies must contain active ingredients that are listed in the

Homeopathic Pharmacopeia of the United States (HPUS). The HPUS lists active ingredients that may be legally included in homeopathic products and standards for strength, quality, and purity of that ingredient. In addition, the FDA requires that the label on the product, outer container, or accompanying leaflet include at least one major indication (i.e., medical problem to be treated), a list of ingredients, the number of times the active ingredient was diluted, and directions for use. If a homeopathic remedy claims to treat a serious disease such as cancer, it must be sold by prescription. Only products for minor health problems, like a cold or a headache, which go away on their own, can be sold without a prescription.

## The Status of Homeopathy Research

Most rigorous clinical trials and systematic analyses of the research on homeopathy have concluded that there is little evidence to support homeopathy as an effective treatment for any specific condition.

A comprehensive assessment of evidence by the Australian government's National Health and Medical Research Council (NHMRC) concluded that there are no health conditions for which there is reliable evidence that homeopathy is effective.

Homeopathy is a controversial topic in complementary medicine research. A number of the key concepts of homeopathy are not consistent with fundamental concepts of chemistry and physics. For example, it is not possible to explain in scientific terms how a remedy containing little or no active ingredient can have any effect. This, in turn, creates major challenges to a rigorous clinical investigation of homeopathic remedies. For example, one cannot confirm that an extremely dilute remedy contains what is listed on the label, or develop objective measures that show effects of extremely dilute remedies in the human body.

Another research challenge is that homeopathic treatments are highly individualized, and there is no uniform prescribing a standard for homeopathic practitioners. There are hundreds of different homeopathic remedies, which can be prescribed in a variety of different dilutions for thousands of symptoms.

## Side Effects and Risks

- Certain homeopathic products (called "nosodes" or "homeopathic immunizations") have been promoted by some as substitutes for conventional immunizations, but data to support such claims is lacking. The National Center for Complementary and Integrative Health (NCCIH) supports the Centers for Disease Control and Prevention's (CDC) recommendations for immunizations/vaccinations.

- While many homeopathic remedies are highly diluted, some products sold or labeled as homeopathic may not be highly diluted; they can contain substantial amounts of active ingredients. Like any drug or dietary supplement that contains chemical ingredients, these homeopathic products may cause side effects or drug interactions. Negative health effects from homeopathic products of this type have been reported.

- A systematic review found that highly diluted homeopathic remedies, taken under the supervision of trained professionals, are generally safe and unlikely to cause severe adverse reactions. However, like any drug or dietary supplement, these products could pose risks if they are improperly manufactured (for example, if they are contaminated with microorganisms or incorrectly diluted).

- A systematic review of case reports and case series concluded that using certain homeopathic treatments (such as those containing heavy metals like mercury or iron that are not highly diluted) or replacing an effective conventional treatment with an ineffective homeopathic one can cause adverse effects, some of which may be serious.

- Liquid homeopathic remedies may contain alcohol. The FDA allows higher levels of alcohol in these remedies than it allows in conventional drugs.

- Homeopathic practitioners expect some of their patients to experience "homeopathic aggravation" (a temporary worsening of existing symptoms after taking a homeopathic prescription). Researchers have not found much evidence of this reaction in clinical studies; however, research on homeopathic aggravations is scarce. Always discuss changes in your symptoms with your healthcare provider.

- The FDA has warned consumers about different products labeled as homeopathic. For example, in 2015, it warned consumers not to rely on asthma products labeled as homeopathic that are sold over-the-counter (OTC). These products have not been evaluated by the FDA for safety and effectiveness.

# If You Are Thinking about Using Homeopathy

- Do not use homeopathy as a replacement for proven conventional care or to postpone seeing a healthcare provider about a medical problem.

- If you are considering using a homeopathic remedy, bring the product with you when you visit your healthcare provider. The provider may be able to help you determine whether the product might pose a risk of side effects or drug interactions.

- Follow the recommended conventional immunization schedules for children and adults. Do not use homeopathic products as a substitute for conventional immunizations.

- Women who are pregnant or nursing, or people who are thinking of using homeopathy to treat a child, should consult their (or their child's) healthcare providers.

- Tell all your healthcare providers about any complementary health practices you use. Give them a full picture of all you do to manage your health. This will ensure coordinated and safe care.

## Licensing and Certification

Laws regulating the practice of homeopathy in the United States vary from state to state. Usually, individuals who are licensed to practice medicine or another healthcare profession can legally practice homeopathy. In some states, nonlicensed professionals may practice homeopathy.

Arizona, Connecticut, and Nevada are the only states with homeopathic licensing boards for doctors of medicine (holders of M.D. degrees) and doctors of osteopathic medicine (holders of D.O. degrees). Arizona and Nevada also license homeopathic assistants, who are allowed to perform medical services under the supervision of a homeopathic physician. Some states explicitly include homeopathy within the scope of practice of chiropractic, naturopathy, and physical therapy.

## Section 13.2

# *Use Caution with Homeopathic Products*

This section includes text excerpted from "Homeopathic Products,"
U.S. Food and Drug Administration (FDA), March 20, 2018.

Homeopathy is an alternative medical practice that was developed in the late 1700s. Homeopathy is generally based on two main principles:

- That a substance that causes symptoms in a healthy person can be used in diluted form to treat symptoms and illnesses, a principle known as "like-cures-like"; and

- The more diluted the substance, the more potent it is, which is known as the "law of infinitesimals."

Historically, homeopathic products have been identified through "provings," in which substances are administered to healthy volunteers in concentrations that cause symptoms. Symptoms experienced by volunteers are recorded to indicate possible therapeutic uses for the substances. In other words, if a substance causes a particular symptom, individuals experiencing that symptom would be treated with a diluted solution made from that substance.

## *What Are Homeopathic Products and How Can You Tell You Are Taking One?*

There are no FDA-approved products labeled as homeopathic; this means that any product labeled as homeopathic is being marketed in the United States. without FDA evaluation for safety or effectiveness. These products are often marketed as natural, safe and effective alternatives to approved prescription and nonprescription products, and are sold online and in major retail stores.

Products labeled as homeopathic can contain a wide range of substances, including ingredients derived from plants, healthy or diseased animal or human sources, minerals, and chemicals.

Products labeled as homeopathic generally include:

- The word "Homeopathic"
- The ingredients listed in terms of dilution, e.g., 1X, 6X, 2C

## Is FDA Concerned about the Safety of Homeopathic Products?

While products labeled as homeopathic are generally labeled as highly diluted, some of these products have been found to contain measurable amounts of active ingredients and, therefore, could cause significant patient harm. Additionally, the FDA has tested products that were improperly manufactured, which can cause incorrect dilutions and increase the potential for contamination. Further, some products labeled as homeopathic are marketed to treat serious diseases or conditions.

## What Should Consumers Know about Homeopathic Products?

Products labeled as homeopathic and currently marketed in the U.S. have not been reviewed by the FDA for safety and effectiveness to diagnose, treat, cure, prevent or mitigate any diseases or conditions. FDA's evidence-based drug reviews play an essential role in ensuring that drugs are made with quality manufacturing processes, and are safe and effective for their intended uses. Products that have not been evaluated for safety and effectiveness may harm consumers who choose to treat serious diseases or conditions with such products, and consumers may be foregoing treatment with a medical product that has been scientifically proven to be safe and effective.

The FDA recommends consumers talk to their doctor or healthcare professional about safe and effective treatments for their disease or condition.

## How Are Homeopathic Products Regulated?

Under the Federal Food, Drug, and Cosmetic Act (FD&C), homeopathic drug products are subject to the same requirements related to approval, adulteration, and misbranding. However, prescription and nonprescription drug products labeled as homeopathic have been manufactured and distributed without FDA approval under the enforcement policies in the FDA's Compliance Policy Guide (CPG) 400.400 since 1988.

This industry has experienced expansive growth since the issuance of the CPG, which has compounded FDA's concerns about the safety of some of the products. FDA held a public hearing in April 2015 to obtain input from stakeholders about the current use of products labeled as homeopathic and the agency's regulatory framework for such products. FDA also sought broad public input on its enforcement policies related to products labeled as homeopathic, to better protect the public health, and received more than 9,000 comments to the docket.

Since homeopathic drug products have not been approved by the FDA for any use, they may not meet modern standards for safety, effectiveness, and quality. The FDA has determined that it is in the best interest of public health to issue a new draft guidance that proposes a comprehensive, risk-based enforcement approach to drug products labeled as homeopathic and marketed without FDA approval.

The FDA's proposed approach prioritizes enforcement and regulatory actions involving unapproved drug products labeled as homeopathic that pose the greatest risk to patients. Under this approach, many homeopathic products will likely fall outside the risk-based categories described in the new draft guidance and will remain available to consumers. FDA intends to focus its enforcement authorities on the following kinds of products:

- With reported safety concerns;

- That contain or claim to contain ingredients associated with potentially significant safety concerns, such as controlled substances;

- With routes of administration other than oral or topical, e.g., for use as an injection or taken nasally;

- That claim to treat or prevent serious and/or life-threatening diseases and conditions, such as cancer;

- Marketed to vulnerable populations, including children, pregnant women and the elderly; or

- That do not meet regulatory standards of quality, strength, or purity as required under the law.

## *Is FDA Going to Remove Homeopathic Products from the Market?*

The FDA's top concern is patient safety. FDA's draft guidance states that it is intended to provide notice that any product labeled as homeopathic that is being marketed illegally is subject to FDA enforcement action at any time. FDA intends to prioritize its enforcement and regulatory actions against products that pose the greatest risks to patients as described above. However, the agency recognizes that many homeopathic products will likely fall outside the risk-based categories described in the guidance and remain available to consumers.

# Chapter 14

# *Native American Medicine*

Native American medicine refers to the healing practices used by the indigenous peoples of North America. Native American medicine originated thousands of years ago, and it encompasses the traditions and beliefs of more than 500 distinct nations that inhabited the continent before the arrival of Europeans. One of the distinguishing features of Native American medicine is its emphasis on spiritual harmony or balance as a key component of individual health.

Native American healers typically employ a holistic approach that not only addresses the patient's specific illness or injury but also seeks to restore the patient's spirit to a state of harmonious balance with the larger world. They view humans as part of a complex, interrelated spiritual web that encompasses the individual, the community, the Creator, and the natural environment. They believe that diseases, trauma, and bad luck are indications that the relationship between these elements has been disrupted. To return a patient to good health, a healer must also restore balance.

Although the general thrust of Native American medicine is clear, the specific techniques and practices are not well known. Since most Native American cultures never developed a written language, healing techniques were usually passed down verbally from one generation to the next. In the centuries following European contact, many Native American nations experienced dramatic population losses as a result of warfare and epidemics of unfamiliar diseases such as smallpox and

"Native American Medicine," © 2015 Omnigraphics. Reviewed May 2018.

measles. As traditional healers died, they often took their knowledge of Native American medicine with them.

The main documentation of Native American medicine was done by people outside of the cultural tradition. Although these people could observe and describe the physical practices, they could not necessarily understand and capture their underlying spiritual meaning. In fact, some Native American healers claim that their medical practices cannot be reduced to an academic body of knowledge and technique. In addition, many Native American elders decline requests to share their healing secrets with nonnatives, out of concern that their sacred practices will be dishonored or exploited and their spiritual power weakened. Some of the knowledge has survived, however, and Native American medicine continues to be practiced in the 21st century.

## Healers

The traditional healers in Native American tribes were known as medicine men and medicine women. They mixed herbs and administered remedies to people who were sick or injured. In addition to practicing medicine, however, the healers were also religious leaders who helped maintain the connection between the tribe and the Creator or Great Spirit. Under the Native American belief system, an illness could have any number of different causes, including demons and evil spirits. The healers often wore grotesque masks to frighten away evil spirits and performed special ceremonies to purge the patient of demonic influences.

Most healers used tools made from natural sources, such as bones, crystals, feathers, fur, roots, shells, skin, and stones. These tools were used in ceremonies to invoke the help of the Great Spirit in healing illnesses and driving away evil. Many healers carried medicines tied in a cloth bundle or thick hide. The contents of these medicine bags were known only to the healer and were considered a sacred source of power.

Each healer was believed to have a unique perspective that grew out of her or his individual skills, abilities, and life experiences. A person in need of medical treatment would seek a healer who had successfully treated other patients with similar conditions. The healer typically established a relationship with each patient in order to gain an understanding of the patient's unique circumstances and preferences. Often the treatment was designed not only to cure a disease, but also to help the patient achieve spiritual growth and find a healthier balance with the larger world.

90

## Healing Practices and Ceremonies

Although the healing methods used by various Native American nations differed, herbal remedies played a major role in medical treatment for all the tribes. Healers collected plants from surrounding areas that were known to be effective in treating certain ailments. They even traded over long distances to obtain herbs that were not available locally. Various herbs could be ground into powders to be inhaled, mashed into pastes to be applied to the skin, or mixed with water or food to be consumed.

Native American healers also conducted special purification rituals, such as sweat lodges and sweat baths, to help remove toxins from a sick person's body. During these rituals, the healer usually prayed, chanted, sang, or played drums to help cleanse the body and increase clarity of thought. Sage, an herb that was believed to have powerful cleansing properties, was burned in a ceremony called "sweeping the smoke" in order to purify the body and soul.

Native American medicine also involved healing rituals and ceremonies in which the entire community participated. Rather than curing an individual patient, many of these rituals were intended to help restore harmony between the tribe and the Great Spirit in order to promote general health and prosperity. The ceremonies, which sometimes took place over several days, might involve prayers, songs and stories, chants, drumming, and various sacred healing objects. Some tribes used the medicine wheel or sacred hoop, which denotes the circle of life. It incorporates the four directions as well as Mother Earth and Father Sky.

## Native American Medicine Today

In the late 1800s, the U.S. government instituted bans on Native American religious practices, which white officials considered "heathen" rituals that interfered with their goal of "civilizing" the tribes. Since these practices were closely linked to Native American medicine, many traditional healing rituals were prohibited or strongly discouraged as well. After being suppressed for decades, many ancient medical practices were forgotten. Meanwhile, in the early 20th century the federal Indian Health Service began opening hospitals and clinics on reservations to bring modern medicine to Native American communities. An increasing number of Native Americans turned to these facilities for their healthcare needs, especially to treat "white man's diseases" that their healers had proven unable to cure.

The passage of the American Indian Religious Freedom Act in 1978 finally lifted the federal ban on Native American religious practices and healing rituals. Since then, mainstream medical theory has shifted toward a more holistic approach that recognizes a patient's mental and spiritual well-being as an important component of their physical health. As a result, Native American medicine has experienced a surge in popularity and interest.

Traditional herbal remedies drawn from Native American traditions, for instance, hold strong appeal for people who are concerned about the toxicity, addictive properties, and side effects of pharmaceutical drugs. Some people believe that these natural remedies, which have been developed over centuries, can be as effective as prescription medications in treating certain conditions.

Many Native American communities face serious health concerns in the 21st century, including high rates of alcoholism, obesity, diabetes, and heart disease. While most Native Americans rely on conventional medicine to treat these health problems, many find that traditional healing practices provide benefits as well. In addition, the holistic approach used by Native American healers has increasingly attracted nonnative adherents. By treating the patient's body, mind, and spirit together, they believe that Native American medicine can improve their chances of healing and maintain good health.

### References

1.  The Center for Health and Healing. "Traditional and Indigenous Healing Systems: Native American Medicine," Mt. Sinai Beth Israel, 2003.

2.  Mehl-Madrona, Lewis. "Traditional (Native American) Indian Medicine Treatment of Chronic Illness," Healing Center Online, 2008.

3.  Weiser, Kathy. "Native American Medicine," *Legends of America*, May 2015.

# Chapter 15

# *Naturopathy*

Naturopathy—also called naturopathic medicine—is a medical system that has evolved from a combination of traditional practices and healthcare approaches popular in Europe during the 19th century.

People visit naturopathic practitioners for various health-related purposes, including primary care, overall well-being, and treatment of illnesses.

In the United States, naturopathy is practiced by naturopathic physicians, traditional naturopaths, and other healthcare providers who also offer naturopathic services.

## *What Naturopathic Practitioners Do*

Naturopathic practitioners use many different treatment approaches. Examples include:

- Dietary and lifestyle changes

- Exercise therapy

- Herbs and other dietary supplements

- Homeopathy

- Manipulative therapies

---

This chapter includes text excerpted from "Naturopathy," National Center for Complementary and Integrative Health (NCCIH), September 24, 2017.

- Practitioner guided detoxification
- Psychotherapy and counseling
- Stress reduction

Some practitioners use other methods as well or, if appropriate, may refer patients to conventional healthcare providers.

## *Education and Licensure of Practitioners*

Education and licensing differ for the three types of naturopathic practitioners:

- **Naturopathic physicians** generally complete a 4-year, graduate-level program at one of the North American naturopathic medical schools accredited by the Council on Naturopathic Medical Education (CNME), an organization recognized for accreditation purposes by the U.S. Department of Education (ED). Some U.S. states and territories have licensing requirements for naturopathic physicians; others don't. In those jurisdictions that have licensing requirements, naturopathic physicians must graduate from a 4-year naturopathic medical college and pass an examination to receive a license. They must also fulfill annual continuing education requirements.

- **Traditional naturopaths,** also known simply as "naturopaths," may receive training in a variety of ways. Training programs vary in length and content and are not accredited by organizations recognized for accreditation purposes by the ED. Traditional naturopaths are often not eligible for licensing.

- **Other healthcare providers** (such as physicians, osteopathic physicians, chiropractors, dentists, and nurses) sometimes offer naturopathic treatments, functional medicine, and other holistic therapies, having pursued additional training in these areas. Training programs vary.

Remember that regulations, licenses, or certificates do not guarantee safe, effective treatment from any healthcare provider—conventional or complementary.

Tell all your healthcare providers about any complementary or integrative health approaches you use. Give them a full picture of what you do to manage your health. This will help ensure coordinated and safe care.

# Chapter 16

# *Traditional Chinese Medicine (TCM)*

Traditional Chinese medicine (TCM) originated in ancient China and has evolved over thousands of years. TCM practitioners use herbal medicines and various mind and body practices, such as acupuncture and tai chi, to treat or prevent health problems. In the United States, people use TCM primarily as a complementary health approach.

## *Is It Safe?*

- Acupuncture is generally considered safe when performed by an experienced practitioner using sterile needles. Improperly performed acupuncture can cause potentially serious side effects.

- Tai chi and qi gong, two mind and body practices used in TCM, are generally safe.

- There have been reports of Chinese herbal products being contaminated with drugs, toxins, or heavy metals or not containing the listed ingredients. Some of the herbs used in Chinese medicine can interact with drugs, have serious side effects, or be unsafe for people with certain medical conditions.

---

This chapter includes text excerpted from "Traditional Chinese Medicine: In Depth," National Center for Complementary and Integrative Health (NCCIH), October 2013. Reviewed May 2018.

## Is It Effective?

For most conditions, there is not enough rigorous scientific evidence to know whether TCM methods work for the conditions for which they are used.

## Keep in Mind

Tell all your healthcare providers about any complementary health approaches you use. Give them a full picture of what you do to manage your health. This will help ensure coordinated and safe care.

## Background

TCM encompasses many different practices, including acupuncture, moxibustion (burning an herb above the skin to apply heat to acupuncture points), Chinese herbal medicine, tui na (Chinese therapeutic massage), dietary therapy, and tai chi and qi gong (practices that combine specific movements or postures, coordinated breathing, and mental focus). TCM is rooted in the ancient philosophy of Taoism and dates back more than 2,500 years. Traditional systems of medicine also exist in other East and South Asian countries, including Japan (where the traditional herbal medicine is called Kampo) and Korea. Some of these systems have been influenced by TCM and are similar to it in some ways, but each has developed distinctive features of its own.

## Side Effects and Risks

- Herbal medicines used in TCM are sometimes marketed in the United States as dietary supplements. The U.S. Food and Drug Administration (FDA) regulations for dietary supplements are not the same as those for prescription or over-the-counter (OTC) drugs; in general, the regulations for dietary supplements are less stringent. For example, manufacturers don't have to prove to the FDA that most claims made for dietary supplements are valid; if the product were a drug, they would have to provide proof.

- Some Chinese herbal products may be safe, but others may not be. There have been reports of products being contaminated with drugs, toxins, or heavy metals or not containing the listed ingredients. Some of the herbs used in Chinese medicine can interact with drugs, can have serious side effects, or may be unsafe for people with certain medical conditions. For example, the Chinese herb ephedra (ma huang) has been linked to serious health complications, including heart attack and stroke. In 2004, the FDA banned the sale of ephedra-containing dietary supplements, but the ban does not apply to TCM remedies.

- The FDA regulates acupuncture needles as medical devices and requires that the needles be sterile, nontoxic, and labeled for single use by qualified practitioners only. Relatively few complications from the use of acupuncture have been reported. However, adverse effects—some of them serious—have resulted from the use of nonsterile needles or improper delivery of acupuncture treatments.

- Tai chi and qi gong are considered to be generally safe practices.

- Information on the safety of other TCM methods is limited. Reported complications of moxibustion include allergic reactions, burns, and infections, but how often these events occur is not known. Both moxibustion and cupping (applying a heated cup to the skin to create a slight suction) may mark the skin, usually temporarily. The origin of these marks should be explained to healthcare providers so that they will not be mistaken for signs of disease or physical abuse.

TCM practitioners use a variety of techniques in an effort to promote health and treat disease. In the United States, the most commonly used approaches include Chinese herbal medicine, acupuncture, and tai chi.

- **Chinese herbal medicine.** The Chinese *Materia Medica* (a pharmacological reference book used by TCM practitioners) describes thousands of medicinal substances—primarily plants, but also some minerals and animal products. Different parts of plants, such as the leaves, roots, stems, flowers, and seeds, are used. In TCM, herbs are often combined in formulas and given as teas, capsules, liquid extracts, granules, or powders.

- **Acupuncture.** Acupuncture is a family of procedures involving the stimulation of specific points on the body using a variety of techniques. The acupuncture technique that has been most often studied scientifically involves penetrating the skin with thin, solid, metal needles that are manipulated by the hands or by electrical stimulation.

- **Tai chi.** Tai chi is a centuries-old mind and body practice. It involves gentle, dance-like body movements with mental focus, breathing, and relaxation.

## Underlying Concepts

When thinking about ancient medical systems such as TCM, it is important to separate questions about traditional theories and concepts of health and wellness from questions about whether specific interventions might be helpful in the context of modern science-based medicine and health promotion practices.

The ancient beliefs on which TCM is based include the following:

- The human body is a miniature version of the larger, surrounding universe.

- Harmony between two opposing yet complementary forces, called *yin* and *yang*, supports health, and disease results from an imbalance between these forces.

- Five elements—fire, earth, wood, metal, and water— symbolically represent all phenomena, including the stages of human life, and explain the functioning of the body and how it changes during disease.

- Qi, a vital energy that flows through the body, performs multiple functions in maintaining health.

## The Status of TCM Research

In spite of the widespread use of TCM in China and its use in the West, rigorous scientific evidence of its effectiveness is limited. TCM can be difficult for researchers to study because its treatments are often complex and are based on ideas very different from those of modern Western medicine.

Most research studies on TCM have focused on specific techniques, primarily acupuncture and Chinese herbal remedies, and there have been many systematic reviews of studies of TCM approaches for various conditions.

- An assessment of the research found that 41 of 70 systematic reviews of the scientific evidence (including 19 of 26 reviews on acupuncture for a variety of conditions and 22 of 42 reviews on Chinese herbal medicine) were unable to reach conclusions about whether the technique worked for the condition under investigation because there was not enough good-quality evidence. The other 29 systematic reviews (including 7 of 26 reviews on acupuncture and 20 of 42 reviews on Chinese herbal medicine) suggested possible benefits but could not reach definite conclusions because of the small quantity or poor quality of the studies.

- In an analysis that combined data on individual participants in 29 studies of acupuncture for pain, patients who received acupuncture for back or neck pain, osteoarthritis, or chronic headache had better pain relief than those who did not receive acupuncture. However, in the same analysis, when actual acupuncture was compared with simulated acupuncture (a sham procedure that resembles acupuncture but in which the needles do not penetrate the skin or penetrate it only slightly), the difference in pain relief between the two treatments was much smaller—so small that it may not have been meaningful to patients.

- Tai chi has not been investigated as extensively as acupuncture or Chinese herbal medicine, but studies, including some supported by the National Center for Complementary and Integrative Health (NCCIH), suggest that practicing tai chi may help to improve balance and stability in people with Parkinson disease (PD); reduce pain from knee osteoarthritis (OA) and fibromyalgia (FM); and promote quality of life and mood in people with heart failure.

## If You Are Thinking about Using TCM

- Do not use TCM to replace effective conventional care or as a reason to postpone seeing a healthcare provider about a medical problem.

- Look for published research studies on TCM for the health condition that interests you.

- It is better to use TCM herbal remedies under the supervision of your healthcare provider or a professional trained in herbal medicine than to try to treat yourself.

- Ask about the training and experience of the TCM practitioner you are considering.

- If you are pregnant or nursing, or are thinking of using TCM to treat a child, you should be especially sure to consult your (or the child's) healthcare provider.

- Tell all your healthcare providers about any complementary health approaches you use. Give them a full picture of what you do to manage your health. This will help ensure coordinated and safe care.

# Part Three

# Dietary Supplements

Chapter 17

# Dietary Supplements: What You Need to Know

## Chapter Contents

## Section 17.1

# *Understanding Dietary Supplements*

This section includes text excerpted from "Information for Consumers—Dietary Supplements: What You Need to Know," U.S. Food and Drug Administration (FDA), November 29, 2017.

Dietary Supplements can be beneficial to your health—but taking supplements can also involve health risks. The U.S. Food and Drug Administration (FDA) does not have the authority to review dietary supplement products for safety and effectiveness before they are marketed.

You've heard about them, may have used them, and may have even recommended them to friends or family. While some dietary supplements are well understood and established, others need further study.

Before making decisions about whether to take a supplement, talk to your healthcare provider. They can help you achieve a balance between the foods and nutrients you personally need.

### *What Are Dietary Supplements?*

Dietary supplements include such ingredients as vitamins, minerals, herbs, amino acids, and enzymes. Dietary supplements are marketed in forms such as tablets, capsules, softgels, gel caps, powders, and liquids.

### *What Are the Benefits of Dietary Supplements?*

Some supplements can help assure that you get enough of the vital substances the body needs to function; others may help reduce the risk of disease. But supplements should not replace complete meals which are necessary for a healthful diet so, be sure you eat a variety of foods as well.

Unlike drugs, supplements are not permitted to be marketed for the purpose of treating, diagnosing, preventing, or curing diseases. That means supplements should not make disease claims, such as "lowers high cholesterol" or "treats heart disease." Claims like these cannot be legitimately made for dietary supplements.

## Are There any Risks in Taking Supplements?

Yes. Many supplements contain active ingredients that have strong biological effects in the body. This could make them unsafe in some situations and hurt or complicate your health. For example, the following actions could lead to harmful—even life-threatening—consequences:

- Combining supplements

- Using supplements with medicines (whether prescription or over-the-counter (OTC))

- Substituting supplements for prescription medicines

- Taking too much of some supplements, such as vitamin A, vitamin D, or iron

Some supplements can also have unwanted effects before, during, and after surgery. So, be sure to inform your healthcare provider, including your pharmacist about any supplements you are taking.

## Common Dietary Supplements

Some of the common dietary supplements include:

- Calcium
- Echinacea
- Fish oil
- Ginseng
- Glucosamine and/or
- Chondroitin sulfate

- Garlic
- Vitamin D
- St. John's Wort
- Saw Palmetto
- Ginkgo
- Green tea

## Who Is Responsible for the Safety of Dietary Supplements?

The FDA is not authorized to review dietary supplement products for safety and effectiveness before they are marketed. The manufacturers and distributors of dietary supplements are responsible for making sure their products are safe before they go to market. If the dietary supplement contains a new ingredient, manufacturers must notify the FDA about that ingredient prior to marketing. However, the notification will only be reviewed by the FDA (not approved) and only for safety, not effectiveness.

Manufacturers are required to produce dietary supplements in a quality manner and ensure that they do not contain contaminants or impurities, and are accurately labeled according to current Good Manufacturing Practice (cGMP) and labeling regulations. If a serious problem associated with a dietary supplement occurs, manufacturers must report it to the FDA as an adverse event. The FDA can take dietary supplements off the market if they are found to be unsafe or if the claims on the products are false and misleading.

## How Can I Find Out More about the Dietary Supplement I'm Taking?

Dietary supplement labels must include name and location information for the manufacturer or distributor. If you want to know more about the product that you are taking, check with the manufacturer or distributor about:

- Information to support the claims of the product

- Information on the safety and effectiveness of the ingredients in the product

## How Can I Be a Smart Supplement Shopper?

Be a savvy supplement user. Here's how:

- When searching for supplements on the Internet, use noncommercial sites (e.g., the National Institutes of Health (NIH), the FDA, the U.S. Department of Agriculture (USDA)) rather than depending on information from sellers.

- If claims sound too good to be true, they probably are. Be mindful of product claims such as "works better than (a prescription drug)," "totally safe," or has "no side effects."

- Be aware that the term "natural" doesn't always mean safe.

- Ask your healthcare provider if the supplement you're considering would be safe and beneficial for you.

- Always remember—safety first!

## Section 17.2

# *Tips for Dietary Supplement Users*

This section includes text excerpted from "Food—Tips for
Dietary Supplement Users," U.S. Food and Drug
Administration (FDA), February 23, 2018.

## *Making Informed Decisions and Evaluating Information*

The U.S. Food and Drug Administration (FDA), as well as health
professionals and their organizations, receive many inquiries each
year from consumers seeking health-related information, especially
about dietary supplements. Clearly, people choosing to supplement
their diets with herbals, vitamins, minerals, or other substances
want to know more about the products they choose so that they can
make informed decisions about them. The choice to use a dietary
supplement can be a wise decision that provides health benefits.
However, under certain circumstances, these products may be
unnecessary for good health or they may even create unexpected
risks.

Given the abundance and conflicting nature of information now
available about dietary supplements, you may need help to sort
the reliable information from the questionable. Below are tips and
resources that will help you be a savvy dietary supplement user. The
principles underlying these tips are similar to those principles a savvy
consumer would use for any product.

## *Basic Points to Consider*

### *Do I Need to Think about My Total Diet?*

Yes. Dietary supplements are intended to supplement the diets
of some people, but not to replace the balance of the variety of foods
important to a healthy diet. While you need enough nutrients, too
much of some nutrients can cause problems.

## *Should I Check with My Doctor or Healthcare Provider before Using a Supplement?*

This is a good idea, especially for certain population groups. Dietary supplements may not be risk-free under certain circumstances. If you are pregnant, nursing a baby, or have a chronic medical condition, such as diabetes, hypertension, or heart disease be sure to consult your doctor or pharmacist before purchasing or taking any supplement.

While vitamin and mineral supplements are widely used and generally considered safe for children, you may wish to check with your doctor or pharmacist before giving these or any other dietary supplements to your child. If you plan to use a dietary supplement in place of drugs or in combination with any drug, tell your healthcare provider first. Many supplements contain active ingredients that have strong biological effects and their safety is not always assured in all users. If you have certain health conditions and take these products, you may be placing yourself at risk.

## *Some Supplements May Interact with Prescription and Over-the-Counter (OTC) Medicines*

Taking a combination of supplements or using these products together with medications (whether prescription or over-the-counter (OTC)) could under certain circumstances produce adverse effects, some of which could be life-threatening. Be alert to advisories about these products, whether taken alone or in combination. For example, Coumadin (a prescription medicine), ginkgo biloba (an herbal supplement), aspirin (an OTC drug) and vitamin E (a vitamin supplement) can each thin the blood, and taking any of these products together can increase the potential for internal bleeding. Combining St. John's Wort with certain human immunodeficiency virus (HIV) drugs significantly reduces their effectiveness. St. John's Wort may also reduce the effectiveness of prescription drugs for heart disease, depression, seizures, certain cancers, or oral contraceptives.

## *Some Supplements Can Have Unwanted Effects during Surgery*

It is important to fully inform your doctor about the vitamins, minerals, herbs, or any other supplements you are taking, especially before elective surgery. You may be asked to stop taking these products at least 2–3 weeks ahead of the procedure to avoid potentially dangerous supplement/drug interactions—such as changes in heart rate, blood pressure, and increased bleeding—that could adversely affect the outcome of your surgery.

### *Adverse Effects from the Use of Dietary Supplements Should Be Reported to MedWatch*

You, your healthcare provider, or anyone may directly to the FDA if you believe it is related to the use of any dietary supplement product, by calling the FDA at 800-FDA-1088 (800-332-1088), by fax at 800-FDA-0178 (800-332-0178) or reporting report a serious adverse event or illness online. FDA would like to know whenever you think a product caused you a serious problem, even if you are not sure that the product was the cause, and even if you do not visit a doctor or clinic. In addition to communicating with the FDA online or by phone, you may use the MedWatch form available from the FDA's website.

### *Who Is Responsible for Ensuring the Safety and Efficacy of Dietary Supplements?*

Under the law, manufacturers of dietary supplements are responsible for making sure their products are safe before they go to market. They are also responsible for determining that the claims on their labels are accurate and truthful. Dietary supplement products are not reviewed by the government before they are marketed, but the FDA has the responsibility to take action against any unsafe dietary supplement product that reaches the market. If the FDA can prove that claims on marketed dietary supplement products are false and misleading, the agency may take action also against products with such claims.

## *Tips on Searching the Web for Information on Dietary Supplements*

When searching on the web, try using directory sites of respected organizations, rather than doing blind searches with a search engine. Ask yourself the following questions:

* **Who operates the site?** Is the site run by the government, a university, or a reputable medical or health-related association (e.g., American Medical Association (AMA), American Diabetes Association (ADA), American Heart Association (AHA), the National Institutes of Health (NIH), the National Academies of Science (NAS), or the FDA)? Is the information written or

reviewed by qualified health professionals, experts in the field, academia, government or the medical community?

- **What is the purpose of the site?** Is the purpose of the site to objectively educate the public or just to sell a product? Be aware of practitioners or organizations whose main interest is in marketing products, either directly or through sites with which they are linked. Commercial sites should clearly distinguish scientific information from advertisements. Most nonprofit and government sites contain no advertising, and access to the site and materials offered are usually free.

- **What is the source of the information and does it have any references?** Has the study been reviewed by recognized scientific experts and published in reputable peer-reviewed scientific journals, like the *New England Journal of Medicine?* Does the information say "some studies show..." or does it state where the study is listed so that you can check the authenticity of the references? For example, can the study be found in the National Library of Medicine's (NLM) database of literature citations?

- **Is the information current?** Check the date when the material was posted or updated. Often new research or other findings are not reflected in old material, e.g., side effects or interactions with other products or new evidence that might have changed earlier thinking. Ideally, health and medical sites should be updated frequently.

- **How reliable is the Internet or e-mail solicitations?** While the Internet is a rich source of health information, it is also an easy vehicle for spreading myths, hoaxes, and rumors about alleged news, studies, products or findings. To avoid falling prey to such hoaxes, be skeptical and watch out for an overly emphatic language with UPPERCASE LETTERS and lots of exclamation points!!!! Beware of such phrases such as: "This is not a hoax" or "Send this to everyone you know."

## More Tips and To-Do's

### Ask Yourself: Does It Sound Too Good to Be True?

Do the claims for the product seem exaggerated or unrealistic? Are there simplistic conclusions being drawn from a complex study to sell a product? While the web can be a valuable source of accurate, reliable information, it also has a wealth of misinformation that may not be obvious. Learn to distinguish hype from evidence-based science. Nonsensical lingo can sound very convincing. Also, be skeptical about anecdotal information from persons who have no formal training in nutrition or botanicals, or from personal testimonials (e.g., from store employees, friends, or online chat rooms and message boards) about incredible benefits or results obtained from using a product. The question these people on their training and knowledge in nutrition or medicine.

## *Think Twice about Chasing the Latest Headline*

Sound health advice is generally based on a body of research, not a single study. Be wary of results claiming a "quick fix" that depart from previous research and scientific beliefs. Keep in mind science does not proceed by dramatic breakthroughs, but by taking many small steps, slowly building towards a consensus. Furthermore, news stories, about the latest scientific study, especially those on TV or radio, are often too brief to include important details that may apply to you or allow you to make an informed decision.

Check your assumptions about the following:

### *Questionable Assumptions*

- "Even if a product may not help me, it at least won't hurt me." It's best not to assume that this will always be true. When consumed in high enough amounts, for a long enough time, or in combination with certain other substances, all chemicals can be toxic, including nutrients, plant components, and other biologically active ingredients.

- "When I see the term 'natural,' it means that a product is healthful and safe." Consumers can be misled if they assume this term assures wholesomeness, or that these food-like substances necessarily have milder effects, which makes them safer to use than drugs. The term "natural" on labels is not well defined and is sometimes used ambiguously to imply unsubstantiated benefits or safety. For example, many weight-loss products claim to be "natural" or "herbal" but this doesn't necessarily make them safe. Their ingredients may interact with drugs or may be dangerous for people with certain medical conditions.

- "A product is safe when there is no cautionary information on the product label." Dietary supplement manufacturers may not necessarily include warnings about potential adverse effects on the labels of their products. If consumers want to know about the safety of a specific dietary supplement, they should contact the manufacturer of that brand directly. It is the manufacturer's responsibility to determine that the supplement it produces or distributes is safe and that there is substantiated evidence that the label claims are truthful and not misleading.

- "A recall of a harmful product guarantees that all such harmful products will be immediately and completely removed from the marketplace." A product recall of a dietary supplement is voluntary and while many manufacturers do their best, a recall does not necessarily remove all harmful products from the marketplace.

**Contact the manufacturer for more information about the specific product that you are purchasing.** If you cannot tell whether the product you are purchasing meets the same standards as those used in the research studies you read about, check with the manufacturer or distributor. Ask to speak to someone who can address your questions, some of which may include:

- What information does the firm have to substantiate the claims made for the product? Be aware that sometimes firms supply so-called "proof" of their claims by citing undocumented reports from satisfied consumers, or "internal" graphs and charts that could be mistaken for evidence-based research.

- Does the firm have information to share about tests it has conducted on the safety or efficacy of the ingredients in the product?

- Does the firm have a quality control system in place to determine if the product actually contains what is stated on the label and is free of contaminants?

- Has the firm received any adverse events reports from consumers using their products?

# Section 17.3

# *Tips for Older Dietary Supplement Users*

This section includes text excerpted from "Information for
Consumers—Tips for Older Dietary Supplement Users,"
U.S. Food and Drug Administration (FDA), November 29, 2017.

## Can Dietary Supplements Help Older Consumers?

Even if you eat a wide variety of foods, how can you be sure that
you are getting all the vitamins, minerals, and other nutrients you
need as you get older? If you are over 50, your nutritional needs may
change. Informed food choices are the first place to start, making sure
you get a variety of foods while watching your calorie intake. Supplements and fortified foods may also help you get appropriate amounts
of nutrients. To help you make informed decisions, talk to your doctor
and/or registered dietitian. They can work together with you to determine if your intake of a specific nutrient might be too low or too high
and then decide how you can achieve a balance between the foods and
nutrients you personally need.

## What Are Dietary Supplements?

* Today's dietary supplements are not only vitamins and
  minerals. They also include other less familiar substances,
  such as herbals, botanicals, amino acids, enzymes, and animal
  extracts. Some dietary supplements are well understood and
  established, but others need further study. Whatever your
  choice, supplements should not replace the variety of foods
  important to a healthful diet.

* Unlike drugs, dietary supplements are not preapproved by the
  government for safety or effectiveness before marketing. Also,
  unlike drugs, supplements are not intended to treat, diagnose,
  prevent, or cure diseases. But some supplements can help assure
  that you get an adequate dietary intake of essential nutrients;
  others may help you reduce your risk of disease. Some older
  people, for example, are tired due to low iron levels. In that case,
  their doctor may recommend an iron supplement.

113

- At times, it can be confusing to tell the difference between a dietary supplement, a food, or over-the-counter (OTC) medicines. This is because supplements, by law, come in a variety of forms that resemble these products, such as tablets, capsules, powders, energy bars, or drinks. One way to know if a product is a dietary supplement is to look for the supplement facts label on the product.

# Supplement Facts

Serving Size 1 Capsule

| Amount Per Capsule | % Daily Value |
|---|---|
| Calories  20 | |
| Calories from Fat  20 | |
| Total Fat  2 g | 3%• |
| Saturated Fat  0.5 g | 3%• |
| Polyunsaturated Fat  1 g | † |
| Monounsaturated Fat  0.5 g | † |
| Vitamin A  4250 IU | 85% |
| Vitamin D  425 IU | 106% |
| Omega-3 fatty acids  0.5 g | † |

• Percent Daily Values are based on a 2,000 calorie diet.
† Daily Value not established.

Ingredients: Cod liver oil, gelatin, water, and glycerin.

**Figure 17.1.** *Supplement Facts Label*

## Are There Any Risks, Especially to Older Consumers?

While certain products may be helpful to some older individuals, there may be circumstances when these products may not benefit your health or when they may create unexpected risks. Many supplements contain active ingredients that have strong biological effects in the body. This could make them unsafe in some situations and hurt or complicate your health. For example:

- Are you taking both medicines and supplements? Are you substituting one for the other? Taking a combination of supplements, using these products together with medications (whether prescription or over-the-counter (OTC)), or substituting them in place of medicines your doctor prescribes could lead to harmful, even life-threatening results. Be alert to any advisories about these products. Coumadin (a prescription medicine), ginkgo biloba (an herbal supplement), aspirin (an OTC drug), and vitamin E (a vitamin supplement) can each thin the blood. Taking any of these products alone or together can increase the potential for internal bleeding or stroke. Another example is St. John's Wort that may reduce the effectiveness of prescription drugs for heart disease, depression, seizures, certain cancers, or human immunodeficiency virus (HIV).

- Are you planning surgery? Some supplements can have unwanted effects before, during, and after surgery. It is important to fully inform your healthcare professional, including your pharmacist, about the vitamins, minerals, herbal, and any other supplements you are taking, especially before surgery. You may be asked to stop taking these products at least 2–3 weeks ahead of the procedure to avoid potentially dangerous supplement/drug interactions such as changes in heart rate, blood pressure, or bleeding risk that could adversely affect the outcome of your surgery.

- Is taking more of a good thing better? Some people might think that if a little is good, taking a lot is even better. But taking too much of some nutrients, even vitamins, and minerals, can also cause problems. Depending on the supplement, your age, and the status of your health, taking more than 100 percent of the Daily Value (DV) of certain vitamins and minerals, e.g., vitamin A, vitamin D, and iron (from supplements and food sources like vitamin-fortified cereals and drinks) may actually harm your health. Large amounts can also interfere with how your medicines work.

**Remember**: Your combined intake of all supplements (including multivitamins, single supplements, and combination products) plus fortified foods, like some cereals, and drinks, could cause health problems.

## Why Speak to My Healthcare Provider about Dietary Supplements?

You and your health professionals (doctors, nurses, registered dietitians, pharmacists, and other caregivers) are a team working

115

toward a common goal—to develop a personalized health plan for you. Your doctor and other members of the health team can help monitor your medical condition and overall health, especially if any problems develop. Although they may not immediately have answers to your questions, these health professionals have access to the most current research on dietary supplements.

There are numerous resources that provide information about dietary supplements. These include TV, radio, newspapers, magazines, store clerks, friends, family, or the Internet. It is important to question recommendations from people who have no formal training in nutrition, botanicals, or medicine. While some of these sources, like the web, may seem to offer a wealth of accurate information, these same sources may contain misinformation that may not be obvious. Given the abundance and conflicting nature of information now available about supplements, it is more important than ever to partner with your healthcare team to sort the reliable information from the questionable.

## *How will I Be Able to Spot False Claims?*

Be savvy! Although the benefits of some dietary supplements have been documented, the claims of others may be unproven. If something sounds too good to be true, it usually is. Here are some signs of a false claim:

- Statements that the product is a quick and effective "cure-all." For example: "Extremely beneficial in the treatment of rheumatism, arthritis, infections, prostate problems, ulcers, cancer, heart trouble, hardening of the arteries, and more."

- Statements that suggest the product can treat or cure diseases. For example: "shrinks tumors" or "cures impotency." Actually, these are drug claims and should not be made for dietary supplements.

- Statements that claim the product is "totally safe," "all natural," or has "definitely no side effects."

- Promotions that use words like "scientific breakthrough," "miraculous cure," "exclusive product," "secret ingredient," or "ancient remedy." For example: "A scientific breakthrough formulated by using proven principles of natural health-based medical science."

- Text that uses overly impressive-sounding terms, like those for a weight-loss product: "hunger stimulation point" and "thermogenesis."

- Personal testimonials from consumers or doctors claiming amazing results. For example: "My husband has Alzheimer. He began eating a teaspoonful of this product each day. And now in just 22 days, he mowed the grass, cleaned out the garage, and weeded the flower beds; we take our morning walk together again."

- Limited availability and advance payment required. For example: "Hurry. This offer will not last. Send us a check now to reserve your supply."

- Promises of no-risk "money-back guarantees." For example: "If after 30 days you have not lost at least 4 pounds each week, your uncashed check will be returned to you."

## What Are the Key "Points to Ponder" before I Buy?

- **Think twice about chasing the latest headline.** Sound health advice is generally based on research over time, not a single study. Be wary of results claiming a "quick fix" that depart from scientific research and established dietary guidance. Keep in mind that science does not generally proceed by dramatic breakthroughs, but rather by taking many small steps, slowly building towards a scientific agreement.

- **We may think, "Even if a product may not help me, it at least won't hurt me."** It's best not to assume that this will always be true. Some product ingredients, including nutrients and plant components, can be toxic based on their activity in your body. Some products may become harmful when consumed in high enough amounts, for a long enough time, or in combination with certain other substances.

- **The term "natural" does not always mean safe.** Do not assume this term assures wholesomeness or that these products have milder effects, making them safer to use than prescribed drugs. For example, many weight-loss products claim to be "natural" or "herbal" but this doesn't necessarily make them safe. The products' ingredients may interact with drugs or may be dangerous for people with certain medical conditions.

- **Spend your money wisely.** Some supplement products may be expensive and may not work, given your specific condition. Be wary of substituting a product or therapy for prescription medicines. Be sure to talk with your healthcare team to help you determine what is best for your overall health.

- **Remember: Safety first.** Resist the pressure to decide "on the spot" about trying an untested product or treatment. Ask for more information and consult your doctor, nurse, dietitian, pharmacist, and/or caregiver about whether the product is right for you and safe for you to use.

## Who Is Responsible for Ensuring the Safety and Efficacy of Dietary Supplements?

Unlike prescription and OTC medicines, dietary supplement products are not reviewed by the government before they are marketed. Under the law, manufacturers of dietary supplements are responsible for making sure their products are safe before they go to market. If you want to know more about the product you are purchasing, check with the manufacturer to find out if the firm:

- Can supply information to support the claims for their products

- Can share information on the safety or efficacy of the ingredients in the product

- Has received any adverse event reports from consumers using their products

## What Is the U.S. Food and Drug Administration's (FDA) Responsibility?

The FDA has the responsibility to take action against unsafe dietary supplement products after they reach the market. The agency may also take legal action against dietary supplement manufacturers if the FDA can prove that claims on marketed dietary supplements are false and misleading.

## What If I Think I Have Had a Reaction to a Dietary Supplement?

Adverse effects from the use of dietary supplements should be reported to the FDA's MedWatch Program. You, your healthcare provider, or anyone should report a serious adverse event or illness directly to the FDA if you believe it is related to the use of any dietary supplement product by calling the FDA at 800-FDA-1088 (800-332-1088), by fax at 800-FDA-0178 (800-332-0178) or reporting online. FDA would like to know whenever you think a product caused you a serious problem, even if you are not sure that the product was the cause, and even if you do not visit a doctor or clinic.

### *Questions to Ask*

- Is taking a dietary supplement an important part of my total diet?
- Are there any precautions or warnings I should know about (e.g., is there an amount or "upper limit" I should not go above)?
- Are there any known side effects (e.g., loss of appetite, nausea, headaches, etc.)? Do they apply to me?
- Are there any foods, medicines (prescription or OTC), or other supplements I should avoid while taking this product?
- If I am scheduled for surgery, should I be concerned about the dietary supplements I am taking?

### *Other Questions to Consider*

- What is this product for?
- What are its intended benefits?
- How, when, and for how long should I take it?

Because many products are marketed as dietary supplements, it is important to remember that supplements include botanical/herbal as well as vitamin/mineral products.

## Section 17.4

# *FAQs on Dietary Supplements*

This section includes text excerpted from "Information for Consumers—Questions and Answers on Dietary Supplements," U.S. Food and Drug Administration (FDA), November 29, 2017.

Congress defined the term "dietary supplement" in the Dietary Supplement Health and Education Act (DSHEA) of 1994. A dietary supplement is a product taken by mouth that contains a "dietary ingredient" intended to supplement the diet. The "dietary ingredients" in these products may include vitamins, minerals, herbs or other botanicals, amino acids, and substances such as enzymes, organ tissues, glandulars, and metabolites. Dietary supplements can also be extracts or concentrates and may be found in many forms such as tablets, capsules, soft gels, gelcaps, liquids, or powders. They can also be in other forms, such as a bar, but if they are, information on their label must not represent the product as a conventional food or a sole item of a meal or diet. Whatever their form may be, DSHEA places dietary supplements in a special category under the general umbrella of "foods," not drugs, and requires that every supplement is labeled a dietary supplement.

## *What Is a "New Dietary Ingredient" in a Dietary Supplement?*

DSHEA of 1994 defined both of the terms "dietary ingredient" and "new dietary ingredient" as components of dietary supplements. In order for an ingredient of a dietary supplement to be a "dietary ingredient," it must be one or any combination of the following substances:

- a vitamin
- a mineral
- an herb or other botanical
- an amino acid

- a dietary substance for use by man to supplement the diet by increasing the total dietary intake (e.g., enzymes or tissues from organs or glands)

- a concentrate, metabolite, constituent, or extract

## What Is the U.S. Food and Drug Administration's (FDA) Role in Regulating Dietary Supplements versus the Manufacturer's Responsibility for Marketing Them?

In October 1994, the DSHEA was signed into law by President Clinton. Before this time, dietary supplements were subject to the same regulatory requirements as were other foods. This new law, which amended the Federal Food, Drug, and Cosmetic Act (FFDCA), created a new regulatory framework for the safety and labeling of dietary supplements. Under DSHEA, a firm is responsible for determining that the dietary supplements it manufactures or distributes are safe and that any representations or claims made about them are substantiated by adequate evidence to show that they are not false or misleading. This means that dietary supplements do not need approval from the FDA before they are marketed. Except in the case of a new dietary ingredient, where premarket review for safety data and other information is required by law, a firm does not have to provide the FDA with the evidence it relies on to substantiate safety or effectiveness before or after it markets its products. Also, manufacturers need to register themselves pursuant to the Bioterrorism Act with the FDA before producing or selling supplements. In June 2007, the FDA published comprehensive regulations for current Good Manufacturing Practices (cGMP) for those who manufacture, package or hold dietary supplement products. These regulations focus on practices that ensure the identity, purity, quality, strength, and composition of dietary supplements.

## When Must a Manufacturer or Distributor Notify the FDA about a Dietary Supplement It Intends to Market in the United States?

DSHEA requires that a manufacturer or distributor notify the FDA if it intends to market a dietary supplement in the United States that contains a "new dietary ingredient." The manufacturer (and distributor) must demonstrate to the FDA why the ingredient is reasonably expected to be safe for use in a dietary supplement unless it has been recognized as a food substance and is present in the food supply. There is no authoritative list of dietary ingredients that were marketed before October 15, 1994. Therefore, manufacturers and distributors are responsible for determining if a dietary ingredient is "new," and if it is not, for documenting that the dietary supplements it sells, containing the dietary ingredient, were marketed before October 15, 1994.

## What Information Must the Manufacturer Disclose on the Label of a Dietary Supplement?

FDA regulations require that certain information appears on dietary supplement labels. Information that must be on a dietary supplement label includes:

- a descriptive name of the product stating that it is a "supplement"

- the name and place of business of the manufacturer, packer, or distributor

- a complete list of ingredients

- the net contents of the product

In addition, each dietary supplement (except for some small volume products or those produced by eligible small businesses) must have nutrition labeling in the form of a "Supplement Facts" panel. This label must identify each dietary ingredient contained in the product.

## Must All Ingredients Be Declared on the Label of a Dietary Supplement?

Yes, ingredients not listed on the "Supplement Facts" panel must be listed in the "other ingredient" statement beneath the panel. The types of ingredients listed there could include the source of dietary ingredients, if not identified in the "Supplement Facts" panel (e.g., rose hips as the source of vitamin C), other food ingredients (e.g., water and sugar), and technical additives or processing aids (e.g., gelatin, starch, colors, stabilizers, preservatives, and flavors).

## Are Dietary Supplement Serving Sizes Standardized or Are There Restrictions on the Amount of a Nutrient That Can Be in One Serving?

Other than the manufacturer's responsibility to ensure safety, there are no rules that limit a serving size or the amount of a nutrient in any form of dietary supplements. This decision is made by the manufacturer and does not require the FDA review or approval.

## Where Can I Get Information about a Specific Dietary Supplement?

Manufacturers and distributors do not need the FDA's approval to sell their dietary supplements. This means that the FDA does not keep a list of manufacturers, distributors or the dietary supplement products they sell. If you want more detailed information than the label tells you about a specific product, you may contact the manufacturer of that brand directly. The name and address of the manufacturer or distributor can be found on the label of the dietary supplement.

## Who Has the Responsibility for Ensuring That a Dietary Supplement Is Safe?

By law (DSHEA), the manufacturer is responsible for ensuring that its dietary supplement products are safe before they are marketed. Unlike drug products that must be proven safe and effective for their intended use before marketing, there are no provisions in the law for the FDA to "approve" dietary supplements for safety or effectiveness before they reach the consumer. Under DSHEA, once the product is marketed, the FDA has the responsibility for showing that a dietary supplement is "unsafe," before it can take action to restrict the product's use or removal from the marketplace. However, manufacturers and distributors of dietary supplements must record, investigate and forward to the FDA any reports they receive of serious adverse events associated with the use of their products that are reported to them directly. FDA is able to evaluate these reports and any other adverse event information reported directly to us by healthcare providers or consumers to identify early signals that a product may present safety risks to consumers.

## Do Manufacturers or Distributors of Dietary Supplements Have to Tell the FDA or Consumers What Evidence They Have about Their Product's Safety or What Evidence They Have to Back Up the Claims They Are Making for Them?

No, except for rules described above that govern "new dietary ingredients," there is no provision under any law or regulation that the FDA enforces that requires a firm to disclose to the FDA or consumers the information they have about the safety or purported benefits of their dietary supplement products. Likewise, there is no prohibition against them making this information available either to the FDA or to their customers. It is up to each firm to set its own policy on disclosure of such information. For more information, see claims that can be made for dietary supplements

## How Can Consumers Inform Themselves about Safety and Other Issues Related to Dietary Supplements?

It is important to be well informed about products before purchasing them. Because it is often difficult to know what information is reliable and what is questionable, consumers may first want to contact the manufacturer about the product they intend to purchase.

## What Is the FDA's Oversight Responsibility for Dietary Supplements?

Because dietary supplements are under the "umbrella" of foods, the FDA's Center for Food Safety and Applied Nutrition (CFSAN) is responsible for the agency's oversight of these products. The FDA's efforts to monitor the marketplace for potential illegal products (that is, products that may be unsafe or make false or misleading claims) include obtaining information from inspections of dietary supplement manufacturers and distributors, the Internet, consumer, and trade complaints, occasional laboratory analyses of selected products, and adverse events associated with the use of supplements that are reported to the agency.

## Does the FDA's Routinely Analyze the Content of Dietary Supplements?

In that the FDA has limited resources to analyze the composition of food products, including dietary supplements, it focuses these resources first on public health emergencies and products that may have caused injury or illness. Enforcement priorities then go to products thought to be unsafe or fraudulent or in violation of the law. The remaining funds are used for routine monitoring of products pulled from store shelves or collected during inspections of manufacturing firms. The agency does not analyze dietary supplements before they are sold to consumers. The manufacturer is responsible for ensuring that the "Supplement Facts" label and ingredient list are accurate, that the dietary ingredients are safe, and that the content matches the amount declared on the label. The FDA does not have resources to analyze dietary supplements sent to the agency by consumers who want to know their content. Instead, consumers may contact the manufacturer or a commercial laboratory for an analysis of the content.

## Is It Legal to Market a Dietary Supplement Product as a Treatment or Cure for a Specific Disease or Condition?

No, a product sold as a dietary supplement and promoted on its label or in labeling* as a treatment, prevention or cure for a specific disease or condition would be considered an unapproved—and thus illegal—drug. To maintain the product's status as a dietary supplement, the label and labeling must be consistent with the provisions in DSHEA of 1994.

*Labeling refers to the label as well as accompanying material that is used by a manufacturer to promote and market a specific product.

## Who Validates Claims and What Kinds of Claims Can Be Made on Dietary Supplement Labels?

The FDA receives many consumer inquiries about the validity of claims for dietary supplements, including product labels, advertisements, media, and printed materials. The responsibility for ensuring the validity of these claims rests with the manufacturer, the FDA, and, in the case of advertising, with the Federal Trade Commission (FTC). By law, manufacturers may make three types of claims for their dietary supplement products:

1. Health claims
2. Structure/function claims
3. Nutrient content claims

Some of these claims describe the link between a food substance and disease or a health-related condition; the intended benefits of using the product; or the amount of a nutrient or dietary substance in a product. Different requirements generally apply to each type of claim and are described in more detail.

## Why Do Some Supplements Have Wording That Says: "This Statement Has Not Been Evaluated by the FDA. This Product Is Not Intended to Diagnose, Treat, Cure, or Prevent Any Disease"?

This statement or "disclaimer" is required by law (DSHEA) when a manufacturer makes a structure/function claim on a dietary supplement label. In general, these claims describe the role of a nutrient or dietary ingredient intended to affect the structure or function of the body. The manufacturer is responsible for ensuring the accuracy and truthfulness of these claims; they are not approved by the FDA. For this reason, the law says that if a dietary supplement label includes such a claim, it must state in a "disclaimer" that the FDA has not evaluated this claim. The disclaimer must also state that this product is not intended to "diagnose, treat, cure, or prevent any disease," because only a drug can legally make such a claim.

### How Are Advertisements for Dietary Supplements Regulated?

The FTC regulates advertising, including infomercials, for dietary supplements and most other products sold to consumers. FDA works closely with FTC in this area, but FTC's work is directed by different laws.

### How Do I, My Healthcare Provider, or Any Informed Individual Report a Problem or Illness Caused by a Dietary Supplement to the FDA?

If you think you have suffered a serious harmful effect or illness from a dietary supplement, the first thing you should do is contact or see your healthcare provider immediately. Then, you or your healthcare provider can report this by submitting a report through the Safety Reporting Portal (SRP). If you do not have access to the Internet, you may submit a report by calling the FDA's MedWatch hotline at 800-FDA-1088 (800-332-1088).

The FDA would like to know when a dietary supplement causes a problem even if you are unsure the product caused the problem or even if you do not visit a doctor or clinic. Anyone may report a serious adverse event or illness thought to be related to a dietary supplement directly to the FDA by accessing the SRP mentioned above.

Consumers are also encouraged to report instances of product problems using the SRP. Examples of product problems are foreign objects in the packaging or other apparent quality defects. In addition to communicating with the FDA online or by phone, you may use the postage-paid MedWatch form available from the FDA's website.

**Note.** The identity of the reporter and/or patient is kept confidential. For a general complaint or concern about food products, including dietary supplements, you may contact the consumer complaint coordinator at the local FDA District Office nearest you.

# Chapter 18

# *Botanical Dietary Supplements*

## *Chapter Contents*

129

# Section 18.1

# *Understanding Botanical Dietary Supplements*

This section includes text excerpted from "Botanical Dietary Supplements," Office of Dietary Supplements (ODS), National Institutes of Health (NIH), June 24, 2011. Reviewed May 2018.

A botanical is a plant or plant part valued for its medicinal or therapeutic properties, flavor, and/or scent. Herbs are a subset of botanicals. Products made from botanicals that are used to maintain or improve health may be called herbal products, botanical products, or phytomedicines.

In naming botanicals, botanists use a Latin name made up of the genus and species of the plant. Under this system the botanical black cohosh is known as *Actaea racemosa L.,* where "L" stands for Linnaeus, who first described the type of plant specimen. The Office of Dietary Supplements (ODS), do not include such initials because they do not appear on most products used by consumers.

## *Can Botanicals Be Dietary Supplements?*

To be classified as a dietary supplement, a botanical must meet the definition given below. Many botanical preparations meet the definition.

As defined by Congress in the Dietary Supplement Health and Education Act (DSHEA), which became law in 1994, a dietary supplement is a product (other than tobacco) that:

- is intended to supplement the diet;

- contains one or more dietary ingredients (including vitamins; minerals; herbs or other botanicals; amino acids; and other substances) or their constituents;

- is intended to be taken by mouth as a pill, capsule, tablet, or liquid; and

- is labeled on the front panel as being a dietary supplement.

## How Are Botanicals Commonly Sold and Prepared?

Botanicals are sold in many forms: as fresh or dried products; liquid or solid extracts; tablets, capsules, powders, tea bags, and other forms. For example, fresh ginger root is often found in the produce section of food stores; dried ginger root is sold packaged in tea bags, capsules, or tablets; and liquid preparations made from ginger root are also sold. A particular group of chemicals or a single chemical may be isolated from a botanical and sold as a dietary supplement, usually in tablet or capsule form. An example is phytoestrogens from soy products.

Common preparations include teas, decoctions, tinctures, and extracts:

- A tea, also known as an infusion, is made by adding boiling water to fresh or dried botanicals and steeping them. The tea may be drunk either hot or cold.

- Some roots, bark, and berries require more forceful treatment to extract their desired ingredients. They are simmered in boiling water for longer periods than teas, making a decoction, which also may be drunk hot or cold.

- A tincture is made by soaking a botanical in a solution of alcohol and water. Tinctures are sold as liquids and are used for concentrating and preserving a botanical. They are made in different strengths that are expressed as botanical-to-extract ratios (i.e., ratios of the weight of the dried botanical to the volume or weight of the finished product).

- An extract is made by soaking the botanicals in a liquid that removes specific types of chemicals. The liquid can be used as is or evaporated to make a dry extract for use in capsules or tablets.

## Are Botanical Dietary Supplements Standardized?

Standardization is a process that manufacturers may use to ensure batch-to-batch consistency of their products. In some cases, standardization involves identifying specific chemicals (also known as markers) that can be used to manufacture a consistent product. The standardization process can also provide a measure of quality control.

Dietary supplements are not required to be standardized in the United States. In fact, no legal or regulatory definition exists for standardization in the United States as it applies to botanical dietary supplements. Because of this, the term "standardization" may mean many different things. Some manufacturers use the term standardization incorrectly to refer to uniform manufacturing practices; following a recipe is not sufficient for a product to be called standardized. Therefore, the presence of the word "standardized" on a supplement label does not necessarily indicate product quality.

Ideally, the chemical markers chosen for standardization would also be the constituents that are responsible for a botanical's effect in the body. In this way, each lot of the product would have a consistent health effect. However, the components responsible for the effects of most botanicals have not been identified or clearly defined. For example, the sennosides in the botanical senna are known to be responsible for the laxative effect of the plant, but many compounds may be responsible for valerian's relaxing effect.

## *Are Botanical Dietary Supplements Safe?*

Many people believe that products labeled "natural" are safe and good for them. This is not necessarily true because the safety of a botanical depends on many things, such as its chemical makeup, how it works in the body, how it is prepared, and the dose used.

The action of botanicals ranges from mild to powerful (potent). A botanical with mild action may have subtle effects. Chamomile and peppermint, both mild botanicals, are usually taken as teas to aid digestion and are generally considered safe for self-administration.

Some mild botanicals may have to be taken for weeks or months before their full effects are achieved. For example, valerian may be effective as a sleep aid after 14 days of use but it is rarely effective after just one dose. In contrast, a powerful botanical produces a fast result. Kava, as one example, is reported to have an immediate and powerful action affecting anxiety and muscle relaxation.

The dose and form of a botanical preparation also play important roles in its safety. Teas, tinctures, and extracts have different strengths. The same amount of a botanical may be contained in a cup of tea, a few teaspoons of tincture, or an even smaller quantity of an extract. Also, different preparations vary in the relative amounts and concentrations of chemical removed from the whole botanical. For example, peppermint tea is generally considered safe to drink but peppermint oil is much more concentrated and can be toxic if used incorrectly. It is important to follow the manufacturer's suggested directions for using a botanical and not exceed the recommended dose without the advice of a healthcare provider.

## Does a Label Indicate the Quality of a Botanical Dietary Supplement Product?

It is difficult to determine the quality of a botanical dietary supplement product from its label. The degree of quality control depends on the manufacturer, the supplier, and others in the production process.

The U.S. Food and Drug Administration (FDA) issued Good Manufacturing Practices (GMPs) for dietary supplements, a set of requirements and expectations by which dietary supplements must be manufactured, prepared, and stored to ensure quality. Manufacturers are now expected to guarantee the identity, purity, strength, and composition of their dietary supplements. For example, the GMPs aim to prevent the inclusion of the wrong ingredients, the addition of too much or too little of a dietary ingredient, the possibility of contamination (by pesticides, heavy metals such as lead, bacteria, etc.), and the improper packaging and labeling of a product.

## What Methods Are Used to Evaluate the Health Benefits and Safety of a Botanical Dietary Supplement?

Like other dietary supplements, botanicals are not required by federal law to be tested for safety and effectiveness before they are marketed, so the amount of scientific evidence available for various botanical ingredients varies widely. Some botanicals have been evaluated in scientific studies. For example, research shows that St. John's wort may be useful for short-term treatment of mild to moderate depression. Other botanical dietary supplements need more study to determine their value.

Scientists can use several approaches to evaluate botanical dietary supplements for their potential health benefits and risks. They may investigate history of use, conduct laboratory studies using cell or tissue cultures, and experiment with animals. Studies on people (e.g., individual case reports, observational studies, and clinical trials) provide the most direct evidence of a botanical supplements' effect on health and patterns of use.

# Section 18.2

# *National Toxicology Program (NTP) and Botanical Dietary Supplements*

This section includes text excerpted from "NTP Botanical Dietary Supplements Program," National Institute of Environmental Health Sciences (NIEHS), April 2016.

Botanical dietary supplements are sometimes referred to as herbals or herbal dietary supplements. Botanical dietary supplements are available to consumers as plants, plant parts, or plant extracts. A dietary supplement is defined, in part, as a product intended for ingestion that may contain one or more dietary ingredients, and is intended to supplement the diet. Dietary supplements may be found in many forms, such as tablets, capsules, softgels, gelcaps, liquids, or powders. Some botanical dietary supplements are used in complementary and alternative medicine, also sometimes called traditional medicine.

## *Why Is the National Toxicology Program (NTP) Studying Botanical Dietary Supplements?*

The National Toxicology Program (NTP) has received a number of nominations to study botanical dietary supplements from the public and other federal agencies, because people are concerned about the safety of these products. Dietary supplements containing ingredients of botanical origin are widely available in the United States. A nationwide government survey found that natural products, including botanical dietary supplements, are frequently used by adults and children. Approximately 18 percent of adults, 18 years or older, and 4 percent of children use natural products, such as botanical dietary supplements. The U.S. Food and Drug Administration (FDA) is responsible for taking action against any unsafe dietary supplement, after it reaches the market. If a manufacturer wants to distribute a supplement containing a new dietary ingredient, they must notify the FDA prior to putting it on the market. However, notification does not mean that the FDA has determined that use of the new dietary ingredient is safe. For these reasons, the NTP is conducting numerous studies in rodents to identify potential adverse effects of these agents after both short- and long-term exposure.

These studies may provide toxicology data that can be used by the FDA, the National Institutes of Health (NIH), the public, and other stakeholders in evaluating the safety of supplements, and may lead to removal of unsafe products from the market.

## How Does the NTP Evaluate Botanical Dietary Supplements?

Researching the potential adverse effects of botanical dietary supplements presents several unique challenges. For example, many supplements contain a complex mixture of ingredients, making it difficult to identify and link active ingredients to observed outcomes. Growing, harvesting, and processing conditions also can affect the chemical makeup of a botanical supplement. Possible contaminants in a botanical dietary supplement, such as metals, molds, and pesticides, may also affect its toxicity. For these reasons, the NTP fully characterizes the chemical and physical composition of the botanical dietary supplements studied in its testing program. the NTP conducts toxicology studies in animal models under strict guidelines, to understand what happens once the supplement enters the body. the NTP also conducts additional studies, including nonanimal-based studies, to learn about the mechanisms of action. These studies focus on characterizing potential adverse health effects, such as cancer. the NTP looks at toxicity that results from short-term exposure to high doses, long-term exposure to lower doses, or a combination of both. the NTP also examines toxicities to specific systems, including the reproductive, neurological, cardiovascular, and immune systems.

## Completed NTP Studies

NTP studies are conducted in male and female rats and mice. Multiple doses are given over two years, with doses that are typically higher than what humans are exposed to. These studies may be used in conjunction with other data to assess cancer and other adverse health risks to humans.

# Chapter 19

# *Adolescents and Supplement Use*

Nearly 12 percent of children (about one in nine) in the United States use a complementary health approach, such as dietary or herbal supplements. Some teens use products advertised as dietary supplements for weight loss or bodybuilding. Increasingly, products sold as dietary supplements, particularly for weight loss and bodybuilding, contain ingredients that could be harmful, including prescription drug ingredients and controlled substances. In addition, many dietary supplements haven't been tested in children. Because children's bodies aren't fully developed, the side effects of these products on children and adults may differ.

Here are ten things to know about dietary supplements for children and teens.

1. Although many dietary supplements come from natural sources, **"natural" does not necessarily mean "safe."**

2. Federal regulations for dietary supplements are less strict than those for prescription and over-the-counter (OTC) drugs.

3. Dietary and herbal supplements may be poor quality and contain contaminants, including drugs, chemicals, or metals. Studies of dietary supplements have found significant

This chapter includes text excerpted from "10 Things to Know about Dietary Supplements for Children and Teens," National Center for Complementary and Integrative Health (NCCIH), March 23, 2017.

differences between what's on the label and what's in the bottle of some supplements.

4. Dietary supplements may interact with other products or medications or have unwanted side effects on their own.

5. About 4,600 children go to the emergency room every year because of dietary supplements. Most took a vitamin or mineral when unsupervised. Child-resistant packaging isn't required for dietary supplements.

6. Certain homeopathic products (called "nosodes" or "homeopathic immunizations") are promoted as substitutes for conventional immunizations, but they haven't been shown to protect children against diseases. Follow the Centers for Disease Control and Prevention's (CDC) vaccination recommendations to safeguard your children against vaccine-preventable diseases. Vaccinating children helps protect our community's and our children's health.

7. Here's safety information for some common supplements:

   • St. John's wort interacts with many medications, including antidepressants, birth control pills, and seizure and cancer treatments.

   • Melatonin, a hormone used as a sleep aid, appears safe for short-term use but not much is known about its long-term effects.

   • Giving probiotics to children doesn't appear to be risky, but conclusive evidence is lacking, particularly for long-term use. Critically ill patients shouldn't use probiotics.

   • Omega-3 supplements may cause minor stomach problems, such as belching, indigestion, or diarrhea.

   • The American Academy of Pediatrics (AAP) doesn't recommend multivitamins for healthy children and teens who eat a varied diet. It's best if they can get their vitamins from foods.

8. Hidden ingredients are increasingly becoming a problem in products promoted for bodybuilding. Some bodybuilding products marketed as dietary supplements contain steroids or steroid-like substances. These could lead to serious liver injury, stroke, kidney failure, or other serious conditions.

9. Dietary supplements marketed for rapid weight loss, such as acai, and hoodie, don't help keep weight off for the long-term and can have side effects. Some supplements have a lot of caffeine or herbs such as guarana that contains caffeine, which can cause life-threatening changes in your heart rhythm. The U.S. Food and Drug Administration (FDA) has also found weight-loss products tainted with potentially dangerous prescription drugs.

10. Ask your child's healthcare provider about the effectiveness and possible risks of any complementary health approaches you are considering or already using for your child. Also, remind your teenagers to talk to their healthcare providers about complementary health approaches they may use or are considering.

Chapter 20

# Antioxidants and Supplements

## Chapter Contents

141

# Section 20.1

# *Antioxidants and Health*

This section includes text excerpted from "Antioxidants:
In Depth," National Center for Complementary and Integrative
Health (NCCIH), November 2013. Reviewed May 2018.

Antioxidants are artificial or natural substances that may prevent or delay some types of cell damage. Diets high in vegetables and fruits, which are good sources of antioxidants, have been found to be healthy; however, research has not shown antioxidant supplements to be beneficial in preventing diseases. Examples of antioxidants include vitamins C and E, selenium, and carotenoids, such as beta carotene, lycopene, lutein, and zeaxanthin. This section provides basic information about antioxidants, summarizes what the science says about antioxidants and health, and ends with details on clinical trials.

- Vegetables and fruits are rich sources of antioxidants. There is good evidence that eating a diet that includes plenty of vegetables and fruits is healthy, and official U.S. government policy urges people to eat more of these foods. Research has shown that people who eat more vegetables and fruits have lower risks of several diseases; however, it is not clear whether these results are related to the amount of antioxidants in vegetables and fruits, to other components of these foods, to other factors in people's diets, or to other lifestyle choices.

- Rigorous scientific studies involving more than 100,000 people combined have tested whether antioxidant supplements can help prevent chronic diseases, such as cardiovascular diseases, cancer, and cataracts. In most instances, antioxidants did not reduce the risks of developing these diseases.

- Concerns have not been raised about the safety of antioxidants in food. However, high-dose supplements of antioxidants may be linked to health risks in some cases. Supplementing with high doses of beta carotene may increase the risk of lung cancer in smokers. Supplementing with high doses of vitamin E may increase risks of prostate cancer and one type of stroke.

- Antioxidant supplements may interact with some medicines.

- Tell all of your healthcare providers about any complementary and integrative health approaches you use. Give them a full picture of what you do to manage your health. This will help ensure coordinated and safe care.

## About Free Radicals, Oxidative Stress, and Antioxidants

Free radicals are highly unstable molecules that are naturally formed when you exercise and when your body converts food into energy. Your body can also be exposed to free radicals from a variety of environmental sources, such as cigarette smoke, air pollution, and sunlight. Free radicals can cause "oxidative stress," a process that can trigger cell damage. Oxidative stress is thought to play a role in a variety of diseases including cancer, cardiovascular diseases, diabetes, Alzheimer disease (AD), Parkinson disease (PD), and eye diseases such as cataracts and age-related macular degeneration (AMD).

Antioxidant molecules have been shown to counteract oxidative stress in laboratory experiments (for example, in cells or animal studies). However, there is debate as to whether consuming large amounts of antioxidants in supplement form actually benefits health. There is also some concern that consuming antioxidant supplements in excessive doses may be harmful.

Vegetables and fruits are healthy foods and rich sources of antioxidants. The official U.S. government policy urges people to eat more vegetables and fruits. Concerns have not been raised about the safety of any amounts of antioxidants in food.

## Use of Antioxidant Supplements in the United States

A 2009 analysis using data from the National Health and Nutrition Examination Survey (NHNES) (1999–2000 and 2001–2002) estimated the amounts of antioxidants adults in the United States get from foods and supplements. Supplements accounted for 54 percent of vitamin C, 64 percent of vitamin E, 14 percent of alpha and beta carotene, and 11 percent of selenium intake.

### Safety

High-dose antioxidant supplements may be harmful in some cases. For example, the results of some studies have linked the use of high-dose beta carotene supplements to an increased risk of lung cancer in smokers and use of high-dose vitamin E supplements to increased risks of hemorrhagic stroke (a type of stroke caused by bleeding in the brain) and prostate cancer.

Like some other dietary supplements, antioxidant supplements may interact with certain medications. For example, vitamin E supplements may increase the risk of bleeding in people who are taking anticoagulant drugs ("blood thinners"). There is conflicting evidence on the effects of taking antioxidant supplements during cancer treatment; some studies suggest that this may be beneficial, but others suggest that it may be harmful. The National Cancer Institute (NCI) recommends that people who are being treated for cancer talk with their healthcare provider before taking supplements.

## What the Science Says

Several decades of dietary research findings suggested that consuming greater amounts of antioxidant-rich foods might help to protect against diseases. Because of these results, there has been a lot of research on antioxidant supplements. Rigorous trials of antioxidant supplements in large numbers of people have not found that high doses of antioxidant supplements prevent disease.

### Observational and Laboratory Studies

Observational studies on the typical eating habits, lifestyles, and health histories of large groups of people have shown that those who ate more vegetables and fruits had lower risks of several diseases, including cardiovascular disease, stroke, cancer, and cataracts. Observational studies can provide ideas about possible relationships between dietary or lifestyle factors and disease risk, but they cannot show that one factor causes another because they cannot account for other factors that may be involved. For example, people who eat more antioxidant-rich foods might also be more likely to exercise and less likely to smoke. It may be that these factors, rather than antioxidants, account for their lower disease risk.

Researchers have also studied antioxidants in laboratory experiments. These experiments showed that antioxidants interacted with free radicals and stabilized them, thus preventing the free radicals from causing cell damage.

## Clinical Trials of Antioxidants

Because the results of such research seemed very promising, large, long-term studies—many of which were funded by the National Institutes of Health (NIH)—were conducted to test whether antioxidant supplements, when taken for periods of at least a few years, could help prevent diseases such as cardiovascular diseases and cancer in people. In these studies, volunteers were randomly assigned to take either an antioxidant or a placebo (an identical-looking product that did not contain the antioxidant). The research was conducted in a double-blind manner (neither the study participants nor the investigators knew which product was being taken). Studies of this type—called clinical trials—are designed to provide clear answers to specific questions about how a substance affects people's health.

Among the earliest of these studies were three large NIH-sponsored trials of high-dose supplements of beta carotene, alone or in combination with other nutrients. These trials showed that beta carotene did not protect against cancer or cardiovascular disease. In one trial, beta carotene supplements increased the risk of lung cancer in smokers, and in another trial, supplements containing both beta carotene and vitamin A had the same effect.

More studies have also found that in most instances antioxidant supplements did not help to prevent disease. For example:

- The Women's Health Study, which included almost 40,000 healthy women at least 45 years of age, found that vitamin E supplements did not reduce the risk of heart attack, stroke, cancer, AMD, or cataracts. Although vitamin E supplements were associated with fewer deaths from cardiovascular causes, they did not reduce the overall death rate of study participants.

- The Women's Antioxidant Cardiovascular Study found no beneficial effects of vitamin C, vitamin E, or beta carotene supplements on cardiovascular events (heart attack, stroke, or death from cardiovascular diseases) or the likelihood of developing diabetes or cancer in more than 8,000 female health professionals, aged 40 years or older, who were at high risk for cardiovascular disease. Antioxidant supplements also did not

145

slow changes in cognitive function among women in this study who were aged 65 or older.

- The Physicians' Health Study II, which included more than 14,000 male physicians aged 50 or older, found that neither vitamin E nor vitamin C supplements reduced the risk of major cardiovascular events (heart attack, stroke, or death from cardiovascular disease), cancer, or cataracts. In fact, vitamin E supplements were associated with an increased risk of hemorrhagic stroke in this study.

- The Selenium and Vitamin E Cancer Prevention Trial (SELECT)—a study of more than 35,000 men aged 50 or older—found that selenium and vitamin E supplements, taken alone or together, did not prevent prostate cancer. A 2011 updated analysis from this trial, based on a longer follow-up period of study participants, concluded that vitamin E supplements increased the occurrence of prostate cancer by 17 percent in men who received the vitamin E supplement alone compared with those who received placebo. There was no increase in prostate cancer when vitamin E and selenium were taken together.

Unlike the studies described above, the Age-Related Eye Disease Study (AREDS), led by the National Eye Institute (NEI) and cosponsored by other components of NIH, including the National Center for Complementary and Integrative Health (NCCIH), found a beneficial effect of antioxidant supplements. This study showed that a combination of antioxidants (vitamin C, vitamin E, and beta carotene) and zinc reduced the risk of developing the advanced stage of AMD by 25 percent in people who had the intermediate stage of this disease or who had the advanced stage in only one eye. Antioxidant supplements used alone reduced the risk by about 17 percent. In the same study, however, antioxidants did not help to prevent cataracts or slow their progression.

A follow-up study, AREDS2, found that adding omega-3 fatty acids (fish oil) to the combination of supplements did not improve its effectiveness. However, adding lutein and zeaxanthin (two carotenoids found in the eye) improved the supplement's effectiveness in people who were not taking beta carotene and those who consumed only small amounts of lutein and zeaxanthin in foods.

# Section 20.2

# Coenzyme $Q_{10}$ (Co$Q_{10}$)

This section includes text excerpted from "Coenzyme $Q_{10}$ (PDQ®)—Patient Version," National Cancer Institute (NCI), March 16, 2018.

$CoQ_{10}$ is a compound that is made in the body. The Q and the 10 in coenzyme $Q_{10}$ refer to the groups of chemicals that make up the product. $CoQ_{10}$ is also known by the following names:

- $Q_{10}$
- Vitamin $Q_{10}$
- Ubiquinone
- Ubidecarenone

A coenzyme helps an enzyme do its job. An enzyme is a protein that speeds up the rate at which chemical reactions take place in cells of the body. The body's cells use $CoQ_{10}$ to make energy needed for the cells to grow and stay healthy. The body also uses $CoQ_{10}$ as an antioxidant. An antioxidant protects cells from chemicals called free radicals.

$CoQ_{10}$ is found in most body tissues. The highest amounts are found in the heart, liver, kidneys, and pancreas. The lowest amounts are found in the lungs. $CoQ_{10}$ decreases in the body as people get older.

## How Co$Q_{10}$ Is Given

$CoQ_{10}$ is taken by mouth as a tablet or capsule. It may also be given by injection into a vein.

## Laboratory or Animal Studies Done Using Co$Q_{10}$

In laboratory studies, tumor cells are used to test a substance to find out if it is likely to have any anticancer effects. In animal studies, tests are done to see if a drug, procedure, or treatment is safe and effective in animals. Laboratory and animal studies are done before a substance is tested in people.

## Human Studies Done Using $CoQ_{10}$

There have been few clinical trials that study the use of $CoQ_{10}$ in patients with cancer. A trial of 236 breast cancer patients were randomized to receive either $CoQ_{10}$ or placebo, each combined with vitamin E, for 24 weeks. The study found that levels of fatigue and quality of life were not improved in patients who received $CoQ_{10}$ compared to patients who received the placebo.

A randomized trial of 20 children treated for acute lymphoblastic leukemia or non-Hodgkin lymphoma looked at whether $CoQ_{10}$ would protect the heart from the damage caused by doxorubicin. The results reported that $CoQ_{10}$ decreased the harmful effects of doxorubicin on the heart.

Clinical trials have been limited to small numbers of people, and it is not clear if the benefits reported were from the $CoQ_{10}$ therapy, other dietary supplements, or standard treatments used before or during the $CoQ_{10}$ therapy.

## Side Effects or Risks from $CoQ_{10}$

Reported side effects from the use of $CoQ_{10}$ include the following:

- High levels of liver enzymes
- Nausea
- Heartburn
- Headache
- Pain in the upper part of the abdomen
- Dizziness
- Rashes
- Unable to fall sleep or stay asleep
- Feeling very tired
- Feeling irritable
- Sensitivity to light

It is important to check with healthcare providers to find out if $CoQ_{10}$ can be safely used with other drugs. Certain drugs, such as those that are used to lower cholesterol, blood pressure, or blood sugar levels, may decrease the effects of $CoQ_{10}$. $CoQ_{10}$ may change the way the body uses warfarin (a drug that prevents the blood from clotting) and insulin.

## $CoQ_{10}$ Use for Cancer Treatment in the United States

The U.S. Food and Drug Administration (FDA) has not approved the use of $CoQ_{10}$ as a treatment for cancer. The FDA does not approve dietary supplements as safe or effective. The company that makes the dietary supplements is responsible for making sure that they are safe and that the claims on the label are true and do not mislead the patient. The way that supplements are made is not regulated, so all batches and brands of $CoQ_{10}$ supplements may not be the same.

# Chapter 21

# *Vitamins and Minerals*

## *Chapter Contents*

# Section 21.1

# *Vitamins and Minerals: An Overview*

This section includes text excerpted from "Vitamins and
Minerals," National Center for Complementary and
Integrative Health (NCCIH), February 9, 2018.

Vitamins and minerals are essential substances that our bodies
need to develop and function normally. The known vitamins include A,
C, D, E, and K, and the B vitamins: thiamin ($B_1$), riboflavin ($B_2$), niacin
($B_3$), pantothenic acid ($B_5$), pyridoxal ($B_6$), cobalamin ($B_{12}$), biotin, and
folate/folic acid. A number of minerals are essential for health: calcium, phosphorus, potassium, sodium, chloride, magnesium, iron, zinc,
iodine, sulfur, cobalt, copper, fluoride, manganese, and selenium. The
*Dietary Guidelines for Americans 2015–2020* recommends that people
should aim to meet their nutrient requirements through a healthy
eating pattern that includes nutrient-dense forms of foods.

## *Multivitamin/Multimineral Supplements (MVMs)*

Multivitamins/multiminerals (MVMs) are the most frequently used
dietary supplements, with close to half of American adults taking
them. MVMs cannot take the place of eating a variety of foods that
are important to a healthy diet. Foods provide more than vitamins and
minerals. Many foods also have fiber and other substances that can
provide health benefits. However, some people who don't get enough
vitamins and minerals from food alone, or who have certain medical
conditions, might benefit from taking one or more of these nutrients
found in single-nutrient supplements or in MVMs. However, evidence
to support their use for overall health or disease prevention in the
general population remains limited.

## *Safety*

- Taking a daily dose of a basic MVM is unlikely to pose a health
  risk for most people. However, if you consume fortified foods and
  beverages (such as cereals or drinks with added vitamins and

minerals) along with dietary supplements, you should make sure that your total intake of vitamins and minerals is not more than the safe upper limits for any nutrients. Read the Nutrition Facts label on packaged foods or the Supplement Facts label of MVMs to see if the level far exceeds 100 percent DV (Daily Value).

- Smokers, and possibly former smokers, should avoid MVM products that provide more than 100 percent DV for vitamin A (either as preformed retinol or beta carotene or some combination of the two) because two studies have linked high supplemental doses of these nutrients with an increased risk of lung cancer in smokers.

- Taking excess amounts of vitamin A (preformed retinol form, not as beta carotene) during pregnancy has been shown to increase the risk of birth defects.

- Except in cases of iron deficiency or inadequacy, or unless a physician recommends otherwise, adult males and postmenopausal women should avoid using iron supplements or MVMs containing more than their recommended daily allowance for iron (8 mg/day). Iron supplements may be recommended for women of childbearing age, pregnant women, preterm infants, older infants, and teenage girls because they are at greater risk of developing deficiency. Yet, iron supplements are a leading cause of poisoning in young children, so parents and guardians should keep iron-containing supplements out of the reach of children.

- MVMs providing nutrients at or up to 100 percent DV do not typically interact with medications. However, if you take a blood thinner, such as warfarin (Coumadin® and other brand names), talk to your healthcare provider before taking any MVM or dietary supplement that contains vitamin K (this vitamin lowers the medicine's effectiveness, and doctors base the medicine's dose partly on the overall amount of vitamin K a person usually consumes in foods and supplements).

## Section 21.2

# *Fortify Your Knowledge about Vitamins*

This section includes text excerpted from "Consumer Updates—Fortify Your Knowledge about Vitamins," U.S. Food and Drug Administration (FDA), November 19, 2017.

Vitamins are essential nutrients that contribute to a healthy life. Although most people get all the vitamins they need from the foods they eat, millions of people worldwide take supplemental vitamins as part of their health regimen.

### *Why Buy Vitamins?*

There are many good reasons to consider taking vitamin supplements, such as over-the-counter (OTC) multivitamins. According to the American Academy of Family Physicians (AAFP), a doctor may recommend that you take them:

- for certain health problems

- if you eat a vegetarian or vegan diet

- if you are pregnant or breastfeeding

### *Vitamin Facts*

Your body uses vitamins for a variety of biological processes, including growth, digestion, and nerve function. There are 13 vitamins that the body absolutely needs: vitamins A, C, D, E, K, and the B vitamins (thiamine, riboflavin, niacin, pantothenic acid, biotin, vitamin $B_6$, vitamin $B_{12}$ and folate). AAFP cites two categories of vitamins:

- **Water-soluble vitamins** are easily absorbed by the body, which doesn't store large amounts. The kidneys remove those vitamins that are not needed.

- **Fat-soluble vitamins** are absorbed into the body with the use of bile acids, which are fluids used to absorb fat. The body stores these for use as needed.

## Develop a Vitamin Strategy

It is important for consumers to have an overall strategy for how they will achieve adequate vitamin intakes. The *Dietary Guidelines for Americans* advises that nutrient needs be met primarily through consuming foods, with supplementation suggested for certain sensitive populations.

These guidelines, published by the U.S. Department of Health and Human Services (HHS) and the U.S. Department of Agriculture (USDA), provide science-based advice to promote health and to reduce the risk for chronic diseases through diet and physical activity. They form the basis for federal food, nutrition education, and information programs.

### Special Nutrient Needs

According to the *Dietary Guidelines for Americans*, many people consume more calories than they need without taking in recommended amounts of a number of nutrients. The *Guidelines* warn that there are numerous nutrients—including vitamins—for which low dietary intake may be a cause for concern. These nutrients are:

- calcium, potassium, fiber, magnesium, and vitamins A (as carotenoids), C, and E (for adults)

- calcium, potassium, fiber, magnesium, and vitamin E (for children and adolescents)

- vitamin $B_{12}$, iron, folic acid, and vitamins E, and D (for specific population groups)

Regarding the use of vitamin supplements, the *Dietary Guidelines* include the following:

- **Consume a variety of nutrient-dense foods and beverages within and among the basic food groups.** At the same time, choose foods that limit the intake of saturated and trans fats, cholesterol, added sugars, salt, and alcohol.

- **Meet recommended nutrient intakes within energy needs by adopting a balanced eating pattern**, such as one of those recommended in the *USDA Food Guide* or the National Institute of Health's (NIH) *Dietary Approaches to Stop Hypertension (DASH)* eating plan.

- **If you're over age 50**, consume vitamin $B_{12}$ in its crystalline form, which is found in fortified foods or supplements.

- **If you're a woman of childbearing age who may become pregnant**, eat foods high in heme-iron and/or consume iron-rich plant foods or iron-fortified foods with an iron-absorption enhancer, such as foods high in vitamin C.

- **If you're a woman of childbearing age who may become pregnant or is in the first trimester of pregnancy**, consume adequate synthetic folic acid daily (from fortified foods or supplements) in addition to food forms of folate from a varied diet.

- **If you are an older adult**, have dark skin, or are exposed to insufficient ultraviolet (UV) band radiation (such as sunlight), consume extra vitamin D from vitamin D-fortified foods and/or supplements.

## How Vitamins Are Regulated

Vitamin products are regulated by FDA as "Dietary Supplements." The law defines dietary supplements, in part, as products taken by mouth that contain a "dietary ingredient" intended to supplement the diet.

Listed in the "dietary ingredient" category are not only vitamins, but minerals, botanicals products, amino acids, and substances such as enzymes, microbial probiotics, and metabolites. Dietary supplements can also be extracts or concentrates and may be found in many forms. The Dietary Supplement Health and Education Act (DSHEA) of 1994 requires that all such products be labeled as dietary supplements.

## Risks of Overdoing It

As is the case with all dietary supplements, the decision to use supplemental vitamins should not be taken lightly, says Vasilios Frankos, Ph.D., Director of FDA's Division of Dietary Supplement Programs.

"Vitamins are not dangerous unless you get too much of them," he says. "More is not necessarily better with supplements, especially if you take fat-soluble vitamins." For some vitamins and minerals, the National Academy of Sciences (NAS) has established upper limits of intake that it recommends not be exceeded during any given day.

## Fat-Soluble Vitamins

- **Vitamin A** (retinol, retinal, retinoic acid). Nausea, vomiting, headache, dizziness, blurred vision, clumsiness, birth defects, liver problems, possible risk of osteoporosis. You may be at greater risk of these effects if you drink high amounts of alcohol or you have liver problems, high cholesterol levels or don't get enough protein.

- **Vitamin D** (calciferol). Nausea, vomiting, poor appetite, constipation, weakness, weight loss, confusion, heart rhythm problems, deposits of calcium and phosphate in soft tissues.

If you take blood thinners, talk to your doctor before taking vitamin E or vitamin K pills.

## Water-Soluble Vitamins

- **B$_3$ (niacin).** Flushing, redness of the skin, upset stomach
- **B$_6$ (pyridoxine, pyridoxal, and pyridoxamine).** Nerve damage to the limbs, which may cause numbness, trouble walking, and pain
- **C (ascorbic acid).** Upset stomach, kidney stones, increased iron absorption
- **Folic acid (folate).** High levels may, especially in older adults, hide signs of B$_{12}$ deficiency, a condition that can cause nerve damage

Taking too much of a vitamin can also cause problems with some medical tests or interfere with how some drugs work.

# Section 21.3

# *Vitamins and Minerals for Women*

This section includes text excerpted from "Vitamins and Minerals for Women," Office on Women's Health (OWH), U.S. Department of Health and Human Services (HHS), March 1, 2018.

Your body needs vitamins and minerals for good health. Each vitamin and mineral has specific benefits and is essential for keeping your body functioning well. Also, there are some vitamins and minerals that women need more of than men do.

## *Vitamins and Minerals That Are Important for Women's Health*

All vitamins and minerals are important for good health. Vitamins and minerals often work together in your body. It's usually best to get your vitamins and minerals from many different types of food in all of the food groups. Fill your plate with fruits, vegetables, dairy, grains, and a variety of protein foods to build a healthy plate.

### *Folic Acid / Folate (Vitamin B₉)*

*Why It's Important*

- Helps your body make blood cells and the deoxyribonucleic acid (DNA) for new cells

- Helps prevent certain birth defects called neural tube defects, which happen in the first three months of pregnancy

- Helps prevent premature births and low birth weight

*Who May Need It*

All women who might get pregnant or are pregnant need to get 400–800 mcg of folic acid each day from either dietary supplements (most prenatal vitamins have this amount) or fortified foods like many breakfast cereals. Nearly half, or 45 percent, of all pregnancies in the United States, are not planned, so it's important to make sure you are getting enough folic acid even if you're not planning on getting pregnant right now.

*Where to Find It in Food*

Spinach and other dark green leafy vegetables, oranges and pure orange juice, nuts, beans, chicken, lean beef, whole grains, and cereals with added folic acid

## Vitamin B$_{12}$

*Why It's Important*

- Helps your body make red blood cells
- Helps your neurons (cells in your brain and nervous system) work correctly

*Who May Need It*

Some women may not get enough B$_{12}$. Talk to your doctor or nurse about taking a B$_{12}$ supplement if you are:

- **Pregnant.** Vitamin B$_{12}$ is very important for your unborn baby's development. Without it, your baby may have a low birth weight or other health problems.

- **Vegetarian.** Because vitamin B$_{12}$ comes mostly from animal products, you may need to take a supplement to make sure you get enough. Also, talk to your doctor or nurse if you are feeding your baby breastmilk only, because your baby may need to take a supplement too.

- **Age 50 or older.** As we age, our bodies cannot absorb vitamin B$_{12}$ as well, so you may need to get more vitamin B$_{12}$ from supplements or fortified foods because it is easier to absorb

*Where to Find It in Food*

Low-fat or fat-free milk, eggs, liver, poultry, clams, sardines, flounder, herring, blue cheese, nutritional yeast, and foods with vitamin B$_{12}$ added, including some cereals, fortified soy beverages, and veggie burgers

## *Vitamin D*

### *Why It's Important*

- With calcium, helps build strong bones and prevent osteoporosis

- Helps reduce inflammation in your cells

- Helps your immune system fight off germs that can make you sick

### *Who May Need It*

Women who:

- Do not get much sunlight (you live in the northern part of the country or are homebound)

- Are African-American, Hispanic, or Asian-American

- Are postmenopausal

- Are obese

- Have inflammatory bowel disease (IBD) or any other disease that makes it harder for the gut to absorb fat (vitamin D is a fat-soluble vitamin, meaning it has to be absorbed by the gut)

- Have had gastric bypass surgery (weight-loss surgery)

Talk to your doctor or nurse if you think you may not get enough vitamin D. Most women do not need testing for vitamin D deficiency.

### *Where to Find It in Food*

Fish like tuna, and salmon, and fortified foods (low-fat, or fat-free milk, and some brands of orange juice, cereals, soy beverages, and yogurt)

## *Calcium*

### *Why It's Important*

- Helps protect and build strong bones and reduce the risk of osteoporosis. Your body stores calcium in your bones, so if you don't get enough calcium from food, your body will take calcium from your bones, making them weak and easily broken.

- Helps messages go between your brain and muscles

*Who May Need It*

- Girls ages 9–18 need 1,300 milligrams (mg) of calcium each day. During this time, bones absorb calcium and build strong bones for adulthood and older age.

- Adult women need 1,000 mg of calcium each day.

- After menopause, you need 1,200 mg of calcium each day to help slow the bone loss that comes with aging

*Where to Find It in Food*

Low-fat or fat-free yogurt, cheese, and milk; foods with calcium added, such as some soy beverages, 100 percent orange juice, tofu, and cereals; canned salmon; and dark green leafy vegetables

## *Iron*

*Why It's Important*

- Builds healthy blood cells that carry oxygen in your body

- Helps make certain hormones and connective tissue in your body

*Who May Need It*

- All women who have menstrual periods. Iron is lost during monthly periods.

- Pregnant women. Women need more iron during pregnancy to supply enough blood for their growing babies.

Many women, especially pregnant women, do not get enough iron from food alone. This can put you at risk for iron-deficiency anemia. This condition causes your heart to work harder to pump blood so that more oxygen can reach all of your body. Anemia can make you feel tired, weak, and dizzy.

The amount of iron you need each day throughout your life is listed below:

- **Ages 19–50:** 18 mg

- **During pregnancy:** 27 mg

- **Ages 51 and older:** 8 mg

*Where to Find It in Food*

Lean red meats and chicken, seafood, cereals/bread with iron added, oysters, beans, dark chocolate, liver, spinach, tofu, and canned tomatoes.

## Should I Take a Vitamin or Mineral Supplement?

Most women do not need a vitamin or mineral supplement. You should be able to get all the nutrients you need, including vitamins and minerals, by choosing healthy foods.

But there are three groups of women who might need a vitamin and mineral supplement:

- **Women who are pregnant or could become pregnant.** A supplement ensures that you get the folic acid you need daily to lower the risk of certain birth defects, including spina bifida. Check the Nutrition Facts label to make sure the supplement has at least 400 micrograms (mcg) of folic acid.

- **Postmenopausal women.** After menopause women lose bone density faster than men because of hormonal changes. Many women do not get enough calcium and vitamin D from the foods they eat. Calcium and vitamin D, along with weight-bearing exercise, help prevent osteoporosis. You may also need to take supplements with vitamin $B_{12}$.

- **Vegetarians.** You can get some vitamins from animal products more easily than from plant sources. For example, vitamin $B_{12}$ is found in many animal products, including eggs and dairy, but it is not found in plants. Also, vegans especially may not get enough of vitamins $B_2$ (riboflavin), $B_{12}$, and D from food alone.

Talk with your doctor or nurse about whether you need a supplement and, if so, how much you should take.

## Dietary Supplements and Safety Concerns

Many dietary supplements are safe, especially those recommended by your doctor or nurse. But dietary supplements are not regulated by the U.S. Food and Drug Administration (FDA) the same way medicines are regulated.

Companies that make vitamins and other types of dietary supplements (such as minerals and herbs) do not have to get approval from the FDA to sell their products. The companies are required to report any negative side effects from supplements. The FDA can take products off the market if they are found to be unsafe, have false or misleading claims on them, contain harmful ingredients (like heavy metals), or have too much or too little of an ingredient.

You should always talk to your doctor or nurse before taking a dietary supplement. Certain supplements can raise your risk for new health problems, especially if you are also taking other medicines. Some supplements can make prescription medicines not work. For example:

- If you take prescription medicine, such as blood thinners, certain supplements may interact with the medicine. When they interact with medicines, supplements can make medicines not work like they should and can lead to serious health problems.

- St. John's wort, an herbal supplement some people take to help with minor depression, can make some medicines break down in your body more quickly than they should, making them less likely to work. These medicines include birth control pills.

- High doses (more than 3,000 micrograms (mcg) or 10,000 international units (IU)) of vitamin A may cause birth defects, bone loss, and liver damage.

# Chapter 22

# *Multivitamin/Mineral (MVM) Supplements*

## What Are Multivitamin/Mineral (MVM) Dietary Supplements?

Multivitamin/mineral (MVM) supplements contain a combination of vitamins and minerals, and sometimes other ingredients as well. They go by many names, including multis and multiples or simply vitamins. The vitamins and minerals in MVMs have unique roles in the body.

## What Kinds of MVM Supplements Are Available?

There are many types of MVMs in the marketplace. Manufacturers choose which vitamins, minerals, and other ingredients, as well as their amounts, to include in their products. Among the most common MVMs are basic, once daily products containing all or most vitamins and minerals, with the majority in amounts that are close to recommended amounts. Higher-potency MVMs often come in packs of two or more pills to take each day. Manufacturers promote other MVMs for special purposes, such as better performance or energy, weight control, or improved immunity. These products usually contain herbal

This chapter includes text excerpted from "Multivitamin/Mineral Supplements," Office of Dietary Supplements (ODS), National Institutes of Health (NIH), February 17, 2016.

and other ingredients (such as echinacea and glucosamine) in addition to vitamins and minerals.

The recommended amounts of nutrients people should get vary by age and gender and are known as recommended dietary allowances (RDA) and adequate intakes (AI). One value for each nutrient, known as the daily value (DV), is selected for the labels of dietary supplements and foods. ADV is often, but not always, similar to one's RDA or AI for that nutrient. The label provides the (%DV) so that you can see how much (what percentage) a serving of the product contributes to reaching the DV.

## Who Takes MVM Supplements?

Research has shown that more than one-third of Americans take MVMs. About one in four young children takes an MVM, but adolescents are least likely to take them. Use increases with age during adulthood so that by age 71 years, more than 40 percent take an MVM. Women; the elderly; people with more education, more income, healthier diets and lifestyles, and lower body weights; and people in the western United States use MVMs most often. Smokers and members of certain ethnic and racial groups (such as African Americans, Hispanics, and Native Americans) are less likely to take a daily MVM.

## What Are Some Effects of MVMs on Health?

People take MVMs for many reasons. Here are some examples of what research has shown about using them to increase nutrient intakes, promote health, and reduce the risk of disease.

### Increase Nutrient Intakes

Taking an MVM increases nutrient intakes and helps people get the recommended amounts of vitamins and minerals when they cannot or do not meet these needs from food alone. But taking an MVM can also raise the chances of getting too much of some nutrients, like iron, vitamin A, zinc, niacin, and folic acid, especially when a person uses more than a basic, once-daily product.

Some people take an MVM as a form of dietary or nutritional "insurance." Ironically, people who take MVMs tend to consume more vitamins and minerals from food than those who don't. Also, the people least likely to get enough nutrients from diet alone who might benefit from MVMs are the least likely to take them.

## Health Promotion and Chronic Disease Prevention

For people with certain health problems, specific MVMs might be helpful. For example, a study showed that a particular high-dose formula of several vitamins and minerals slowed vision loss in some people with age-related macular degeneration. Although a few studies show that MVMs might reduce the overall risk of cancer in certain men, most research shows that healthy people who take an MVM do not have a lower chance of getting cancer, heart disease, or diabetes. Based on current research, it's not possible to recommend for or against the use of MVMs to stay healthier longer. One reason we know so little about whether MVMs have health benefits is that studies often use different products, making it hard to compare their results to find patterns. Many MVMs are available, and manufacturers can change their composition at will. It is, therefore, difficult for researchers to study whether a specific combination of vitamins and minerals affects health. Also, people with healthier diets and lifestyles are more likely to take dietary supplements, making it hard to identify any benefits from the MVMs.

## Should I Take an MVM?

MVMs cannot take the place of eating a variety of foods that are important to a healthy diet. Foods provide more than vitamins and minerals. They also have fiber and other ingredients that may have positive health effects. But people who don't get enough vitamins and minerals from food alone, are on low-calorie diets, have a poor appetite, or avoid certain foods (such as strict vegetarians and vegans) might consider taking an MVM. Healthcare providers might also recommend MVMs to patients with certain medical problems.

Some people might benefit from taking certain nutrients found in MVMs. For example:

- Women who might become pregnant should get 400 mcg/day of folic acid from fortified foods and/or dietary supplements to reduce the risk of birth defects of the brain and spine in their newborn babies.

- Pregnant women should take an iron supplement as recommended by their healthcare provider. A prenatal MVM is likely to provide iron.

- Breastfed and partially breastfed infants should receive vitamin D supplements of 400 international units (IU)/day, as should nonbreastfed infants who drink less than about 1 quart per day of vitamin D-fortified formula or milk.

- In postmenopausal women, calcium, and vitamin D supplements may increase bone strength and reduce the risk of fractures.

- People over age 50 should get recommended amounts of vitamin $B_{12}$ from fortified foods and/or dietary supplements because they might not absorb enough of the $B_{12}$ that is naturally found in food.

### Can MVMs Be Harmful?

Taking a basic MVM is unlikely to pose any risks to health. But if you consume fortified foods and drinks (such as cereals or beverages with added vitamins and minerals) or take other dietary supplements, make sure that the MVM you take doesn't cause your intake of any vitamin or mineral to go above the upper levels.

Pay particular attention to the amounts of vitamin A, beta carotene (which the body can convert to vitamin A), and iron in the MVM.

- Women who get too much vitamin A during pregnancy can increase the risk of birth defects in their babies. This risk does not apply to beta carotene, though. Smokers, and perhaps former smokers, should avoid MVMs with large amounts of beta carotene and vitamin A because these ingredients might increase the risk of developing lung cancer.

- Adult men and postmenopausal women should avoid taking MVMs that contain 18 mg or more of iron unless their doctor has told them that they have iron deficiency or inadequacy. When the body takes in much more iron than it can eliminate, the iron can collect in body tissues and organs, such as the liver and heart, and damage them. Iron supplements are a leading cause of poisoning in children under age 6, so keep any products containing iron (such as children's chewable MVMs or adults' iron supplements) out of children's reach.

### Are There Any Interactions with MVMs That I Should Know about?

MVMs with recommended intake levels of nutrients don't usually interact with medications, with one important exception. If you take medicine to reduce blood clotting, such as warfarin (Coumadin® and other brand names), talk to your healthcare provider before taking any MVM or dietary supplement with vitamin K. Vitamin K lowers the drug's effectiveness and doctors base the medicine dose partly on the amount of vitamin K you usually consume in foods and supplements.

## Which Kind of MVM Should I Choose?

Talk to a healthcare provider to help you figure out whether you should take an MVM and, if so, which one is best for you. Consider basic MVMs whose amounts of most or all vitamins and minerals do not go above the DVs. These MVMs usually have low amounts of calcium and magnesium, so some people might need to take one or both minerals separately. Make sure that the product does not have too much vitamin A and iron.

Also consider choosing an MVM designed for your age, sex, and other factors (like pregnancy). MVMs for men often contain little or no iron, for example. MVMs for seniors usually provide more calcium and vitamins D and $B_{12}$ and less iron than MVMs for younger adults. Prenatal MVMs for pregnant women often provide vitamin A as beta carotene.

## MVMs and Healthful Eating

People should get most of their nutrients from food, advises the federal government's *Dietary Guidelines for Americans*. Foods contain vitamins, minerals, dietary fiber, and other substances that benefit health. In some cases, fortified foods and dietary supplements may provide nutrients that otherwise may be consumed in less than recommended amounts.

# Chapter 23

# *Vitamin A and Carotenoids*

Vitamin A is the name of a group of fat-soluble retinoids, including retinol, retinal, and retinyl esters. Vitamin A is involved in immune function, vision, reproduction, and cellular communication. Vitamin A is critical for vision as an essential component of rhodopsin, a protein that absorbs light in the retinal receptors, and because it supports the normal differentiation and functioning of the conjunctival membranes and cornea. Vitamin A also supports cell growth and differentiation, playing a critical role in the normal formation and maintenance of the heart, lungs, kidneys, and other organs.

Two forms of vitamin A are available in the human diet: preformed vitamin A (retinol and its esterified form, retinyl ester) and provitamin A carotenoids. Preformed vitamin A is found in foods from animal sources, including dairy products, fish, and meat (especially liver). By far the most important provitamin A carotenoid is beta carotene; other provitamins A carotenoids are alpha carotene and beta cryptoxanthin. The body converts these plant pigments into vitamin A. Both provitamin A and preformed vitamin A must be metabolized intracellularly to retinal and retinoic acid, the active forms of vitamin A, to support the vitamins' important biological functions. Other carotenoids found in food, such as lycopene, lutein, and zeaxanthin, are not converted into vitamin A.

The various forms of vitamin A are solubilized into micelles in the intestinal lumen and absorbed by duodenal mucosal cells. Both retinyl esters and provitamin A carotenoids are converted to retinol, which is

This chapter includes text excerpted from "Vitamin A," Office of Dietary Supplements (ODS), National Institutes of Health (NIH), March 2, 2018.

171

oxidized to retinal and then to retinoic acid. Most of the body's vitamin A is stored in the liver in the form of retinyl esters.

Retinol and carotenoid levels are typically measured in plasma, and plasma retinol levels are useful for assessing vitamin A inadequacy. However, their value for assessing marginal vitamin A status is limited because they do not decline until vitamin A levels in the liver are almost depleted. Liver vitamin A reserves can be measured indirectly through the relative dose-response test, in which plasma retinol levels are measured before and after the administration of a small amount of vitamin A. A plasma retinol level increase of at least 20 percent indicates an inadequate vitamin A level. For clinical practice purposes, plasma retinol levels alone are sufficient for documenting significant deficiency.

A plasma retinol concentration lower than 0.70 micromoles/L (or 20 micrograms [mcg]/dL) reflects vitamin A inadequacy in a population, and concentrations of 0.70–1.05 micromoles/L could be marginal in some people. In some studies, high plasma or serum concentrations of some provitamin A carotenoids have been associated with a lower risk of various health outcomes, but these studies have not definitively demonstrated that this relationship is causal.

## Recommended Intakes

Intake recommendations for vitamin A and other nutrients are provided in the Dietary Reference Intakes (DRI) developed by the Food and Nutrition Board (FNB) at the Institute of Medicine of the National Academies (IMNA) (formerly National Academy of Sciences (NAS)). DRI is the general term for a set of reference values used for planning and assessing nutrient intakes of healthy people. These values, which vary by age and gender, include:

- **Recommended dietary allowance (RDA).** Average daily level of intake sufficient to meet the nutrient requirements of nearly all (97–98%) healthy individuals; often used to plan nutritionally adequate diets for individuals.

- **Adequate intake (AI).** Intake at this level is assumed to ensure nutritional adequacy; established when evidence is insufficient to develop an RDA.

- **Estimated average requirement (EAR).** Average daily level of intake estimated to meet the requirements of 50 percent of healthy individuals; usually used to assess the nutrient intakes of groups of people and to plan nutritionally adequate diets for them; can also be used to assess the nutrient intakes of individuals.

- **Tolerable upper intake level (UL).** Maximum daily intake unlikely to cause adverse health effects.

RDAs for vitamin A are given as mcg of retinol activity equivalents (RAE) to account for the different bioactivities of retinol and provitamin A carotenoids. Because the body converts all dietary sources of vitamin A into retinol, 1 mcg of physiologically available retinol is equivalent to the following amounts from dietary sources: 1 mcg of retinol, 12 mcg of beta carotene, and 24 mcg of alpha carotene or beta cryptoxanthin. From dietary supplements, the body converts 2 mcg of beta carotene to 1 mcg of retinol.

Currently, vitamin A is listed on food and supplement labels in international units (IU) even though nutrition scientists rarely use this measure. Conversion rates between mcg RAE and IU are as follows:

- 1 IU retinol = 0.3 mcg RAE
- 1 IU beta carotene from dietary supplements = 0.15 mcg RAE
- 1 IU beta carotene from food = 0.05 mcg RAE
- 1 IU alpha carotene or beta cryptoxanthin = 0.025 mcg RAE

However, for the manufacture and addition of preformed vitamin A and provitamin A carotenoids to dietary supplements and foods, as well as for labeling the vitamin A content of these products, the U.S. Food and Drug Administration (FDA) mandates that older conversion factors published by the FNB in 1968 be used: 1 IU = 0.3 mcg as retinol = 0.6 mcg as beta carotene. Under FDA's new labeling regulations for foods and dietary supplements that take effect by July 26, 2018 (for companies with annual sales of $10 million or more) or July 26, 2019 (for smaller companies), vitamin A will be listed only in mcg and not IUs.

An RAE cannot be directly converted into an IU without knowing the source(s) of vitamin A. For example, the RDA of 900 mcg RAE for adolescent and adult men is equivalent to 3,000 IU if the food or supplement source is preformed vitamin A (retinol). However, this RDA is also equivalent to 6,000 IU of beta carotene from supplements, 18,000 IU of beta carotene from food, or 36,000 IU of alpha carotene or beta cryptoxanthin from food. So a mixed diet containing 900 mcg RAE provides between 3,000–36,000 IU of vitamin A, depending on the foods consumed.

## Sources of Vitamin A

### *Food*

Concentrations of preformed vitamin A are highest in liver and fish oils. Other sources of preformed vitamin A are milk and eggs, which also include some provitamin A. Most dietary provitamin A comes from leafy green vegetables, orange and yellow vegetables, tomato products, fruits, and some vegetable oils. The top food sources of vitamin A in the U.S. diet include dairy products, liver, fish, and fortified cereals; the top sources of provitamin A include carrots, broccoli, cantaloupe, and squash.

Table 23.1 suggests many dietary sources of vitamin A. The foods from animal sources in table 23.1 contain primarily preformed vitamin A, the plant-based foods have provitamin A, and the foods with a mixture of ingredients from animals and plants contain both preformed vitamin A and provitamin A.

**Table 23.1.** Selected Food Sources of Vitamin A

| Food | mcg RAE per Serving | IU per Serving | Percent DV |
|---|---|---|---|
| Sweet potato, baked in skin, 1 whole | 1403 | 28058 | 561 |
| Beef liver, pan-fried, 3 ounces | 6582 | 22175 | 444 |
| Spinach, frozen, boiled, ½ cup | 573 | 11458 | 229 |
| Carrots, raw, ½ cup | 459 | 9189 | 184 |
| Pumpkin pie, commercially prepared, 1 piece | 488 | 3743 | 249 |
| Cantaloupe, raw, ½ cup | 135 | 2706 | 54 |
| Peppers, sweet, red, raw, ½ cup | 117 | 2332 | 47 |
| Mangos, raw, 1 whole | 112 | 2240 | 45 |
| Black-eyed peas (cowpeas), boiled, 1 cup | 66 | 1305 | 26 |
| Apricots, dried, sulfured, 10 halves | 63 | 1261 | 25 |
| Broccoli, boiled, ½ cup | 60 | 1208 | 24 |
| Ice cream, French vanilla, soft serve, 1 cup | 278 | 1014 | 20 |
| Cheese, ricotta, part skim, 1 cup | 263 | 945 | 19 |
| Tomato juice, canned, ¾ cup | 42 | 821 | 16 |

**Table 23.1.** Continued

| Food | mcg RAE per Serving | IU per Serving | Percent DV |
|---|---|---|---|
| Herring, Atlantic, pickled, 3 ounces | 219 | 731 | 15 |
| Ready-to-eat cereal, fortified with 10% of the DV for vitamin A, ¾–1 cup (more heavily fortified cereals might provide more of the DV) | 127–149 | 500 | 10 |
| Milk, fat-free or skim, with added vitamin A and vitamin D, 1 cup | 149 | 500 | 10 |
| Baked beans, canned, plain or vegetarian, 1 cup | 13 | 274 | 5 |
| Egg, hard-boiled, 1 large | 75 | 260 | 5 |
| Summer squash, all varieties, boiled, ½ cup | 10 | 191 | 4 |
| Salmon, sockeye, cooked, 3 ounces | 59 | 176 | 4 |
| Yogurt, plain, low fat, 1 cup | 32 | 116 | 2 |
| Pistachio nuts, dry roasted, 1 ounce | 4 | 73 | 1 |
| Tuna, light, canned in oil, drained solids, 3 ounces | 20 | 65 | 1 |
| Chicken, breast meat, and skin, roasted, ½ breast | 5 | 18 | 0 |

\*\*DV = Daily Value. DVs were developed by the FDA to help consumers compare the nutrient contents of products within the context of a total diet. The DV for vitamin A is 5,000 IU for adults and children age 4 and older. Foods providing 20 percent or more of the DV are considered to be high sources of a nutrient. The U.S. Department of Agriculture's (USDA) Nutrient lists the nutrient content of many foods and provides a comprehensive list of foods containing vitamin A in IUs arranged by nutrient content and by food name, and foods containing beta carotene in mcg arranged by nutrient content and by food name.

### Dietary Supplements

Vitamin A is available in multivitamins and as a stand-alone supplement, often in the form of retinyl acetate or retinyl palmitate. A portion of the vitamin A in some supplements is in the form of beta carotene and the remainder is performed vitamin A; others contain only preformed vitamin A or only beta carotene. Supplement labels usually indicate the percentage of each form of the vitamin. The amounts of vitamin A in stand-alone supplements range widely. Multivitamin supplements typically contain 2,500–10,000 IU vitamin A, often in the form of both retinol and beta carotene.

About 28–37 percent of the general population uses supplements containing vitamin A. Adults aged 71 years or older and children younger than 9 are more likely than members of other age groups to take supplements containing vitamin A.

## Vitamin A Intakes and Status

According to an analysis of data the National Health and Nutrition Examination Survey (NHANES), the average daily dietary vitamin A intake in Americans aged 2 years and older is 607 mcg RAE. Adult men have slightly higher intakes (649 mcg RAE) than adult women (580 mcg RAE). Although these intakes are lower than the RDAs for individual men and women, these intake levels are considered to be adequate for population groups.

The adequacy of vitamin A intake decreases with age in children. Furthermore, girls and African-American children have a higher risk of consuming less than two-thirds of the vitamin A RDA than other children.

## Vitamin A Deficiency

Frank vitamin A deficiency is rare in the United States. However, vitamin A deficiency is common in many developing countries, often because residents have limited access to foods containing preformed vitamin A from animal-based food sources and they do not commonly consume available foods containing beta carotene due to poverty. According to the World Health Organization (WHO), 190 million pre-school-aged children and 19.1 million pregnant women around the world have a serum retinol concentration below 0.70 micromoles/L. In these countries, low vitamin A intake is most strongly associated with health consequences during periods of high nutritional demand, such as during infancy, childhood, pregnancy, and lactation.

In developing countries, vitamin A deficiency typically begins during infancy, when infants do not receive adequate supplies of colostrum or breast milk. Chronic diarrhea also leads to excessive loss of vitamin A in young children, and vitamin A deficiency increases the risk of diarrhea. The most common symptom of vitamin A deficiency in young children and pregnant women is xerophthalmia. One of the early signs of xerophthalmia is night blindness, or the inability to see in low light or darkness. Vitamin A deficiency is one of the top causes of preventable blindness in children. People with vitamin A deficiency (and, often, xerophthalmia with its characteristic Bitot's spots) tend to have low iron status, which can lead to anemia. Vitamin A deficiency also increases the severity and mortality risk of infections (particularly diarrhea and measles) even before the onset of xerophthalmia.

## Groups at Risk of Vitamin A Inadequacy

The following groups are among those most likely to have inadequate intakes of vitamin A.

### Premature Infants

In developed countries, clinical vitamin A deficiency is rare in infants and occurs only in those with malabsorption disorders. However, preterm infants do not have adequate liver stores of vitamin A at birth and their plasma concentrations of retinol often remain low throughout the first year of life. Preterm infants with vitamin A deficiency have an increased risk of eye, chronic lung, and gastrointestinal diseases.

### Infants and Young Children in Developing Countries

In developed countries, the amounts of vitamin A in breast milk are sufficient to meet infants' needs for the first 6 months of life. But in women with vitamin A deficiency, breast milk volume and vitamin A content are suboptimal and not sufficient to maintain adequate vitamin A stores in infants who are exclusively breastfed. The prevalence of vitamin A deficiency in developing countries begins to increase in young children just after they stop breastfeeding. The most common and readily recognized symptom of vitamin A deficiency in infants and children is xerophthalmia.

### Pregnant and Lactating Women in Developing Countries

Pregnant women need extra vitamin A for fetal growth and tissue maintenance and for supporting their own metabolism. The WHO estimates that 9.8 million pregnant women around the world have xerophthalmia as a result of vitamin A deficiency. Other effects of vitamin A deficiency in pregnant and lactating women include increased maternal and infant morbidity and mortality, increased anemia risk, and slower infant growth and development.

177

## People with Cystic Fibrosis (CF)

Most people with cystic fibrosis (CF) have pancreatic insufficiency, increasing their risk of vitamin A deficiency due to difficulty absorbing fat. Several cross-sectional studies found that 15–40 percent of patients with CF have vitamin A deficiency. However, improved pancreatic replacement treatments, better nutrition, and caloric supplements have helped most patients with CF become vitamin A sufficient. Several studies have shown that oral supplementation can correct low serum beta carotene levels in people with CF but no controlled studies have examined the effects of vitamin A supplementation on clinical outcomes in patients with CF.

## Vitamin A and Health

This chapter focuses on three diseases and disorders in which vitamin A might play a role: cancer, age-related macular degeneration (AMD), and measles.

### Cancer

Because of the role vitamin A plays in regulating cell growth and differentiation, several studies have examined the association between vitamin A and various types of cancer. However, the relationship between serum vitamin A levels or vitamin A supplementation and cancer risk is unclear.

Several prospective and retrospective observational studies in current and former smokers, as well as in people who have never smoked, found that higher intakes of carotenoids, fruits, and vegetables, or both are associated with a lower risk of lung cancer. However, clinical trials have not shown that supplemental beta carotene and/or vitamin A helps prevent lung cancer. In the Carotene and Retinol Efficacy Trial (CARET), 18,314 current and former smokers (including some males who had been occupationally exposed to asbestos) took daily supplements containing 30 mg beta carotene and 25,000 IU retinyl palmitate for 4 years, on average. In the Alpha Tocopherol, Beta Carotene (ATBC) Cancer Prevention Study, 29,133 male smokers took 50 mg/day alpha tocopherol, 20 mg/day beta carotene, 50 mg/day alpha tocopherol and 20 mg/day beta carotene, or placebo for 5–8 years. In the beta carotene component of the Physicians' Health Study, 22,071 male physicians took 325 mg aspirin plus 50 mg beta carotene, 50 mg beta carotene plus aspirin placebo, 325 mg aspirin plus beta carotene placebo, or both placebos every other day for 12 years. In all three of these studies, taking very high doses of beta carotene, with or without 25,000 IU retinyl palmitate or 325 mg aspirin, did not prevent lung cancer. In fact, both the CARET and ATBC studies showed a significant increase in lung cancer risk among study participants taking beta carotene supplements or beta carotene and retinyl palmitate supplements. The Physicians' Health Study did not find an increased lung cancer risk in participants taking beta carotene supplements, possibly because only 11 percent of physicians in the study were current or former smokers.

The evidence on the relationship between beta carotene and prostate cancer is mixed. CARET study participants who took daily supplements of beta carotene and retinyl palmitate had a 35 percent lower risk of nonaggressive prostate cancer than men not taking the supplements. However, the ATBC study found that baseline serum beta carotene and retinol levels and supplemental beta carotene had no effect on survival. Moreover, men in the highest quintile of baseline serum retinol levels were 20 percent more likely to develop prostate cancer than men in the lowest quintile.

The ATBC and CARET study results suggest that large supplemental doses of beta carotene with or without retinyl palmitate have detrimental effects in current or former smokers and workers exposed to asbestos. The relevance of these results to people who have never smoked or to the effects of beta carotene or retinol from food or multivitamins (which typically have modest amounts of beta carotene) is not known. More research is needed to determine the effects of vitamin A on prostate, lung, and other types of cancer.

## Age-Related Macular Degeneration (AMD)

AMD is a major cause of significant vision loss in older people. AMD's etiology is usually unknown, but the cumulative effect of oxidative stress is postulated to play a role. If so, supplements containing carotenoids with antioxidant functions, such as beta carotene lutein, and zeaxanthin, might be useful for preventing or treating this condition. Lutein and zeaxanthin, in particular, accumulate in the retina, the tissue in the eye that is damaged by AMD.

The Age-Related Eye Disease Study (AREDS), a large randomized clinical trial, found that participants at high risk of developing advanced AMD (i.e., those with intermediate AMD or those with advanced AMD in one eye) reduced their risk of developing advanced AMD by 25 percent by taking a daily supplement containing beta carotene (15 mg), vitamin E (400 IU dl-alpha-tocopheryl acetate), vitamin

C (500 mg), zinc (80 mg), and copper (2 mg) for 5 years compared to participants taking a placebo.

A follow-up AREDS2 study confirmed the value of this supplement in reducing the progression of AMD over a median follow-up period of 5 years but found that adding lutein (10 mg) and zeaxanthin (2 mg) or omega-3 fatty acids to the formulation did not confer any additional benefits. Importantly, the study revealed that beta carotene was not a required ingredient; the original AREDS formulation without beta carotene provided the same protective effect against developing advanced AMD. In a more detailed analysis of results, supplementation with lutein and zeaxanthin reduced the risk of advanced AMD by 26 percent in participants with the lowest dietary intakes of these two carotenoids who took a supplement containing them compared to those who did not take a supplement with these carotenoids. The risk of advanced AMD was also 18 percent lower in participants who took the modified AREDS supplement containing lutein and zeaxanthin but not beta carotene than in participants who took the formulation with beta carotene but not lutein or zeaxanthin.

Individuals who have or are developing AMD should talk to their healthcare provider about taking one of the supplement formulations used in AREDS.

### Measles

Measles is a major cause of morbidity and mortality in children in developing countries. About half of all measles deaths happen in Africa, but the disease is not limited to low-income countries. Vitamin A deficiency is a known risk factor for severe measles. The WHO recommends high oral doses (200,000 IU) of vitamin A for two days for children over age 1 with measles who live in areas with a high prevalence of vitamin A deficiency.

A Cochrane review of eight randomized controlled trials of treatment with vitamin A for children with measles found that 200,000 IU of vitamin A on each of two consecutive days reduced mortality from measles in children younger than 2 and mortality due to pneumonia in children. Vitamin A also reduced the incidence of croup but not pneumonia or diarrhea, although the mean duration of fever, pneumonia, and diarrhea was shorter in children who received vitamin A supplements. A meta-analysis of six high-quality randomized controlled trials of measles treatment also found that two doses of 100,000 IU in infants and 200,000 IU in older children significantly reduced measles mortality. The vitamin A doses used in these studies are much higher than the UL. The effectiveness of vitamin A supplementation to treat measles in countries, such as the United States, where vitamin A intakes are usually adequate is uncertain.

The body needs vitamin A to maintain the corneas and other epithelial surfaces, so the lower serum concentrations of vitamin A associated with measles, especially in people with protein-calorie malnutrition, can lead to blindness. None of the studies evaluated in a Cochrane review evaluated blindness as a primary outcome. However, a careful clinical investigation of 130 African children with measles revealed that half of all corneal ulcers in these children, and nearly all bilateral blindness, occurred in those with vitamin A deficiency.

## Health Risks from Excessive Vitamin A

Because vitamin A is fat soluble, the body stores excess amounts, primarily in the liver, and these levels can accumulate. Although excess preformed vitamin A can have significant toxicity (known as hypervitaminosis A), large amounts of beta carotene and another provitamin A carotenoids are not associated with major adverse effects. The manifestations of hypervitaminosis A depend on the size and rapidity of the excess intake. The symptoms of hypervitaminosis A following sudden, massive intakes of vitamin A, as with Arctic explorers who ate polar bear liver, are acute. Chronic intakes of excess vitamin A lead to increased intracranial pressure (pseudotumor cerebri), dizziness, nausea, headaches, skin irritation, pain in joints and bones, coma, and even death. Although hypervitaminosis A can be due to excessive dietary intakes, the condition is usually a result of consuming too much-preformed vitamin A from supplements or therapeutic retinoids. When people consume too much vitamin A, their tissue levels take a long time to fall after they discontinue their intake, and the resulting liver damage is not always reversible.

Observational studies have suggested an association between high intakes of preformed vitamin A (more than 1,500 mcg daily—only slightly higher than the RDA), reduced bone mineral density, and increased fracture risk. However, the results of studies on this risk have been mixed, so the safe retinol intake level for this association is unknown.

Total intakes of preformed vitamin A that exceed the UL and some synthetic retinoids used as topical therapies (such as isotretinoin and etretinate) can cause congenital birth defects. These birth defects can include malformations of the eye, skull, lungs, and heart. Women who might be pregnant should not take high doses of vitamin A supplements.

Unlike preformed vitamin A, beta carotene is not known to be teratogenic or lead to reproductive toxicity. And even large supplemental doses (20–30 mg/day) of beta carotene or diets with high levels of carotenoid-rich food for long periods are not associated with toxicity. The most significant effect of long-term, excess beta carotene is carotenodermia, a harmless condition in which the skin becomes yellow-orange. This condition can be reversed by discontinuing beta carotene ingestion.

Supplementation with beta carotene, with or without retinyl palmitate, for 5–8 years has been associated with an increased risk of lung cancer and cardiovascular disease in current and former male and female smokers and in male current and former smokers occupationally exposed to asbestos. In the ATBC study, beta carotene supplements (20 mg daily) were also associated with increased mortality, mainly due to lung cancer and ischemic heart disease. The CARET study ended early after the investigators found that daily beta carotene (30 mg) and retinyl palmitate (25,000 IU) supplements increased the risk of lung cancer and cardiovascular disease mortality.

The FNB has established ULs for preformed vitamin A that apply to both food and supplement intakes. The FNB based these ULs on the amounts associated with an increased risk of liver abnormalities in men and women, teratogenic effects, and a range of toxic effects in infants and children. The FNB also considered levels of preformed vitamin A associated with decreased bone mineral density but did not use these data as the basis for its ULs because the evidence was conflicting. The FNB has not established ULs for beta carotene and another provitamin A carotenoids. The FNB advises against beta carotene supplements for the general population, except as a provitamin A source to prevent vitamin A deficiency.

## Interactions with Medications

Vitamin A can interact with certain medications, and some medications can have an adverse effect on vitamin A levels. A few examples are provided below. Individuals taking these and other medications on a regular basis should discuss their vitamin A status with their healthcare providers.

### Orlistat

Orlistat (Alli®, Xenical®), a weight-loss treatment, can decrease the absorption of vitamin A, other fat-soluble vitamins, and beta carotene, causing low plasma levels in some patients. The manufacturers of Alli and Xenical recommend encouraging patients on orlistat to take a multivitamin supplement containing vitamin A and beta carotene, as well as other fat-soluble vitamins.

### Retinoids

Several synthetic retinoids derived from vitamin A are used orally as prescription medicines. Examples include the psoriasis treatment acitretin (Soriatane®) and bexarotene (Targretin®), used to treat the skin effects of T-cell lymphoma. Retinoids can increase the risk of hypervitaminosis A when taken in combination with vitamin A supplements.

### Vitamin A and Healthful Diets

The federal government's 2015–2020 *Dietary Guidelines for Americans* notes that "Nutritional needs should be met primarily from foods. Foods in nutrient-dense forms contain essential vitamins and minerals and also dietary fiber and other naturally occurring substances that may have positive health effects. In some cases, fortified foods and dietary supplements may be useful in providing one or more nutrients that otherwise may be consumed in less-than-recommended amounts."

# Chapter 24

# Vitamin $B_6$

## What Is Vitamin $B_6$ and What Does It Do?

Vitamin $B_6$ is a vitamin that is naturally present in many foods. The body needs vitamin $B_6$ for more than 100 enzyme reactions involved in metabolism. Vitamin $B_6$ is also involved in brain development during pregnancy and infancy as well as immune function.

## How Much Vitamin $B_6$ Do I Need?

The amount of vitamin $B_6$ you need depends on your age. Average daily recommended amounts are listed below in milligrams (mg).

**Table 24.1.** Vitamin $B_6$ Intake: Recommended Amount

| Life Stage | Recommended Amount |
|---|---|
| Birth to 6 months | 0.1 mg |
| Infants 7–12 months | 0.3 mg |
| Children 1–3 years | 0.5 mg |
| Children 4–8 years | 0.6 mg |
| Children 9–13 years | 1.0 mg |
| Teens 14–18 years (boys) | 1.3 mg |
| Teens 14–18 years (girls) | 1.2 mg |

This chapter includes text excerpted from "Vitamin $B_6$," Office of Dietary Supplements (ODS), National Institutes of Health (NIH), February 17, 2016.

**Table 24.1.** Continued

| Life Stage | Recommended Amount |
|---|---|
| Adults 19–50 years | 1.3 mg |
| Adults 51+ years (men) | 1.7 mg |
| Adults 51+ years (women) | 1.5 mg |
| Pregnant teens and women | 1.9 mg |
| Breastfeeding teens and women | 2.0 mg |

## What Foods Provide Vitamin B₆?

Vitamin $B_6$ is found naturally in many foods and is added to other foods. You can get recommended amounts of vitamin $B_6$ by eating a variety of foods, including the following:

- Poultry, fish, and organ meats, all rich in vitamin $B_6$

- Potatoes and other starchy vegetables, which are some of the major sources of vitamin $B_6$ for Americans

- Fruits (other than citrus), which are also among the major sources of vitamin $B_6$ for Americans

## What Kinds of Vitamin B₆ Dietary Supplements Are Available?

Vitamin $B_6$ is available in dietary supplements, usually in the form of pyridoxine. Most multivitamin-mineral (MVM) supplements contain vitamin $B_6$. Dietary supplements that contain only vitamin $B_6$, or vitamin $B_6$ with other B vitamins, are also available.

## Am I Getting Enough Vitamin B₆?

Most people in the United States get enough vitamin $B_6$ from the foods they eat. However, certain groups of people are more likely than others to have trouble getting enough vitamin $B_6$:

- People whose kidneys do not work properly, including people who are on kidney dialysis and those who have had a kidney transplant

- People with autoimmune disorders, which cause their immune system to mistakenly attack their own healthy tissues. For example, people with rheumatoid arthritis (RA), celiac disease,

Crohn's disease, ulcerative colitis (UC), or inflammatory bowel disease (IBD) sometimes have low vitamin B$_6$ levels.

• People with alcohol dependence

## What Happens If I Don't Get Enough Vitamin B$_6$?

Vitamin B$_6$ deficiency is uncommon in the United States. People who don't get enough vitamin B$_6$ can have a range of symptoms, including anemia, itchy rashes, scaly skin on the lips, cracks at the corners of the mouth, and a swollen tongue. Other symptoms of very low vitamin B$_6$ levels include depression, confusion, and a weak immune system. Infants who do not get enough vitamin B$_6$ can become irritable or develop extremely sensitive hearing or seizures.

## What Are Some Effects of Vitamin B$_6$ on Health?

Scientists are studying vitamin B$_6$ to understand how it affects health. Here are some examples of what this research has shown.

### Heart Disease

Some scientists had thought that certain B vitamins (such as folic acid, vitamin B$_{12}$, and vitamin B$_6$) might reduce heart disease risk by lowering levels of homocysteine, an amino acid in the blood. Although vitamin B supplements do lower blood homocysteine, research shows that they do not actually reduce the risk or severity of heart disease or stroke.

### Cancer

People with low levels of vitamin B$_6$ in the blood might have a higher risk of certain kinds of cancer, such as colorectal cancer. But studies to date have not shown that vitamin B$_6$ supplements can help prevent cancer or lower the chances of dying from this disease.

### Cognitive Function

Some research indicates that elderly people who have higher blood levels of vitamin B$_6$ have a better memory. However, taking vitamin B$_6$ supplements (alone or combined with vitamin B$_{12}$ and/or folic acid) does not seem to improve cognitive function or mood in healthy people or in people with dementia.

187

### Premenstrual Syndrome (PMS)

Scientists aren't yet certain about the potential benefits of taking vitamin $B_6$ for premenstrual syndrome (PMS). But some studies show that vitamin $B_6$ supplements could reduce PMS symptoms, including moodiness, irritability, forgetfulness, bloat, and anxiety.

### Nausea and Vomiting in Pregnancy

At least half of all women experience nausea, vomiting, or both in the first few months of pregnancy. Based on the results of several studies, the American Congress of Obstetricians and Gynecologists (ACOG) recommends taking vitamin $B_6$ supplements under a doctor's care for nausea and vomiting during pregnancy.

## Can Vitamin $B_6$ Be Harmful?

People almost never get too much vitamin $B_6$ from food. But taking high levels of vitamin $B_6$ from supplements for a year or longer can cause severe nerve damage, leading people to lose control of their bodily movements. The symptoms usually stop when they stop taking the supplements. Other symptoms of too much vitamin $B_6$ include painful, unsightly skin patches, extreme sensitivity to sunlight, nausea, and heartburn.

The upper limits for vitamin $B_6$ are listed below. These levels do not apply to people who are taking vitamin $B_6$ for medical reasons under the care of a doctor.

**Table 24.2.** Vitamin $B_6$ Intake: Upper Limit

| Life Stage | Upper Limit |
|---|---|
| Birth to 12 months | Not established |
| Children 1–3 years | 30 mg |
| Children 4–8 years | 40 mg |
| Children 9–13 years | 60 mg |
| Teens 14–18 years | 80 mg |
| Adults | 100 mg |

## Are There Any Interactions with Vitamin $B_6$ That I Should Know about?

Yes, vitamin $B_6$ supplements can interact or interfere with medicines that you take.

Here are several examples:

- Vitamin B$_6$ supplements might interact with cycloserine (Seromycin®), an antibiotic used to treat tuberculosis (TB), and worsen any seizures and nerve cell damage that the drug might cause.

- Taking certain epilepsy drugs could decrease vitamin B$_6$ levels and reduce the drugs' ability to control seizures.

- Taking theophylline (Aquaphyllin®, Elixophyllin®, Theolair®, Truxophyllin®, and many others) for asthma or another lung disease can reduce vitamin B$_6$ levels and cause seizures.

Tell your doctor, pharmacist, and other healthcare providers about any dietary supplements and medicines you take. They can tell you if those dietary supplements might interact or interfere with your prescription or over-the-counter (OTC) medicines or if the medicines might interfere with how your body absorbs, uses, or breaks down nutrients.

## Vitamin B$_6$ and Healthful Eating

People should get most of their nutrients from food, advises the federal government's *Dietary Guidelines for Americans*. Foods contain vitamins, minerals, dietary fiber and other substances that benefit health. In some cases, fortified foods and dietary supplements may provide nutrients that otherwise may be consumed in less-than-recommended amounts.

# Chapter 25

# Vitamin B$_{12}$

## What Is Vitamin B$_{12}$ and What Does It Do?

Vitamin B$_{12}$ is a nutrient that helps keep the body's nerve and blood cells healthy and helps make deoxyribonucleic acid (DNA), the genetic material in all cells. Vitamin B$_{12}$ also helps prevent a type of anemia called megaloblastic anemia that makes people tired and weak.

Two steps are required for the body to absorb vitamin B$_{12}$ from food. First, hydrochloric acid in the stomach separates vitamin B$_{12}$ from the protein to which vitamin B$_{12}$ is attached to food. After this, vitamin B$_{12}$ combines with a protein made by the stomach called intrinsic factor and is absorbed by the body. Some people have pernicious anemia, a condition in which they cannot make intrinsic factor. As a result, they have trouble absorbing vitamin B$_{12}$ from all foods and dietary supplements.

## How Much Vitamin B$_{12}$ Do I Need?

The amount of vitamin B$_{12}$ you need each day depends on your age. Average daily recommended amounts for different ages are listed below in micrograms (mcg):

This chapter includes text excerpted from "Vitamin B$_{12}$," Office of Dietary Supplements (ODS), National Institutes of Health (NIH), June 24, 2011. Reviewed May 2018.

**Table 25.1.** Vitamin B$_{12}$ Intake: Recommended Amount

| Life Stage | Recommended Amount |
|---|---|
| Birth to 6 months | 0.4 mcg |
| Infants 7–12 months | 0.5 mcg |
| Children 1–3 years | 0.9 mcg |
| Children 4–8 years | 1.2 mcg |
| Children 9–13 years | 1.8 mcg |
| Teens 14–18 years | 2.4 mcg |
| Adults | 2.4 mcg |
| Pregnant teens and women | 2.6 mcg |
| Breastfeeding teens and women | 2.8 mcg |

## What Foods Provide Vitamin B$_{12}$?

Vitamin B$_{12}$ is found naturally in a wide variety of animal foods and is added to some fortified foods. Plant foods have no vitamin B$_{12}$ unless they are fortified. You can get recommended amounts of vitamin B$_{12}$ by eating a variety of foods including the following:

- Beef liver and clams are the best sources of vitamin B$_{12}$.

- Fish, meat, poultry, eggs, milk, and other dairy products, contains vitamin B$_{12}$.

- Some breakfast cereals, nutritional yeasts, and other food products that are fortified with vitamin B$_{12}$. To find out if vitamin B$_{12}$ has been added to a food product, check the product labels.

## What Kinds of Vitamin B$_{12}$ Dietary Supplements Are Available?

Vitamin B$_{12}$ is found in almost all multivitamins. Dietary supplements that contain only vitamin B$_{12}$, or vitamin B$_{12}$ with nutrients such as folic acid, and other B vitamins, are also available. Vitamin B$_{12}$ is also available in sublingual forms (which are dissolved under the tongue). There is no evidence that sublingual forms are better absorbed than pills that are swallowed.

A prescription form of vitamin B$_{12}$ can be administered as a shot. This is usually used to treat vitamin B$_{12}$ deficiency. Vitamin B$_{12}$ is also available as a prescription medication in nasal gel form (for use in the nose).

## Am I Getting Enough Vitamin B$_{12}$?

Most people in the United States get enough vitamin B$_{12}$ from the foods they eat. But some people have trouble absorbing vitamin B$_{12}$ from food. As a result, vitamin B$_{12}$ deficiency affects between 1.5 percent and 15 percent of the public. Your doctor can test your vitamin B$_{12}$ level to see if you have a deficiency.

Certain groups may not get enough vitamin B$_{12}$ or have trouble absorbing it:

- Many older adults, who do not have enough hydrochloric acid in their stomach to absorb the vitamin B$_{12}$ naturally present in food. People over 50 should get most of their vitamin B$_{12}$ from fortified foods or dietary supplements because, in most cases, their bodies can absorb vitamin B$_{12}$ from these sources.

- People with pernicious anemia whose bodies do not make the intrinsic factor needed to absorb vitamin B$_{12}$. Doctors usually treat pernicious anemia with vitamin B$_{12}$ shots, although very high oral doses of vitamin B$_{12}$ might also be effective.

- People who have had gastrointestinal surgery, such as weight loss surgery, or who have digestive disorders, such as celiac disease or Crohn's disease. These conditions can decrease the amount of vitamin B$_{12}$ that the body can absorb.

- Some people who eat little or no animal foods such as vegetarians and vegans. Only animal foods have vitamin B$_{12}$ naturally. When pregnant women and women who breastfeed their babies are strict vegetarians or vegans, their babies might also not get enough vitamin B$_{12}$.

## What Happens If I Don't Get Enough Vitamin B$_{12}$?

Vitamin B$_{12}$ deficiency causes tiredness, weakness, constipation, loss of appetite, weight loss, and megaloblastic anemia. Nerve problems, such as numbness and tingling in the hands and feet, can also occur. Other symptoms of vitamin B$_{12}$ deficiency include problems with balance, depression, confusion, dementia, poor memory, and soreness of the mouth or tongue. Vitamin B$_{12}$ deficiency can damage the nervous system even in people who don't have anemia, so it is important to treat a deficiency as soon as possible.

In infants, signs of a vitamin B$_{12}$ deficiency include failure to thrive, problems with movement, delays in reaching the typical developmental milestones, and megaloblastic anemia.

193

Large amounts of folic acid can hide a vitamin $B_{12}$ deficiency by correcting megaloblastic anemia, a hallmark of vitamin $B_{12}$ deficiency. But folic acid does not correct the progressive damage to the nervous system that vitamin $B_{12}$ deficiency also causes. For this reason, healthy adults should not get more than 1,000 mcg of folic acid a day.

## What Are Some Effects of Vitamin $B_{12}$ on Health?

Scientists are studying vitamin $B_{12}$ to understand how it affects health. Here are several examples of what this research has shown:

### Heart Disease

Vitamin $B_{12}$ supplements (along with folic acid and vitamin $B_6$) do not reduce the risk of getting heart disease. Scientists had thought that these vitamins might be helpful because they reduce blood levels of homocysteine, a compound linked to an increased risk of having a heart attack or stroke.

### Dementia

As they get older, some people develop dementia. These people often have high levels of homocysteine in the blood. Vitamin $B_{12}$ (with folic acid and vitamin $B_6$) can lower homocysteine levels, but scientists don't know yet whether these vitamins actually help prevent or treat dementia.

### Energy and Athletic Performance

Advertisements often promote vitamin $B_{12}$ supplements as a way to increase energy or endurance. Except in people with a vitamin $B_{12}$ deficiency, no evidence shows that vitamin $B_{12}$ supplements increase energy or improve athletic performance.

## Can Vitamin $B_{12}$ Be Harmful?

Vitamin $B_{12}$ has not been shown to cause any harm.

## Are There Any Interactions with Vitamin $B_{12}$ That I Should Know About?

Yes. Vitamin $B_{12}$ can interact or interfere with medicines that you take, and in some cases, medicines can lower vitamin $B_{12}$ levels in the body. Here are several examples of medicines that can interfere with the body's absorption or use of vitamin B$_{12}$:

- Chloramphenicol (Chloromycetin®), an antibiotic that is used to treat certain infections

- Proton pump inhibitors, such as omeprazole (Prilosec®) and lansoprazole (Prevacid®), that are used to treat acid reflux, and peptic ulcer disease

- Histamine H2 receptor antagonists, such as cimetidine (Tagamet®), famotidine (Pepcid®), and ranitidine (Zantac®), that are used to treat peptic ulcer disease

- Metformin, a drug used to treat diabetes

Tell your doctor, pharmacist, and other healthcare providers about any dietary supplements and medicines you take. They can tell you if those dietary supplements might interact or interfere with your prescription or over-the-counter (OTC) medicines or if the medicines might interfere with how your body absorbs, uses, or breaks down nutrients.

## Vitamin B$_{12}$ and Healthful Eating

People should get most of their nutrients from food, advises the federal government's *Dietary Guidelines for Americans*. Foods contain vitamins, minerals, dietary fiber and other substances that benefit health. In some cases, fortified foods and dietary supplements may provide nutrients that otherwise may be consumed in less-than-recommended amounts.

# Chapter 26

# *Vitamin D*

## *Chapter Contents*

## Section 26.1

# *Vitamin D: Basics*

This section includes text excerpted from "Vitamin D,"
Office of Dietary Supplements (ODS), National
Institutes of Health (NIH), April 15, 2016.

## *What Is Vitamin D and What Does It Do?*

Vitamin D is a nutrient found in some foods that is needed for health and to maintain strong bones. It does so by helping the body absorb calcium (one of the bone's main building blocks) from food and supplements. People who get too little vitamin D may develop soft, thin, and brittle bones, a condition known as rickets in children and osteomalacia in adults.

Vitamin D is important to the body in many other ways as well. Muscles need it to move, for example, nerves need it to carry messages between the brain and every body part, and the immune system needs vitamin D to fight off invading bacteria and viruses. Together with calcium, vitamin D also helps protect older adults from osteoporosis. Vitamin D is found in cells throughout the body.

## *How Much Vitamin D Do I Need?*

The amount of vitamin D you need each day depends on your age. Average daily recommended amounts from the Food and Nutrition Board (FNB) (a national group of experts) for different ages are listed below in International Units (IU):

**Table 26.1.** Vitamin D Intake: Recommended Amount

| Life Stage | Recommended Amount |
|---|---|
| Birth to 12 months | 400 IU |
| Children 1–13 years | 600 IU |
| Teens 14–18 years | 600 IU |
| Adults 19–70 years | 600 IU |

**Table 26.1.** Continued

| Life Stage | Recommended Amount |
|---|---|
| Adults 71 years and older | 800 IU |
| Pregnant and breastfeeding women | 600 IU |

## What Foods Provide Vitamin D?

Very few foods naturally have vitamin D. Fortified foods provide most of the vitamin D in American diets.

- Fatty fish such as salmon, tuna, and mackerel are among the best sources.

- Beef liver, cheese, and egg yolks provide small amounts.

- Mushrooms provide some vitamin D. In some mushrooms that are newly available in stores, the vitamin D content is being boosted by exposing these mushrooms to ultraviolet light.

- Almost all of the U.S. milk supply is fortified with 400 IU of vitamin D per quart. But foods made from milk, like cheese, and ice cream, are usually not fortified.

- Vitamin D is added to many breakfast bowls of cereal and to some brands of orange juice, yogurt, margarine, and soy beverages; check the labels.

## Can I Get Vitamin D from the Sun?

The body makes vitamin D when skin is directly exposed to the sun, and most people meet at least some of their vitamin D needs this way. Skin exposed to sunshine indoors through a window will not produce vitamin D. Cloudy days, shade, and having dark-colored skin also cut down on the amount of vitamin D the skin makes.

However, despite the importance of the sun to vitamin D synthesis, it is prudent to limit exposure of skin to sunlight in order to lower the risk for skin cancer. When out in the sun for more than a few minutes, wear protective clothing and apply sunscreen with a sun protection factor (SPF) of 8 or more. Tanning beds also cause the skin to make vitamin D but pose similar risks for skin cancer.

People who avoid the sun or who cover their bodies with sunscreen or clothing should include good sources of vitamin D in their diets or take a supplement. Recommended intakes of vitamin D are set on the assumption of little sun exposure.

## What Kinds of Vitamin D Dietary Supplements Are Available?

Vitamin D is found in supplements (and fortified foods) in two different forms: D2 (ergocalciferol) and D3 (cholecalciferol). Both increase vitamin D in the blood.

## Am I Getting Enough Vitamin D?

Because vitamin D can come from sun, food, and supplements, the best measure of one's vitamin D status is blood levels of a form known as 25-hydroxyvitamin D. Levels are described in either nanomoles per liter (nmol/L) or nanograms per milliliter (ng/mL), where 1 nmol/L=0.4 ng/mL.

In general, levels below 30 nmol/L (12 ng/mL) are too low for bone or overall health, and levels above 125 nmol/L (50 ng/mL) are probably too high. Levels of 50 nmol/L or above (20 ng/mL or above) are sufficient for most people.

By these measures, some Americans are vitamin D deficient and almost no one has levels that are too high. In general, young people have higher blood levels of 25-hydroxyvitamin D than older people and males have higher levels than females. By race, non-Hispanic blacks tend to have the lowest levels and non-Hispanic whites the highest. The majority of Americans have blood levels lower than 75 nmol/L (30 ng/mL).

Certain other groups may not get enough vitamin D:

- Breastfed infants, because human milk is a poor source of the nutrient. Breastfed infants should be given a supplement of 400 IU of vitamin D each day.

- Older adults, because their skin doesn't make vitamin D when exposed to sunlight as efficiently as when they were young, and their kidneys are less able to convert vitamin D to its active form

- People with dark skin, because their skin has less ability to produce vitamin D from the sun

- People with disorders such as Crohn's disease or celiac disease who don't handle fat properly, because vitamin D needs fat to be absorbed

- Obese people, because their body fat binds to some vitamin D and prevents it from getting into the blood

## What Happens If I Don't Get Enough Vitamin D?

People can become deficient in vitamin D because they don't consume enough or absorb enough from food, their exposure to sunlight is limited, or their kidneys cannot convert vitamin D to its active form in the body. In children, vitamin D deficiency causes rickets, a condition in which the bones become soft and bend. It's a rare disease but still occurs, especially among African American infants and children. In adults, vitamin D deficiency leads to osteomalacia, causing bone pain and muscle weakness.

## What Are Some Effects of Vitamin D on Health?

Vitamin D is being studied for its possible connections to several diseases and medical problems, including diabetes, hypertension, and autoimmune conditions such as multiple sclerosis (MS). Two of them discussed below are bone disorders and some types of cancer.

### Bone Disorders

As they get older, millions of people (mostly women, but men too) develop or are at risk of, osteoporosis, a condition in which bones become fragile and may fracture if one falls. It is one consequence of not getting enough calcium and vitamin D over the long term. Supplements of both vitamin D3 (at 700–800 IU/day) and calcium (500–1,200 mg/day) have been shown to reduce the risk of bone loss and fractures in elderly people aged 62–85 years. Men and women should talk with their healthcare providers about their needs for vitamin D (and calcium) as part of an overall plan to prevent or treat osteoporosis.

### Cancer

Some studies suggest that vitamin D may protect against colon cancer and perhaps even cancers of the prostate and breast. But higher levels of vitamin D in the blood have also been linked to higher rates of pancreatic cancer. At this time, it's too early to say whether low vitamin D status increases cancer risk and whether higher levels protect or even increase risk in some people.

## Can Vitamin D Be Harmful?

Yes, when amounts in the blood become too high. Signs of toxicity include nausea, vomiting, poor appetite, constipation, weakness, and weight loss. And by raising blood levels of calcium, too much vitamin D can cause confusion, disorientation, and problems with heart rhythm. Excess vitamin D can also damage the kidneys.

The upper limit for vitamin D is 1,000–1,500 IU/day for infants, 2,500–3,000 IU/day for children 1–8 years, and 4,000 IU/day for children 9 years and older, adults, and pregnant, and lactating teens, and women. Vitamin D toxicity almost always occurs from overuse of supplements. Excessive sun exposure doesn't cause vitamin D poisoning because the body limits the amount of this vitamin it produces.

## Are There Any Interactions with Vitamin D That I Should Know about?

Like most dietary supplements, vitamin D may interact or interfere with other medicines or supplements you might be taking. Here are several examples:

- Prednisone and other corticosteroid medicines to reduce inflammation impair how the body handles vitamin D, which leads to lower calcium absorption and loss of bone over time.

- Both, the weight-loss drug orlistat (brand names Xenical® and Alli®) and the cholesterol-lowering drug cholestyramine (brand names Questran®, LoCholest®, and Prevalite®), can reduce the absorption of vitamin D and other fat-soluble vitamins (A, E, and K).

- Both, phenobarbital and phenytoin (brand name Dilantin®), used to prevent and control epileptic seizures, increase the breakdown of vitamin D and reduce calcium absorption.

Tell your doctor, pharmacist, and other healthcare providers about any dietary supplements and medicines you take. They can tell you if those dietary supplements might interact or interfere with your prescription or over-the-counter medicines (OTC), or if the medicines might interfere with how your body absorbs, uses, or breaks down nutrients.

## Vitamin D and Healthful Eating

People should get most of their nutrients from food, advises the federal government's *Dietary Guidelines for Americans*. Foods contain vitamins, minerals, dietary fiber, and other substances that benefit health. In some cases, fortified foods and dietary supplements may provide nutrients that otherwise may be consumed in less-than-recommended amounts.

## Section 26.2

# *Calcium and Vitamin D: Important at Every Age*

This section includes text excerpted from "Calcium and Vitamin D: Important at Every Age," National Institutes of Health (NIH), May 2015.

The foods we eat contain a variety of vitamins, minerals, and other important nutrients that help keep our bodies healthy. Two nutrients, in particular, calcium, and vitamin D, are needed for strong bones.

## *The Role of Calcium*

Calcium is needed for our heart, muscles, and nerves to function properly and for blood to clot. Inadequate calcium significantly contributes to the development of osteoporosis. Many published studies show that low calcium intake throughout life is associated with low bone mass and high fracture rates. National nutrition surveys have shown that most people are not getting the calcium they need to grow and maintain healthy bones.

**Table 26.2.** Calcium Intake: Recommended Amount

| Life-Stage Group | Mg/Day |
|---|---|
| Infants 0–6 months | 200 |
| Infants 6–12 months | 260 |
| 1–3 years old | 700 |
| 4–8 years old | 1000 |
| 9–13 years old | 1300 |
| 14–18 years old | 1300 |
| 19–30 years old | 1000 |
| 31–50 years old | 1000 |
| 51–70-year-old males | 1000 |
| 51–70-year-old females | 1200 |

## Table 26.2. Continued

| Life-Stage Group | Mg/Day |
|---|---|
| 70 years old | 1200 |
| 14–18 years old, pregnant/lactating | 1300 |
| 19–50 years old, pregnant/lactating | 1000 |

To learn how easily you can include more calcium in your diet without adding much fat, see the list below.

## Table 26.3. Selected Calcium-Rich Foods

| Food | Calcium (mg) |
|---|---|
| Fortified oatmeal, 1 packet | 350 |
| Sardines, canned in oil, with edible bones, 3 oz. | 324 |
| Cheddar cheese, 1½ oz. shredded | 306 |
| Milk, nonfat, 1 cup | 302 |
| Milkshake, 1 cup | 300 |
| Yogurt, plain, low-fat, 1 cup | 300 |
| Soybeans, cooked, 1 cup | 261 |
| Tofu, firm, with calcium, ½ cup | 204 |
| Orange juice, fortified with calcium, 6 oz. | 200–260 (varies) |
| Salmon, canned, with edible bones, 3 oz. | 181 |
| Pudding, instant (chocolate, banana, etc.) made with 2 percent milk, ½ cup | 153 |
| Baked beans, 1 cup | 142 |
| Cottage cheese, 1 percent milk fat, 1 cup | 138 |
| Spaghetti, lasagna, 1 cup | 125 |
| Frozen yogurt, vanilla, soft-serve, ½ cup | 103 |
| Ready-to-eat cereal, fortified with calcium, 1 cup | 100–1,000 (varies) |
| Cheese pizza, 1 slice | 100 |
| Fortified waffles, 2 | 100 |
| Turnip greens, boiled, ½ cup | 99 |
| Broccoli, raw, 1 cup | 90 |
| Ice cream, vanilla, ½ cup | 85 |
| Soy or rice milk, fortified with calcium, 1 cup | 80–500 (varies) |

## Calcium Culprits

Although a balanced diet aids calcium absorption, high levels of protein and sodium (salt) in the diet are thought to increase calcium excretion through the kidneys. Excessive amounts of these substances should be avoided, especially in those with low calcium intake.

Lactose intolerance also can lead to inadequate calcium intake. Those who are lactose intolerant have insufficient amounts of the enzyme lactase, which is needed to break down the lactose found in dairy products. To include dairy products in the diet, dairy foods can be taken in small quantities or treated with lactase drops, or lactase can be taken as a pill. Some milk products on the market already have been treated with lactase.

## Calcium Supplements

If you have trouble getting enough calcium in your diet, you may need to take a calcium supplement. The amount of calcium you will need from a supplement depends on how much calcium you obtain from food sources. There are several different calcium compounds from which to choose, such as calcium carbonate, and calcium citrate, among others. Except in people with the gastrointestinal disease, all major forms of calcium supplements are absorbed equally well when taken with food.

Calcium supplements are better absorbed when taken in small doses (500 mg or less) several times throughout the day. In many individuals, calcium supplements are better absorbed when taken with food. It is important to check supplement labels to ensure that the product meets United States Pharmacopeia (USP) standards.

## Vitamin D

The body needs vitamin D to absorb calcium. Without enough vitamin D, one can't form enough of the hormone calcitriol (known as the "active vitamin D"). This in turn leads to insufficient calcium absorption from the diet. In this situation, the body must take calcium from its stores in the skeleton, which weakens existing bone and prevents the formation of strong, new bone.

You can get vitamin D in three ways: through the skin, from the diet, and from supplements. Experts recommend a daily intake of 600 IU (International Units) of vitamin D up to age 70. Men and women over age 70 should increase their uptake to 800 IU daily, which also can be obtained from supplements or vitamin D-rich foods such as egg yolks, saltwater fish, liver, and fortified milk. The Institute of Medicine recommends no more than 4,000 IU per day for adults. However, sometimes doctors prescribe higher doses for people who are deficient in vitamin D.

## *A Complete Osteoporosis Program*

Remember, a balanced diet rich in calcium and vitamin D is only one part of an osteoporosis prevention or treatment program. Like exercise, getting enough calcium is a strategy that helps strengthen bones at any age. But these strategies may not be enough to stop bone loss caused by lifestyle, medications, or menopause. Your doctor can determine the need for an osteoporosis medication in addition to diet and exercise.

# Section 26.3

# *Vitamin D and Cancer Prevention*

This section includes text excerpted from "Vitamin D and Cancer Prevention," National Cancer Institute (NCI), October 21, 2013. Reviewed May 2018.

## *What Is Vitamin D?*

Vitamin D is the name given to a group of fat-soluble prohormones (substances that usually have little hormonal activity by themselves but that the body can turn into hormones). Vitamin D helps the body use calcium, and phosphorus to make strong bones and teeth. Skin exposed to sunshine can make vitamin D, and vitamin D can also be obtained from certain foods. Vitamin D deficiency can cause a weakening of the bones that is called rickets in children and osteomalacia in adults.

Two major forms of vitamin D that are important to humans are vitamin D2, or ergocalciferol, and vitamin D3, or cholecalciferol. Vitamin D2 is made naturally by plants, and vitamin D3 is made naturally by the body when skin is exposed to ultraviolet radiation in sunlight. Both forms are converted to 25-hydroxyvitamin D in the liver. 25-Hydroxyvitamin D then travels through the blood to the kidneys, where it is further modified to 1,25-dihydroxyvitamin D, or calcitriol, the active form of vitamin D in the body. The most accurate method of evaluating a person's vitamin D status is to measure the level of 25-hydroxyvitamin D in the blood.

Most people get at least some of the vitamin D they need through sunlight exposure. Dietary sources include a few foods that naturally contain vitamin D, such as fatty fish, fish liver oil, and eggs. However, most dietary vitamin D comes from foods fortified with vitamin D, such as milk, juices, and breakfast cereals. Vitamin D can also be obtained through dietary supplements.

The Institute of Medicine (IOM) of the National Academies has developed the following recommended daily intakes of vitamin D, assuming minimal sun exposure:

- For those between 1–70 years of age, including women who are pregnant or lactating, the recommended dietary allowance (RDA) is 15 micrograms ($\mu$g) per day. Because 1 $\mu$g is equal to 40 International Units (IU), this RDA can also be expressed as 600 IU per day.

- For those 71 years or older, the RDA is 20 $\mu$g per day (800 IU per day).

- For infants, the IOM could not determine an RDA due to a lack of data. However, the IOM set an Adequate Intake level of 10 $\mu$g per day (400 IU per day), which should provide sufficient vitamin D.

Although the average dietary intakes of vitamin D in the United States are below guideline levels, data from the National Health and Nutrition Examination Survey (NHANES) revealed that more than 80 percent of Americans had adequate vitamin D levels in their blood.

Even though most people are unlikely to have high vitamin D intakes, it is important to remember that excessive intake of any nutrient, including vitamin D, can cause toxic effects. Too much vitamin D can be harmful because it increases calcium levels, which can lead to calcinosis (the deposit of calcium salts in soft tissues, such as the kidneys, heart, or lungs) and hypercalcemia (high blood levels of calcium). The safe upper intake level of vitamin D for adults and children older than 8 years of age is 100 $\mu$g per day (4000 IU per day). Toxicity from too much vitamin D is more likely to occur from high intakes of dietary supplements than from high intakes of foods that contain vitamin D. Excessive sun exposure does not cause vitamin D toxicity. However, the IOM states that people should not try to increase vitamin

D production by increasing their exposure to sunlight because this will also increase their risk of skin cancer.

## Why Are Cancer Researchers Studying a Possible Connection between Vitamin D and Cancer Risk?

Early epidemiologic research showed that incidence and death rates for certain cancers were lower among individuals living in southern latitudes, where levels of sunlight exposure are relatively high than among those living at northern latitudes. Because exposure to ultraviolet light from sunlight leads to the production of vitamin D, researchers hypothesized that variation in vitamin D levels might account for this association. However, additional research based on stronger study designs is required to determine whether higher vitamin D levels are related to lower cancer incidence or death rates.

Experimental evidence has also suggested a possible association between vitamin D and cancer risk. In studies of cancer cells and of tumors in mice, vitamin D has been found to have several activities that might slow or prevent the development of cancer, including promoting cellular differentiation, decreasing cancer cell growth, stimulating cell death (apoptosis), and reducing tumor blood vessel formation (angiogenesis).

## What Is the Evidence That Vitamin D Can Help Reduce the Risk of Cancer in People?

A number of epidemiologic studies have investigated whether people with higher vitamin D intakes or higher blood levels of vitamin D have lower risks of specific cancers. The results of these studies have been inconsistent, possibly because of the challenges in carrying out such studies. For example, dietary studies do not account for vitamin D made in the skin from sunlight exposure, and the level of vitamin D measured in the blood at a single point in time (as in most studies) may not reflect a person's true vitamin D status. Also, it is possible that people with higher vitamin D intakes or blood levels are more likely to have other healthy behaviors. It may be one of these other behaviors, rather than vitamin D intake, that influences cancer risk.

Several randomized trials of vitamin D intake have been carried out, but these were designed to assess bone health or other noncancer outcomes. Although some of these trials have yielded information on cancer incidence and mortality, the results need to be confirmed by additional research because the trials were not designed to study cancer specifically.

The cancers for which the most human data are available are colorectal, breast, prostate, and pancreatic cancer. Numerous epidemiologic studies have shown that higher intake or blood levels of vitamin D are associated with a reduced risk of colorectal cancer. In contrast, the Women's Health Initiative randomized trial found that healthy women who took vitamin D and calcium supplements for an average of 7 years did not have a reduced incidence of colorectal cancer. Some scientists have pointed out that the relatively low level of vitamin D supplementation (10 $\mu$g, or 400 IU, once a day), the ability of participants to take additional vitamin D on their own, and the short duration of participant follow-up in this trial might explain why no reduction in colorectal cancer risk was found. Evidence on the association between vitamin D and the risks of all other malignancies studied is inconclusive.

## How Is Vitamin D Being Studied Now in Clinical Cancer Research?

Taken together, the available data are not comprehensive enough to establish whether taking vitamin D can prevent cancer. To fully understand the effects of vitamin D on cancer and other health outcomes, new randomized trials need to be conducted. However, the appropriate dose of vitamin D to use in such trials is still not clear. Other remaining questions include when to start taking vitamin D, and for how long, to potentially see a benefit.

To begin addressing these issues, researchers are conducting two phase I trials to determine what dose of vitamin D may be useful for chemoprevention of prostate, colorectal, and lung cancers (trial descriptions here and here). In addition, larger randomized trials have been initiated to examine the potential role of vitamin D in the prevention of cancer. The Vitamin D/Calcium Polyp Prevention Study (PPS), which has finished recruiting approximately 2,200 participants, is testing whether vitamin D supplements, given alone or with calcium, can prevent the development of colorectal adenomas (precancerous growths) in patients who previously had an adenoma removed. The Vitamin D and Omega-3 Trial (VITAL) will examine whether vitamin D supplements can prevent the development of a variety of cancer types in healthy older men and women. Researchers are also beginning to study vitamin D analogs—chemicals with structures similar to that of vitamin D—which may have the anticancer activity of vitamin D but not its ability to increase calcium levels.

# Section 26.4

# *Infant Overdose Risk with Liquid Vitamin D*

This section includes text excerpted from "Consumer
Updates—Infant Overdose Risk with Liquid Vitamin D,"
U.S. Food and Drug Administration (FDA), December 18, 2017.

The U.S. Food and Drug Administration (FDA) is warning of the
potential risk of overdosing infants with liquid vitamin D. Some liquid
vitamin D supplement products on the market come with droppers
that could allow parents and caregivers to accidentally give harmful
amounts of the vitamin to an infant. These droppers can hold a greater
amount of liquid vitamin D than an infant should receive.

"It is important that infants not get more than the recommended
daily amount of vitamin D," says Linda M. Katz, M.D., M.P.H.,
an interim chief medical officer in FDA's Center for Food Safety
and Applied Nutrition (CFSAN). "Parents and caregivers should
only use the dropper that comes with the vitamin D supplement
purchased."

Vitamin D promotes calcium absorption in the gut and plays a key
role in the development of strong bones. Vitamin D supplements are
recommended for some infants—especially those that are breastfed—
because deficiency of this vitamin can lead to bone problems such as
thinning, soft, and mis-shaped bones, as is seen with the condition
known as rickets.

However, excessive vitamin D can cause nausea and vomiting, loss
of appetite, excessive thirst, frequent urination, constipation, abdominal pain, muscle weakness, muscle and joint aches, confusion, and
fatigue, as well as more serious consequences like kidney damage.

## *FDA's Recommendations*

- Ensure that your infant does not receive more than 400
  international units (IUs) of vitamin D a day, which is the daily
  dose of vitamin D supplement that the American Academy
  of Pediatrics (AAP) recommends for breastfed and partially
  breastfed infants.

- Keep the vitamin D supplement product with its original package so that you and other caregivers can follow the instructions. Follow these instructions carefully so that you use the dropper correctly and give the right dose.

- Use only the dropper that comes with the product; it is manufactured specifically for that product. Do not use a dropper from another product.

- Ensure the dropper is marked so that the units of measure are clear and easy to understand. Also, make sure that the units of measure correspond to those mentioned in the instructions.

- If you cannot clearly determine the dose of vitamin D delivered by the dropper, talk to a healthcare professional before giving the supplement to the infant.

- If your infant is being fully or partially fed with infant formula, check with your pediatrician or another healthcare professional before giving the child vitamin D supplements.

**Remember:** Any type of medication or dietary supplement can have adverse effects and must be taken according to the manufacturer's directions.

# Chapter 27

# *Vitamin E*

## *What Is Vitamin E and What Does It Do?*

Vitamin E is a fat-soluble nutrient found in many foods. In the body, it acts as an antioxidant, helping to protect cells from the damage caused by free radicals. Free radicals are compounds formed when our bodies convert the food we eat into energy. People are also exposed to free radicals in the environment from cigarette smoke, air pollution, and ultraviolet (UV) light from the sun.

The body also needs vitamin E to boost its immune system so that it can fight off invading bacteria and viruses. It helps to widen blood vessels and keep blood from clotting within them. In addition, cells use vitamin E to interact with each other and to carry out many important functions.

## *How Much Vitamin E Do I Need?*

The amount of vitamin E you need each day depends on your age. Average daily recommended intakes are listed below in milligrams (mg) and in international units (IU). Package labels list the amount of vitamin E in foods and dietary supplements in IU.

---

This chapter includes text excerpted from "Vitamin E," Office of Dietary Supplements (ODS), National Institutes of Health (NIH), May 9, 2016.

**Table 27.1.** Vitamin E Intake: Recommended Amount

| Life Stage | Recommended Amount |
|---|---|
| Birth to 6 months | 4 mg (6 IU) |
| Infants 7–12 months | 5 mg (7.5 IU) |
| Children 1–3 years | 6 mg (9 IU) |
| Children 4–8 years | 7 mg (10.4 IU) |
| Children 9–13 years | 11 mg (16.4 IU) |
| Teens 14–18 years | 15 mg (22.4 IU) |
| Adults | 15 mg (22.4 IU) |
| Pregnant teens and women | 15 mg (22.4 IU) |
| Breastfeeding teens and women | 19 mg (28.4 IU) |

## What Foods Provide Vitamin E?

Vitamin E is found naturally in foods and is added to some fortified foods. You can get recommended amounts of vitamin E by eating a variety of foods including the following:

- Vegetable oils like wheat germ, sunflower, and safflower oils are among the best sources of vitamin E. Corn and soybean oils also provide some vitamin E.

- Nuts (such as peanuts, hazelnuts, and, especially, almonds) and seeds (like sunflower seeds) are also among the best sources of vitamin E.

- Green vegetables, such as spinach and broccoli, provide some vitamin E.

- Food companies add vitamin E to some breakfast cereals, fruit juices, margarine, and spreads, and other foods. To find out which ones have vitamin E, check the product labels.

## What Kinds of Vitamin E Dietary Supplements Are Available?

Vitamin E supplements come in different amounts and forms. Two main things to consider when choosing a vitamin E supplement are:

1. **The amount of vitamin E.** Most once-daily multivitamin-mineral (MVM) supplements provides about 30 IU of vitamin E, whereas vitamin E-only supplements usually contain 100–1,000 IU per pill. The doses of vitamin E-only supplements are

much higher than the recommended amounts. Some people take large doses because they believe or hope that doing so will keep them healthy or lower their risk of certain diseases.

2. **The form of vitamin E.** Although vitamin E sounds like a single substance, it is actually the name of eight related compounds in food, including alpha-tocopherol. Each form has a different potency or level of activity in the body.

Vitamin E from natural (food) sources is commonly listed as "*d*-alpha-tocopherol" on food packaging and supplement labels. Synthetic (laboratory-made) vitamin E is commonly listed as "*dl*-alpha-tocopherol." The natural form is more potent. For example, 100 IU of natural vitamin E is equal to about 150 IU of the synthetic form.

Some vitamin E supplements provide other forms of the vitamin, such as gammatocopherol, tocotrienols, and mixed tocopherols. Scientists do not know if any of these forms are superior to alpha-tocopherol in supplements.

## Am I Getting Enough Vitamin E?

The diets of most Americans provide less than the recommended amounts of vitamin E. Nevertheless, healthy people rarely show any clear signs that they are not getting enough vitamin E.

## What Happens If I Don't Get Enough Vitamin E?

Vitamin E deficiency is very rare in healthy people. It is almost always linked to certain diseases in which fat is not properly digested or absorbed. Examples include Crohn disease, cystic fibrosis, and certain rare genetic diseases such as abetalipoproteinemia and ataxia with vitamin E deficiency (AVED). Vitamin E needs some fat for the digestive system to absorb it.

Vitamin E deficiency can cause nerve and muscle damage that results in loss of feeling in the arms and legs, loss of body movement control, muscle weakness, and vision problems. Another sign of deficiency is a weakened immune system.

## What Are Some Effects of Vitamin E on Health?

Scientists are studying vitamin E to understand how it affects health. Here are several examples of what the research has shown.

### Heart Disease

Some studies link higher intakes of vitamin E from supplements to lower chances of developing heart disease. But the best research finds no benefit. People in these studies are randomly assigned to take vitamin E or a placebo (dummy pill with no vitamin E or active ingredients) and they don't know which they are taking. Vitamin E supplements do not seem to prevent heart disease, reduce its severity, or affect the risk of death from this disease. Scientists do not know whether high intakes of vitamin E might protect the heart in younger, healthier people who do not have a high risk of heart disease.

### Cancer

Most research indicates that vitamin E does not help prevent cancer and may be harmful in some cases. Large doses of vitamin E have not consistently reduced the risk of colon and breast cancer in studies, for example. A large study found that taking vitamin E supplements (400 IU/day) for several years increased the risk of developing prostate cancer in men. Two studies that followed middle-aged men and women for 7 or more years found that extra vitamin E (300–400 IU/day, on average) did not protect them from any form of cancer. However, one study found a link between the use of vitamin E supplements for 10 years or more and a lower risk of death from bladder cancer.

Vitamin E dietary supplements and other antioxidants might interact with chemotherapy and radiation therapy. People undergoing these treatments should talk with their doctor or oncologist before taking vitamin E or other antioxidant supplements, especially in high doses.

### Eye Disorders

Age-related macular degeneration (AMD), or the loss of central vision in older people, and cataracts are among the most common causes of vision loss in older people. The results of research on whether vitamin E can help prevent these conditions are inconsistent. Among people with AMD who were at high risk of developing advanced AMD, a supplement containing large doses of vitamin E combined with other antioxidants, zinc, and copper showed promise for slowing down the rate of vision loss.

### Mental Function

Several studies have investigated whether vitamin E supplements might help older adults remain mentally alert and active as well as prevent or slow the decline of mental function and Alzheimer disease (AD). So far, the research provides little evidence that taking vitamin E supplements can help healthy people or people with mild mental functioning problems to maintain brain health.

### Can Vitamin E Be Harmful?

Eating vitamin E in foods is not risky or harmful. In supplement form, however, high doses of vitamin E might increase the risk of bleeding (by reducing the blood's ability to form clots after a cut or injury) and of serious bleeding in the brain (known as hemorrhagic stroke). Because of this risk, the upper limit for adults is 1,500 IU/day for supplements made from the natural form of vitamin E and 1,100 IU/day for supplements made from synthetic vitamin E. The upper limits for children are lower than those for adults. Some research suggests that taking vitamin E supplements even below these upper limits might cause harm. In one study, for example, men who took 400 IU of vitamin E each day for several years had an increased risk of prostate cancer.

### Are There Any Interactions with Vitamin E That I Should Know About?

Vitamin E dietary supplements can interact or interfere with certain medicines that you take. Here are some examples:

- Vitamin E can increase the risk of bleeding in people taking anticoagulant or antiplatelet medicines, such as warfarin (Coumadin®).

- In a study, vitamin E plus other antioxidants (such as vitamin C, selenium, and beta carotene) reduced the heart-protective effects of two drugs taken in combination (a statin and niacin) to affect blood cholesterol levels.

- Taking antioxidant supplements while undergoing chemotherapy or radiation therapy for cancer could alter the effectiveness of these treatments.

Tell your doctor, pharmacist, and other healthcare providers about any dietary supplements and medicines you take. They can tell you if those dietary supplements might interact or interfere with your prescription or over-the-counter (OTC) medicines, or if the medicines might interfere with how your body absorbs, uses, or breaks down nutrients.

## *Vitamin E and Healthful Eating*

People should get most of their nutrients from food, advises the federal government's *Dietary Guidelines for Americans*. Foods contain vitamins, minerals, dietary fiber, and other substances that benefit health. In some cases, fortified foods and dietary supplements may provide nutrients that otherwise may be consumed in less-than-recommended amounts.

# Chapter 28

# *Chromium*

Chromium is a mineral that humans require in trace amounts, although its mechanisms of action in the body and the amounts needed for optimal health are not well defined. It is found primarily in two forms:

1. Trivalent (chromium 3+), which is biologically active and found in food, and

2. Hexavalent (chromium 6+), a toxic form that results from industrial pollution

This chapter focuses exclusively on trivalent (3+) chromium.

Chromium is known to enhance the action of insulin, a hormone critical to the metabolism and storage of carbohydrate, fat, and protein in the body. It also appears to be directly involved in carbohydrate, fat, and protein metabolism, but more research is needed to determine the full range of its roles in the body. The challenges to meeting this goal include:

- **Recommended dietary allowance (RDA).** Average daily level of intake sufficient to meet the nutrient requirements of nearly all (97–98%) healthy individuals; often used to plan nutritionally adequate diets for individuals.

- **Adequate intake (AI).** Intake at this level is assumed to ensure nutritional adequacy; established when evidence is insufficient to develop an RDA.

---

This chapter includes text excerpted from "Chromium," Office of Dietary Supplements (ODS), National Institutes of Health (NIH), March 2, 2018.

- **Estimated average requirement (EAR).** Average daily level of intake estimated to meet the requirements of 50 percent of healthy individuals; usually used to assess the nutrient intakes of groups of people and to plan nutritionally adequate diets for them; can also be used to assess the nutrient intakes of individuals.

- **Tolerable upper intake level (UL).** Maximum daily intake unlikely to cause adverse health effects.

## *Foods That Provide Chromium*

Chromium is widely distributed in the food supply, but most foods provide only small amounts (less than 2 micrograms (mcg) per serving). Meat and whole-grain products, as well as some fruits, vegetables, and spices, are relatively good sources. In contrast, foods high in simple sugars (like sucrose and fructose) are low in chromium.

Dietary intakes of chromium cannot be reliably determined because the content of the mineral in foods is substantially affected by agricultural and manufacturing processes and perhaps by contamination with chromium when the foods are analyzed. Therefore, table 28.1, and food-composition databases generally, provide approximate values of chromium in foods that should only serve as a guide.

**Table 28.1.** Selected Food Sources of Chromium

| Food | Chromium (mcg) |
|---|---|
| Broccoli, ½ cup | 11 |
| Grape juice, 1 cup | 8 |
| English muffin, whole wheat, 1 | 4 |
| Potatoes, mashed, 1 cup | 3 |
| Garlic, dried, 1 teaspoon | 3 |
| Basil, dried, 1 tablespoon | 2 |
| Beef cubes, 3 ounces | 2 |
| Orange juice, 1 cup | 2 |
| Turkey breast, 3 ounces | 2 |
| Whole wheat bread, 2 slices | 2 |
| Red wine, 5 ounces | 1–13 |
| Apple, unpeeled, 1 medium | 1 |
| Banana, 1 medium | 1 |
| Green beans, ½ cup | 1 |

## Recommended Intakes of Chromium

Recommended chromium intakes are provided in the Dietary Reference Intakes (DRIs) developed by the Institute of Medicine of the National Academy of Sciences (IMNAS). DRI is the general term for a set of reference values to plan and assess the nutrient intakes of healthy people. These values include the RDA and the Adequate Intake (AI). The RDA is the average daily intake that meets a nutrient requirement of nearly all (97–98%), healthy individuals. An AI is established when there is insufficient research to establish an RDA; it is generally set at a level that healthy people typically consume.

In 1989, the National Academy of Sciences (NAS) established an "estimated safe and adequate daily dietary intake" range for chromium. For adults and adolescents that range was 50–200 mcg. In 2001, DRIs for chromium was established. The research base was insufficient to establish RDAs, so AIs were developed based on average intakes of chromium from food as found in several studies.

Adult women in the United States consume about 23–29 mcg of chromium per day from food, which meets their AIs unless they're pregnant or lactating. In contrast, adult men average 39–54 mcg per day, which exceeds their AIs.

The average amount of chromium in the breast milk of healthy, well-nourished mothers is 0.24 mcg per quart, so infants exclusively fed breast milk obtain about 0.2 mcg (based on an estimated consumption of 0.82 quarts per day). Infant formula provides about 0.5 mcg of chromium per quart. No studies have compared how well infants absorb and utilize chromium from human milk and formula.

## Factors That Affect Chromium Levels in the Body

Absorption of chromium from the intestinal tract is low, ranging from less than 0.4–2.5 percent of the amount consumed, and the remainder is excreted in the feces. Enhancing the mineral's absorption are vitamin C (found in fruits and vegetables and their juices) and the B vitamin niacin (found in meats, poultry, fish, and grain products). Absorbed chromium is stored in the liver, spleen, soft tissue, and bone.

The body's chromium content may be reduced under several conditions. Diets high in simple sugars (comprising more than 35% of calories) can increase chromium excretion in the urine. Infection, acute exercise, pregnancy and lactation, and stressful states (such as physical trauma) increase chromium losses and can lead to deficiency, especially if chromium intakes are already low.

## Conditions That Lead to Chromium Deficiency

In the 1960s, chromium was found to correct glucose intolerance and insulin resistance in deficient animals, two indicators that the body is failing to properly control blood-sugar levels and which are precursors of type 2 diabetes. However, reports of actual chromium deficiency in humans are rare. Three hospitalized patients who were fed intravenously (IV) showed signs of diabetes (including weight loss, neuropathy, and impaired glucose tolerance) until chromium was added to their feeding solution. The chromium added at doses of 150–250 mcg/day for up to two weeks, corrected their diabetes symptoms. Chromium is now routinely added to intravenous solutions.

## Need for Extra Chromium

There are reports of significant age-related decreases in the chromium concentrations of hair, sweat, and blood, which might suggest that older people are more vulnerable to chromium depletion than younger adults. One cannot be sure, however, as chromium status is difficult to determine. That's because blood, urine, and hair levels do not necessarily reflect body stores. Furthermore, no chromium-specific enzyme or other biochemical marker has been found to reliably assess a person's chromium status.

There is considerable interest in the possibility that supplemental chromium may help to treat impaired glucose tolerance and type 2 diabetes, but the research to date is inconclusive. No large, randomized, controlled clinical trials testing this hypothesis have been reported in the United States. Nevertheless, this is an active area of research.

## Issues and Controversies about Chromium

Chromium has long been of interest for its possible connection to various health conditions. Among the most active areas of chromium, research is its use in supplement form to treat diabetes, lower blood lipid levels, promote weight loss, and improve body composition.

### Type 2 Diabetes and Glucose Intolerance

In type 2 diabetes, the pancreas is usually producing enough insulin but, for unknown reasons, the body cannot use the insulin effectively.

The disease typically occurs, in part, because the cells comprising muscle and other tissues become resistant to insulin's action, especially among the obese. Insulin permits the entry of glucose into most cells, where this sugar is used for energy, stored in the liver and muscles (as glycogen), and converted to fat when present in excess. Insulin resistance leads to higher than normal levels of glucose in the blood (hyperglycemia).

Chromium deficiency impairs the body's ability to use glucose to meet its energy needs and raises insulin requirements. Therefore, it has been suggested that chromium supplements might help to control type 2 diabetes or the glucose and insulin responses in persons at high risk of developing the disease. A review of randomized controlled clinical trials evaluated this hypothesis. This meta-analysis assessed the effects of chromium supplements on three markers of diabetes in the blood: glucose, insulin, and glycated hemoglobin (which provides a measure of long-term glucose levels; also known as hemoglobin A1C). It summarized data from 15 trials on 618 participants, of which 425 were in good health or had impaired glucose tolerance and 193 had type 2 diabetes. Chromium supplementation had no effect on glucose or insulin concentrations in subjects without diabetes nor did it reduce these levels in subjects with diabetes, except in one study. However, that study, conducted in China (in which 155 subjects with diabetes were given either 200 or 1,000 mcg/day of chromium or a placebo) might simply show the benefits of supplementation in a chromium-deficient population.

Overall, the value of chromium supplements for diabetes is inconclusive and controversial. Randomized controlled clinical trials in well-defined, at-risk populations where dietary intakes are known are necessary to determine the effects of chromium on markers of diabetes. The American Diabetes Association (ADA) states that there is insufficient evidence to support the routine use of chromium to improve glycemic control in people with diabetes. It further notes that there is no clear scientific evidence that vitamin and mineral supplementation benefits people with diabetes who do not have underlying nutritional deficiencies.

### Lipid Metabolism

The effects of chromium supplementation on blood lipid levels in humans are also inconclusive. In some studies, 150–1,000 mcg/day has decreased total and low-density-lipoprotein (LDL or "bad") cholesterol and triglyceride levels and increased concentrations of apolipoprotein A (a component of high-density-lipoprotein cholesterol known as HDL or "good" cholesterol) in subjects with atherosclerosis or elevated cholesterol or among those taking a beta blocker drug. These findings are consistent with the results of earlier studies.

However, chromium supplements have shown no favorable effects on blood lipids in other studies. The mixed research findings may be due to difficulties in determining the chromium status of subjects at the start of the trials and the researchers' failure to control for dietary factors that influence blood lipid levels.

### Body Weight and Composition

Chromium supplements are sometimes claimed to reduce body fat and increase lean (muscle) mass. Yet a review of 24 studies that examined the effects of 200–1,000 mcg/day of chromium (in the form of chromium picolinate) on body mass or composition found no significant benefits. Another recent review of randomized, controlled clinical trials did find supplements of chromium picolinate to help with weight loss when compared with placebos, but the differences were small and of debatable clinical relevance. In several studies, chromium's effects on body weight and composition may be called into question because the researchers failed to adequately control for the participants' food intakes. Furthermore, most studies included only a small number of subjects and were of short duration.

## What Are the Health Risks of Too Much Chromium?

Few serious adverse effects have been linked to high intakes of chromium, so the Institute of Medicine (IOM) has not established a Tolerable Upper Intake Level (UL) for this mineral. A UL is the maximum daily intake of a nutrient that is unlikely to cause adverse health effects. It is one of the values (together with the RDA and AI) that comprise the DRIs for each nutrient.

### Chromium and Medication Interactions

Certain medications may interact with chromium, especially when taken on a regular basis (see table 28.2). Before taking dietary supplements, check with your doctor or another qualified healthcare provider, especially if you take prescription or over-the-counter (OTC) medications.

**Table 28.2.** Interactions between Chromium and Medications

| Medications | Nature of Interaction |
|---|---|
| Antacids | These medications alter stomach acidity and may impair chromium absorption or enhance excretion |
| Corticosteroids | |
| H2 blockers (such as cimetidine, famotidine, nizatidine, and ranitidine) | |
| Proton-pump inhibitors (such as omeprazole, lansoprazole, rabeprazole, pantoprazole, and esomeprazole) | |
| Beta blockers (such as atenolol or propranolol) | These medications may have their effects enhanced if taken together with chromium or they may increase chromium absorption |
| Corticosteroids | |
| Insulin | |
| Nicotinic acid | |
| Nonsteroidal anti-inflammatory drugs (NSAIDS) | |
| Prostaglandin inhibitors (such as ibuprofen, indomethacin, naproxen, piroxicam, and aspirin) | |

## Supplemental Sources of Chromium

Chromium is a widely used supplement. Estimated sales to consumers were $85 million in 2002, representing 5.6 percent of the total mineral-supplement market. Chromium is sold as a single-ingredient supplement as well as in combination formulas, particularly those marketed for weight loss and performance enhancement. Supplement doses typically range from 50–200 mcg.

The safety and efficacy of chromium supplements need more investigation. Please consult with a doctor or other trained healthcare professional before taking any dietary supplements.

Chromium supplements are available as chromium chloride, chromium nicotinate, chromium picolinate, high-chromium yeast, and chromium citrate. Chromium chloride, in particular, appears to have poor bioavailability. However, given the limited data on chromium absorption in humans, it is not clear which forms are best to take.

## Chromium and Healthful Diets

The federal government's *2015–2020 Dietary Guidelines for Americans* notes that "Nutritional needs should be met primarily from foods.

Foods in nutrient-dense forms contain essential vitamins and minerals and also dietary fiber and other naturally occurring substances that may have positive health effects. In some cases, fortified foods and dietary supplements may be useful in providing one or more nutrients that otherwise may be consumed in less-than-recommended amounts."

The *Dietary Guidelines for Americans* describes a healthy eating pattern as one that:

- Includes a variety of vegetables, fruits, whole grains, fat-free or low-fat milk, and milk products, and oils

- Whole grain products and certain fruits and vegetables like broccoli, potatoes, grape juice, and oranges are sources of chromium. Ready-to-eat bran cereals can also be a relatively good source of chromium.

- Includes a variety of protein foods, including seafood, lean meats and poultry, eggs, legumes (beans and peas), nuts, seeds, and soy products

- Lean beef, oysters, eggs, and turkey are sources of chromium.

- Limits saturated and *trans* fats, added sugars, and sodium

- Stays within your daily calorie needs

# Chapter 29

# *Folate (Folic Acid)*

Folic acid is the manufactured form of folate, a B vitamin. Folate is found naturally in certain fruits, vegetables, and nuts. Folic acid is found in vitamins and fortified foods.

Folic acid and folate help the body make healthy new red blood cells. Red blood cells carry oxygen to all the parts of your body. If your body does not make enough red blood cells, you can develop anemia. Anemia happens when your blood cannot carry enough oxygen to your body, which makes you pale, tired, or weak. Also, if you do not get enough folic acid, you could develop a type of anemia called folate-deficiency anemia.

## *Women Need Folic Acid*

Everyone needs folic acid to be healthy. But it is especially important for women:

- **Before and during pregnancy.** Folic acid protects unborn children against serious birth defects called neural tube defects. These birth defects happen in the first few weeks of pregnancy, often before a woman knows she is pregnant. Folic acid might also help prevent other types of birth defects and early pregnancy loss (miscarriage). Since about half of all pregnancies in the United States are unplanned, experts recommend all

This chapter includes text excerpted from "Folic Acid," Office on Women's Health (OWH), U.S. Department of Health and Human Services (HHS), March 1, 2018.

women get enough folic acid even if you are not trying to get pregnant.

- **To keep the blood healthy by helping red blood cells (RBC) form and grow.** Not getting enough folic acid can lead to a type of anemia called folate-deficiency anemia. Folate-deficiency anemia is more common in women of childbearing age than in men.

## Sources of Folic Acid

You can get folic acid in two ways.

1. **Through the foods, you eat.** Folate is found naturally in some foods, including spinach, nuts, and beans. Folic acid is found in fortified foods (called "enriched foods"), such as bread, pasta, and cereals. Look for the term "enriched" on the ingredients list to find out whether the food has added folic acid.

2. **As a vitamin.** Most multivitamins sold in the United States contain 400 micrograms, or 100 percent of the daily value, of folic acid. Check the label to make sure.

## How Much Folic Acid a Woman Needs

All women need 400 micrograms of folic acid every day. Women who can get pregnant should get 400–800 micrograms of folic acid from a vitamin or from food that has added folic acid, such as breakfast cereal. This is in addition to the folate you get naturally from food. Some women may need more folic acid each day. See the chart to find out how much folic acid you need.

**Table 29.1.** Folic Acid Requirement

| If You: | Amount of Folic Acid You May Need Daily |
|---|---|
| Could get pregnant or are pregnant | 400–800 micrograms. Your doctor may prescribe a prenatal vitamin with more. |
| Had a baby with a neural tube defect (such as spina bifida) and want to get pregnant again | 4,000 micrograms. Your doctor may prescribe this amount. Research shows taking this amount may lower the risk of having another baby with spina bifida. |
| Have a family member with spina bifida and could get pregnant | 4,000 micrograms. Your doctor may prescribe this amount. |

**Table 29.1.** Continued

| If You: | Amount of Folic Acid You May Need Daily |
|---|---|
| Have spina bifida and want to get pregnant | 4,000 micrograms. Your doctor may prescribe this amount. Women with spina bifida have a higher risk of having children with the condition. |
| Take medicines to treat epilepsy, type 2 diabetes, rheumatoid arthritis, or lupus | Talk to your doctor or nurse. Folic acid supplements can interact with these medicines. |
| Are on dialysis for kidney disease | Talk to your doctor or nurse |
| Have a health condition, such as inflammatory bowel disease (IBD) or celiac disease, that affects how your body absorbs folic acid | Talk to your doctor or nurse |

## Some Women Are at Risk for Not Getting Enough Folic Acid

Certain groups of women do not get enough folic acid each day:

- Women who can get pregnant need more folic acid (400–800 micrograms)

- Nearly one in three African-American women does not get enough folic acid each day.

- Spanish-speaking Mexican-American women often do not get enough folic acid. However, Mexican-Americans who speak English usually gets enough folic acid.

Not getting enough folic acid can cause health problems, including folate-deficiency anemia, and problems during pregnancy for you and your unborn baby.

## Risks of Not Getting Enough Folic Acid during Pregnancy

If you do not get enough folic acid before and during pregnancy, your baby is at higher risk for neural tube defects. Neural tube defects are serious birth defects that affect the spine, spinal cord, or brain and may cause death. These include:

- **Spina bifida.** This condition happens when an unborn baby's spinal column does not fully close during development in the womb, leaving the spinal cord exposed. As a result, the nerves that control the legs and other organs do not work. Children with spina bifida often have lifelong disabilities. They may also need many surgeries.

- **Anencephaly.** This means that most or all of the brain and skull does not develop in the womb. Almost all babies with this condition die before or soon after birth.

## Need to Take Folic Acid Every Day Even If You Are Not Planning to Get Pregnant

All women who can get pregnant need to take 400–800 micrograms of folic acid every day, even if you're not planning to get pregnant. There are several reasons why:

- Your birth control may not work or you may not use birth control correctly every time you have sex. In a survey by the Centers for Disease Control and Prevention (CDC), almost 40 percent of women with unplanned pregnancies were using birth control.

- Birth defects of the brain and spine can happen in the first few weeks of pregnancy, often before you know you are pregnant. By the time you find out you are pregnant, it might be too late to prevent the birth defects.

- You need to take folic acid every day because it is a water-soluble B-vitamin. Water soluble means that it does not stay in the body for a long time. Your body metabolizes (uses) folic acid quickly, so your body needs folic acid each day to work properly.

## Foods That Contain Folate

Folate is found naturally in some foods. Foods that are naturally high in folate include:

- Spinach and other dark green, leafy vegetables
- Oranges and orange juice
- Nuts
- Beans
- Poultry (chicken, turkey, etc.) and meat
- Whole grains

## Foods That Contain Folic Acid

Folic acid is added to foods that are refined or processed (not whole grain):

- Breakfast cereals (some have 100% of the recommended daily value—or 400 micrograms—of folic acid in each serving.)
- Bread and pasta
- Flours
- Cornmeal
- White rice

Since 1998, the U.S. Food and Drug Administration (FDA) has required food manufacturers to add folic acid to processed bread, cereals, flours, cornmeal, pasta, rice, and other grains. For other foods, check the Nutrition Facts label on the package to see if it has folic acid. The label will also tell you how much folic acid is in each serving. Sometimes, the label will say "folate" instead of folic acid.

## Making Sure That You Get Enough Folic Acid

You can get enough folic acid from food alone. Many breakfast cereals have 100 percent of your recommended daily value (400 micrograms) of folic acid. If you are at risk for not getting enough folic acid, your doctor or nurse may recommend that you take a vitamin with folic acid every day. Most U.S. multivitamins have at least 400 micrograms of folic acid. Check the label on the bottle to be sure. You can also take a pill that contains only folic acid.

If swallowing pills is hard for you, try a chewable or liquid product with a folic acid.

## Things to Look for When Buying Vitamins with Folic Acid

Look for the United States Pharmacopeia (USP) or the National Sanitation Foundation (NSF) on the label when choosing vitamins. These "seals of approval" mean the pills are made properly and have the amounts of vitamins it says on the label. Also, make sure the pills have not expired. If the bottle has no expiration date, do not buy it.

Ask your pharmacist for help with selecting a vitamin or folic acid-only pill. If you are pregnant and already take a daily prenatal vitamin, you probably get all the folic acid you need. Check the label to be sure.

231

## Vitamin Label

- Check the "Supplement Facts" label to be sure you are getting 400–800 micrograms (mcg) of folic acid.

| Supplement Facts | | |
|---|---|---|
| Serving Size: 1 tablet | | |
| **Amount Per Serving** | **% Daily Value** | |
| Vitamin A | 5000IU | 100 |
| Vitamin C | 60mg | 100 |
| Vitamin D | 400IU | 100 |
| Vitamin E | 30IU | 100 |
| Thiamin | 1.5mg | 100 |
| Riboflavin | 1.7mg | 100 |
| Niacin | 20mg | 100 |
| Vitamin B6 | 2mg | 100 |
| Folic Acid | 400mcg | 100 |
| Vitamin B12 | 6mcg | 100 |
| Biotin | 30mg | 10 |
| Pantothenic Acid | 10mg | 100 |
| Calcium | 162mg | 16 |
| Iron | 18mg | 100 |
| Iodine | 150mcg | 100 |
| Magnesium | 100mg | 25 |
| Zinc | 15mg | 100 |
| Selenium | 20mcg | 100 |
| Copper | 2mg | 100 |
| Manganese | 3.5mg | 175 |
| Chromium | 65mcg | 54 |
| Molybdenum | 150mcg | 200 |
| Chloride | 72mg | 2 |
| Potassium` | 80mg | 2 |

Find **folic acid:** Choose a vitamin that says "400mcg" or "100%" next to folic acid

**Figure 29.1.** *Folic Acid in Supplement Facts Label*

## Food and Folic Acid

Many people get enough folic acid from food alone. Some foods have high amounts of folic acid. For example, many breakfast cereals have 100 percent of the recommended daily value (400 micrograms) of folic acid in each serving. Check the label to be sure.

Some women, especially women who could get pregnant, may not get enough folic acid from food. African-American women and Mexican Americans are also at higher risk for not getting enough folic acid each day. Talk to your doctor or nurse about whether you should take a vitamin to get the 400 micrograms of folic acid you need each day.

## Folate-Deficiency Anemia

Folate-deficiency anemia is a type of anemia that happens when you do not get enough folate. Folate-deficiency anemia is most common during pregnancy. Other causes of folate-deficiency anemia include alcoholism and certain medicines to treat seizures, anxiety, or arthritis.

The symptoms of folate-deficiency anemia include:

- Fatigue

- A headache

- Pale skin

- Sore mouth and tongue

If you have folate-deficiency anemia, your doctor may recommend taking folic acid vitamins and eating more foods with folate.

## Getting Too Much Folic Acid

You can get too much folic acid, but only from manufactured products such as multivitamins and fortified foods, such as breakfast cereals. You can't get too much from foods that naturally contain folate. You should not get more than 1,000 micrograms of folic acid a day unless your doctor prescribes a higher amount. Too much folic acid can hide signs that you lack vitamin $B_{12}$, which can cause nerve damage.

## Need for Folic Acid after Menopause

Yes. Women who have gone through menopause still need 400 micrograms of folic acid every day for good health. Talk to your doctor or nurse about how much folic acid you need.

## Folic Acid Pills and Insurance Coverage

Under the Affordable Care Act (ACA) (the healthcare law), all health insurance marketplace plans and most other insurance plans cover folic acid pills for women who could get pregnant at no cost to you. Check with your insurance provider to find out what's included in your plan.

233

# Chapter 30

# *Magnesium*

## What Is Magnesium and What Does It Do?

Magnesium is a nutrient that the body needs to stay healthy. Magnesium is important for many processes in the body, including regulating muscle and nerve function, blood sugar levels, and blood pressure and making protein, bone, and deoxyribonucleic acid (DNA).

## How Much Magnesium Do I Need?

The amount of magnesium you need depends on your age and sex. Average daily recommended amounts are listed below in milligrams (mg):

**Table 30.1.** Magnesium Intake: Recommended Amount

| Life Stage | Recommended Amount |
|---|---|
| Birth to 6 months | 30 mg |
| Infants 7–12 months | 75 mg |
| Children 1–3 years | 80 mg |
| Children 4–8 years | 130 mg |
| Children 9–13 years | 240 mg |
| Teen boys 14–18 years | 410 mg |

This chapter includes text excerpted from "Magnesium," Office of Dietary Supplements (ODS), National Institutes of Health (NIH), February 17, 2016.

**Table 30.1.** Continued

| Life Stage | Recommended Amount |
|---|---|
| Teen girls 14–18 years | 360 mg |
| Men | 400–420 mg |
| Women | 310–320 mg |
| Pregnant teens | 400 mg |
| Pregnant women | 350–360 mg |
| Breastfeeding teens | 360 mg |
| Breastfeeding women | 310–320 mg |

## What Foods Provide Magnesium?

Magnesium is found naturally in many foods and is added to some fortified foods. You can get recommended amounts of magnesium by eating a variety of foods, including the following:

- Legumes, nuts, seeds, whole grains, and green leafy vegetables (such as spinach)

- Fortified breakfast cereals, and other fortified foods

- Milk, yogurt, and some other milk products

## What Kinds of Magnesium Dietary Supplements Are Available?

Magnesium is available in multivitamin-mineral (MVM) supplements and other dietary supplements. Forms of magnesium in dietary supplements that are more easily absorbed by the body are magnesium aspartate, magnesium citrate, magnesium lactate, and magnesium chloride.

Magnesium is also included in some laxatives and some products for treating heartburn and indigestion.

## Am I Getting Enough Magnesium?

The diets of most people in the United States provide less than the recommended amounts of magnesium. Men older than 70 and teenage girls are most likely to have low intakes of magnesium. When the number of magnesium people gets from food and dietary supplements are combined, however, total intakes of magnesium are generally above recommended amounts.

## What Happens If I Don't Get Enough Magnesium?

In the short term, getting too little magnesium does not produce obvious symptoms. When healthy people have low intakes, the kidneys help retain magnesium by limiting the amount lost in urine. Low magnesium intakes for a long period of time, however, can lead to magnesium deficiency. In addition, some medical conditions and medications interfere with the body's ability to absorb magnesium or increase the amount of magnesium that the body excretes, which can also lead to magnesium deficiency. Symptoms of magnesium deficiency include loss of appetite, nausea, vomiting, fatigue, and weakness. Extreme magnesium deficiency can cause numbness, tingling, muscle cramps, seizures, personality changes, and an abnormal heart rhythm.

The following groups of people are more likely than others to get too little magnesium:

- People with gastrointestinal diseases (such as Crohn's disease and celiac disease)
- People with type 2 diabetes
- People with long-term alcoholism
- Older people

## What Are Some Effects of Magnesium on Health?

Scientists are studying magnesium to understand how it affects health. Here are some examples of what this research has shown.

### High Blood Pressure and Heart Disease

High blood pressure is a major risk factor for heart disease and stroke. Magnesium supplements might decrease blood pressure, but only by a small amount. Some studies show that people who have more magnesium in their diets have a lower risk of some types of heart disease and stroke. But in many of these studies, it's hard to know how much of the effect was due to magnesium as opposed to other nutrients.

### Type 2 Diabetes

People with higher amounts of magnesium in their diets tend to have a lower risk of developing type 2 diabetes. Magnesium helps the body break down sugars and might help reduce the risk of insulin resistance (a condition that leads to diabetes). Scientists are studying whether magnesium supplements might help people who already have type 2 diabetes control their disease. More research is needed to better understand whether magnesium can help treat diabetes.

### Osteoporosis

Magnesium is important for healthy bones. People with higher intakes of magnesium have a higher bone mineral density, which is important in reducing the risk of bone fractures and osteoporosis. Getting more magnesium from foods or dietary supplements might help older women improve their bone mineral density. More research is needed to better understand whether magnesium supplements can help reduce the risk of osteoporosis or treat this condition.

### Migraine Headaches

People who have migraine headaches sometimes have low levels of magnesium in their blood and other tissues. Several small studies found that magnesium supplements can modestly reduce the frequency of migraines. However, people should only take magnesium for this purpose under the care of a healthcare provider. More research is needed to determine whether magnesium supplements can help reduce the risk of migraines or ease migraine symptoms.

## Can Magnesium Be Harmful?

Magnesium that is naturally present in food is not harmful and does not need to be limited. In healthy people, the kidneys can get rid of any excess in the urine. But magnesium in dietary supplements and medications should not be consumed in amounts above the upper limit unless recommended by a healthcare provider.

The upper limits for magnesium from dietary supplements and/or medications are listed below. For many age groups, the upper limit appears to be lower than the recommended amount. This occurs because the recommended amounts include magnesium from **all** sources-food, dietary supplements, and medications. The upper limits include magnesium from **only** dietary supplements and medications; they do **not** include magnesium found naturally in food.

**Table 30.2.** Magnesium Intake: Upper Limit

| Ages | Upper Limit for Magnesium in Dietary Supplements and Medications |
|---|---|
| Birth to 12 months | Not established |
| Children 1–3 years | 65 mg |
| Children 4–8 years | 110 mg |
| Children 9–18 years | 350 mg |
| Adults | 350 mg |

High intakes of magnesium from dietary supplements and medications can cause diarrhea, nausea, and abdominal cramping. Extremely high intakes of magnesium can lead to irregular heartbeat and cardiac arrest.

## Are There Any Interactions with Magnesium That I Should Know About?

Yes. Magnesium supplements can interact or interfere with some medicines. Here are several examples:

- **Bisphosphonates**, used to treat osteoporosis, are not well absorbed when taken too soon before or after taking dietary supplements or medications with high amounts of magnesium.

- **Antibiotics** might not be absorbed if taken too soon before or after taking a dietary supplement that contains magnesium.

- **Diuretics** can either increase or decrease the loss of magnesium through urine, depending on the type of diuretic.

- **Prescription drugs** used to ease symptoms of acid reflux or treat peptic ulcers can cause low blood levels of magnesium when taken over a long period of time

- Very high doses of **zinc supplements** can interfere with the body's ability to absorb and regulate magnesium.

Tell your doctor, pharmacist, and other healthcare providers about any dietary supplements and prescription or over-the-counter (OTC) medicines you take. They can tell you if the dietary supplements might interact with your medicines or if the medicines might interfere with how your body absorbs, uses, or breaks down nutrients.

## *Magnesium and Healthful Eating*

People should get most of their nutrients from food, advises the federal government's *Dietary Guidelines for Americans*. Foods contain vitamins, minerals, dietary fiber, and other substances that benefit health. In some cases, fortified foods and dietary supplements may provide nutrients that otherwise may be consumed in less-than-recommended amounts.

# Chapter 31

# *Melatonin Supplements*

Melatonin is a natural hormone that plays a role in sleep. Melatonin production and release in the brain is related to the time of day, rising in the evening and falling in the morning. Light at night blocks its production. Melatonin dietary supplements have been studied for sleep disorders, such as jet lag, disruptions of the body's internal "clock," insomnia, and problems with sleep among people who work night shifts. It has also been studied for dementia symptoms.

## *What the Science Says about the Effectiveness of Melatonin*

### *For Sleep Disorders*

Studies suggest that melatonin may help with certain sleep disorders, such as jet lag, delayed sleep phase disorder (DSPD) (a disruption of the body's biological clock in which a person's sleep-wake timing cycle is delayed by 3–6 hours), sleep problems related to shift work, and some sleep disorders in children. It's also been shown to be helpful for a sleep disorder that causes changes in blind people's sleep and wake times. Study results are mixed on whether melatonin is effective for insomnia in adults, but some studies suggest it may slightly reduce the time it takes to fall asleep.

---

This chapter includes text excerpted from "Melatonin: In Depth," National Center for Complementary and Integrative Health (NCCIH), September 24, 2017.

241

### Jet Lag

Jet lag is caused by rapid travel across several time zones; its symptoms include disturbed sleep, daytime fatigue, indigestion, and a general feeling of discomfort.

- In a research review, results from six small studies and two large studies suggested that melatonin may ease jet lag.

- In a clinical practice guideline, the American Academy of Sleep Medicine (AASM) supported using melatonin to reduce jet lag symptoms and improve sleep after traveling across more than one time zone.

### Delayed Sleep Phase Disorder

Adults and teens with this sleep disorder have trouble falling asleep before 2 a.m. and have trouble waking up in the morning.

- In a review of the literature, researchers suggested that a combination of melatonin supplements, a behavioral approach to delay sleep and wake times until the desired sleep time is achieved, and reduced evening light may even out sleep cycles in people with this sleep disorder.

- In a clinical practice guideline, the AASM recommended timed melatonin supplementation for this sleep disorder.

### Shift Work Disorder

Shift work refers to job-related duties conducted outside of morning to evening working hours. About 2 million Americans who work afternoon to nighttime or nighttime to early morning hours are affected by shift work disorder.

- The clinical practice guideline and a review of the evidence concluded that melatonin may improve daytime sleep quality and duration, but not nighttime alertness, in people with shift work disorder.

- The AASM recommended taking melatonin prior to daytime sleep for night shift workers with shift work disorder to enhance daytime sleep.

### Insomnia

Insomnia is a general term for a group of problems characterized by an inability to fall asleep and stay asleep.

- **In adults.** A 2013 analysis of 19 studies of people with primary sleep disorders found that melatonin slightly improved time to fall asleep, total sleep time, and overall sleep quality. In a study of people with insomnia, aged 55 years or older, researchers found that prolonged-release melatonin significantly improved quality of sleep and morning alertness.

- **In children.** There's limited evidence from rigorous studies of melatonin for sleep disorders among young people. A 2011 literature review suggested a benefit with minimal side effects in healthy children as well as youth with attention deficit hyperactivity disorder (ADHD), autism, and several other populations. There's insufficient information to make conclusions about the safety and effectiveness of long-term melatonin use.

### *For Other Conditions*

While there hasn't been enough research to support melatonin's use for other conditions:

- Researchers are investigating whether adding melatonin to standard **cancer care** can improve response rates, survival time, and quality of life.

- Results from a few small studies in people (clinical trials) have led investigators to propose additional research on whether melatonin may help to improve mild cognitive impairment in patients with Alzheimer disease (AD) and prevent cell damage associated with amyotrophic lateral sclerosis (ALS), also known as Lou Gehrig disease. An analysis of the research suggested that adding sustained-release melatonin (but not fast-release melatonin) to high blood pressure management reduced elevated nighttime blood pressure.

## What the Science Says about Safety and Side Effects of Melatonin

Melatonin appears to be safe when used short term, but the lack of long-term studies means we don't know if it's safe for extended use.

- In a study, researchers noted that melatonin supplements may worsen mood in people with dementia.

243

- In 2011, the U.S. Food and Drug Administration (FDA) issued a warning to a company that makes and sells "relaxation brownies," stating that the melatonin in them hasn't been deemed a safe food additive.

- Side effects of melatonin are uncommon but can include drowsiness, headache, dizziness, or nausea. There have been no reports of significant side effects of melatonin in children.

# Chapter 32

# *Omega-3 Fatty Acid Supplements*

## *Chapter Contents*

# Section 32.1

# *Omega-3 Fatty Acids: An Overview*

This section includes text excerpted from "Omega-3
Supplements: In Depth," National Center for Complementary
and Integrative Health (NCCIH), August 2015.

Omega-3 fatty acids (omega-3s) are a group of polyunsaturated fatty acids that are important for a number of functions in the body. Some types of omega-3s are found in foods such as fatty fish and shellfish. Another type is found in some vegetable oils. Omega-3s are also available as dietary supplements. This section provides basic information about omega-3s—with a focus on dietary supplements, summarizes scientific research on effectiveness and safety.

- There has been a substantial amount of research on supplements of omega-3s, particularly those found in seafood and fish oil, and heart disease. The findings of individual studies have been inconsistent. In 2012, two combined analyses of the results of these studies did not find convincing evidence these omega-3s protect against heart disease.

- There is some evidence that omega-3s found in seafood and fish oil may be modestly helpful in relieving symptoms in rheumatoid arthritis (RA). For most other conditions for which omega-3s have been studied, definitive conclusions cannot yet be reached, or studies have not shown omega-3s to be beneficial.

- Omega-3 supplements may interact with drugs that affect blood clotting.

- It is uncertain whether people with fish or shellfish allergies can safely consume fish oil supplements.

- Fish liver oils (which are not the same as fish oils) contain vitamins A and D as well as omega-3 fatty acids; these vitamins can be toxic in high doses.

- Tell all your healthcare providers about any complementary health approaches you use. Give them a full picture of what you do to manage your health. This will help ensure coordinated and safe care.

## *About Omega-3 Fatty Acids*

The three principal omega-3 fatty acids are alpha-linolenic acid (ALA), eicosapentaenoic acid (EPA), and docosahexaenoic acid (DHA). The main sources of ALA in the U.S. diet are vegetable oils, particularly canola and soybean oils; flaxseed oil is richer in ALA than soybean and canola oils but is not commonly consumed. ALA can be converted, usually in small amounts, into EPA and DHA in the body. EPA and DHA are found in seafood, including fatty fish (e.g., salmon, tuna, and trout) and shellfish (e.g., crab, mussels, and oysters).

Commonly used dietary supplements that contain omega-3s include fish oil (which provides EPA and DHA) and flaxseed oil (which provides ALA). Algae oils are a vegetarian source of DHA.

Omega-3 fatty acids are important for a number of bodily functions, including muscle activity, blood clotting, digestion, fertility, and cell division and growth. DHA is important for brain development and function. ALA is an "essential" fatty acid, meaning that people must obtain it from food or supplements because the human body cannot manufacture it.

### *Safety*

- Omega-3 fatty acid supplements usually do not have negative side effects. When side effects do occur, they typically consist of minor gastrointestinal symptoms, such as belching, indigestion, or diarrhea.

- It is uncertain whether people with fish or shellfish allergies can safely consume fish oil supplements.

- Omega-3 supplements may extend bleeding time (the time it takes for a cut to stop bleeding). People who take drugs that affect bleeding time, such as anticoagulants ("blood thinners") or nonsteroidal anti-inflammatory drugs (NSAIDs), should discuss the use of omega-3 fatty acid supplements with a healthcare provider.

- Fish liver oils, such as cod liver oil, are not the same as fish oil. Fish liver oils contain vitamins A and D as well as omega-3 fatty acids. Both of these vitamins can be toxic in large doses. The amounts of vitamins in fish liver oil supplements vary from one product to another.

- There is conflicting evidence about whether omega-3 fatty acids found in seafood and fish oil might increase the risk of prostate cancer. Additional research on the association of omega-3 consumption and prostate cancer risk is underway.

## Use of Omega-3 Supplements in the United States

According to the 2012 National Health Interview Survey (NHIS), which included a comprehensive survey on the use of complementary health approaches in the United States, fish oil supplements are the nonvitamin/nonmineral natural product most commonly taken by both adults and children. The survey findings indicated that about 7.8 percent of adults (18.8 million) and 1.1 percent of children age 4–17 (664,000) had taken a fish oil supplement in the previous 30 days.

### *About Scientific Evidence on Complementary Health Approaches*

Scientific evidence on complementary health approaches includes results from laboratory research as well as clinical trials (studies in people). It provides information on whether an approach is helpful and safe. Scientific journals publish study results, as well as review articles that evaluate the evidence as it accumulates.

## What the Science Says

Moderate evidence has emerged about the health benefits of eating seafood. The health benefits of omega-3 dietary supplements are unclear.

### *Cardiovascular Disease*

Evidence suggests that seafood rich in omega-3 fatty acids should be included in a heart-healthy diet. However, omega-3s in supplement form has not been shown to protect against heart disease.

- Epidemiological studies done more than 30 years ago noted relatively low death rates due to cardiovascular disease in Eskimo populations with high seafood consumption. Since then, much research has been done on seafood and heart disease. The results provide moderate evidence that people who eat seafood at least once a week are less likely to die of heart disease than those who rarely or never eat seafood.

- The federal government's *Dietary Guidelines for Americans* includes a new recommendation that adults eat 8 or more ounces of a variety of seafood (fish or shellfish) per week because it provides a range of nutrients, including omega-3 fatty acids. (Smaller amounts are recommended for young children.)

- Many studies have evaluated the effects of supplements rich in EPA, and DHA, such as fish oil, on heart disease risk.

- In these studies, researchers compared the number of cardiovascular events (such as heart attacks or strokes) or the number of deaths in people who were given the supplements with those in people who were given inactive substances (placebos) or standard care. Most of these studies involved people who already had evidence of heart disease. A smaller number of studies included people with no history of heart disease.

- The results of individual studies were inconsistent; some indicated that the supplements were protective, but others did not.

- In 2012, two groups of scientists conducted meta-analyses of these studies; one group analyzed only studies in people with a history of heart disease, and the other group analyzed studies in people both with and without a history of heart disease. Neither meta-analysis found convincing evidence of a protective effect.

- In 2014, researchers examined the results of the newest high-quality studies of omega-3s. Of nine studies that examined the effects of omega-3s on outcomes related to heart diseases, such as heart attacks or abnormal heart rhythms, only one found evidence of a beneficial effect.

- There are several reasons why supplements that contain eicosapentaenoic acid and docosahexaenoic acid may not help to prevent heart disease even though a diet rich in seafood may. Eating seafood a few times a week might provide enough of these omega-3s to protect the heart; more may not be better. Some of the benefits of seafood may result from people eating it in place of less healthful foods. There is also evidence that people who eat seafood have generally healthier lifestyles, and these other lifestyle characteristics may be responsible for the lower incidence of cardiovascular disease.

## Rheumatoid Arthritis (RA)

A 2012 systematic review concluded that the types of omega-3s found in seafood and fish oil may be modestly helpful in relieving symptoms of rheumatoid arthritis. In the studies included in the review, many of the participants reported that when they were taking fish oil they had briefer morning stiffness, less joint swelling and pain, and less need for anti-inflammatory drugs to control their symptoms.

## Infant Development

The nutritional value of seafood is particularly important during early development. The *Dietary Guidelines* recommend that women who are pregnant or breastfeeding consume at least 8 ounces but no more than 12 ounces of seafood each week and not eat certain types of seafood that are high in mercury—a toxin that can harm the nervous system of a fetus or young child.

## Diseases of the Brain and the Eye

DHA plays important roles in the functioning of the brain and the eye. Research is being conducted on DHA and other omega-3 fatty acids and diseases of the brain and eye, but there is not enough evidence to draw conclusions about the effectiveness of omega-3s for these conditions.

Research is looking at:

- Diseases of the eye, such as age-related macular degeneration (AMD); an eye disease that can cause vision loss in older people and dry eye syndrome (DES). Studies have shown that people who eat diets rich in seafood are less likely to develop the advanced stage of AMD. However, a large National Institutes of Health (NIH)—sponsored study, called Age-Related Eye Disease Study 2 (AREDS2), indicated that supplements containing EPA and DHA did not slow the progression of AMD in people who were at high risk of developing the advanced stage of this disease.

- Diseases of the brain or nervous system, such as cognitive decline (CD), and multiple sclerosis (MS). Study results published in 2015 indicated that taking EPA and DHA supplements did not slow cognitive decline in older adults. The people who were studied were participants in AREDS2, and therefore, all of them had the eye disease AMD.

- Mental and behavioral health problems, such as depression, attention deficit hyperactivity disorder (ADHD), autism, bipolar disorder, borderline personality disorder, and schizophrenia

### Other Conditions

Omega-3 supplements (primarily fish oil supplements) also have been studied for preventing or treating a variety of other conditions such as allergies, asthma, cachexia (severe weight loss) associated with advanced cancer, Crohn's disease, cystic fibrosis, diabetes, kidney disease, lupus, menstrual cramps, obesity, osteoporosis, and ulcerative colitis (UC), as well as organ transplantation outcomes (e.g., decreasing the likelihood of rejection). No conclusions can be drawn about whether omega-3s are helpful for these conditions based on currently available evidence.

## Plan to Use Omega-3 Supplements

If you are considering omega-3 supplements:

- Do not use omega-3 supplements to replace conventional care or to postpone seeing a healthcare provider about a health problem.

- Consult your healthcare provider before using omega-3 supplements. If you are pregnant, trying to become pregnant, or breastfeeding; if you take medicine that affects blood clotting; if you are allergic to fish or shellfish; or if you are considering giving a child an omega-3 supplement, it is especially important to consult your (or your child's) healthcare provider.

- Look for published research studies on omega-3 supplements for the health condition that interests you. Information on evidence-based studies is available from the National Center for Complementary and Integrative Health (NCCIH).

- Tell all your healthcare providers about any complementary health approaches you use. Give them a full picture of what you do to manage your health. This will help ensure coordinated and safe care.

## Section 32.2

# *Seven Things to Know about Omega-3 Fatty Acids*

This section includes text excerpted from "7 Things to Know about
Omega-3 Fatty Acids," National Center for Complementary and
Integrative Health (NCCIH), September 24, 2015.

Omega-3 fatty acids are a group of polyunsaturated fatty acids that
are important for a number of functions in the body. The omega-3 fatty
acids eicosapentaenoic acid (EPA) and docosahexaenoic acid (DHA) are
found in seafood, such as fatty fish (e.g., salmon, tuna, and trout) and
shellfish (e.g., crab, mussels, and oysters). A different kind of omega-3,
called alpha-lipoic acid (ALA), is found in other foods, including some
vegetable oils (e.g., canola and soy). Omega-3s are also available as
dietary supplements; for example, fish oil supplements contain EPA
and DHA, and flaxseed oil supplements contain ALA. Moderate evidence has emerged about the health benefits of consuming seafood.
The health benefits of omega-3 dietary supplements are unclear.

## *What You Should Know about Omega-3 Fatty Acid*

There are seven things you should know about omega-3s:

1. **Results of studies on diets rich in seafood (fish and
   shellfish) and heart disease provide moderate evidence
   that people who eat seafood at least once a week are
   less likely to die of heart disease than those who rarely
   or never eat seafood.** The *Dietary Guidelines for Americans*
   includes a new recommendation that adults eat 8 or more
   ounces of a variety of seafood per week because it provides a
   range of nutrients, including omega-3 fatty acids. (Smaller
   amounts are recommended for young children, and there are
   special recommendations for pregnant or breastfeeding women.

2. **Evidence suggests that seafood rich in EPA and DHA
   should be included in a heart-healthy diet; however,
   supplements of EPA and DHA have not been shown**

**to protect against heart disease.** In 2012, two groups of scientists analyzed the research on the effects of EPA/DHA supplements on heart disease risk. One group analyzed only studies in people with a history of heart disease, and the other group analyzed studies in people both with and without a history of heart disease. Neither review found strong evidence of a protective effect of the supplements.

3. **A 2012 review of the scientific literature concluded that EPA and DHA, the types of omega-3s found in seafood, and fish oil, may be modestly helpful in relieving symptoms of rheumatoid arthritis (RA).** In the studies included in the review, many of the participants reported that when they were taking fish oil they had briefer morning stiffness, less joint swelling and pain, and less need for anti-inflammatory drugs to control their symptoms.

4. **The nutritional value of seafood is of particular importance during fetal growth and development, as well as in early infancy and childhood.** Women who are pregnant or breastfeed should consume 8–12 ounces of seafood per week from a variety of seafood types that are low in methylmercury as part of a healthy eating pattern and while staying within their calorie needs. Pregnant or breastfeeding women should limit the amount of white tuna (labeled as "albacore") to no more than 6 ounces per week. They should not eat tilefish, shark, swordfish, and king mackerel because they are high in methylmercury.

5. **There is ongoing research on omega-3 fatty acids and diseases of the brain and eye, but there is not enough evidence to draw conclusions about the effectiveness of omega-3s for these conditions.** DHA plays important roles in the functioning of the brain and the eye. Researchers are actively investigating the possible benefits of DHA and other omega-3 fatty acids in preventing or treating a variety of brain and eye-related conditions.

6. **There is conflicting evidence about whether a link might exist between the omega-3 fatty acids found in seafood and fish oil (EPA/DHA) and an increased risk of prostate cancer.** Additional research on the association of omega-3 consumption and prostate cancer risk is underway.

253

7. **The bottom line.** Including seafood in your diet is healthful. Whether omega-3 supplements are beneficial is uncertain. If you are considering omega-3 supplements, talk to your healthcare provider. It's especially important to consult your (or your child's) healthcare provider if you are pregnant or breastfeeding if you take medicine that affects blood clotting, if you are allergic to seafood, or if you are considering giving a child an omega-3 supplement.

# Chapter 33

# *Selenium*

Selenium is a nutrient that the body needs to stay healthy. Selenium is important for reproduction, thyroid gland function, deoxyribonucleic acid (DNA) production, and protecting the body from damage caused by free radicals and from infection.

## *How Much Selenium Do I Need?*

The amount of selenium that you need each day depends on your age. Average daily recommended amounts are listed below in micrograms (mcg).

**Table 33.1.** Selenium Intake: Recommended Amount

| Life Stage | Recommended Amount |
|---|---|
| Birth to 6 months | 15 mcg |
| Infants 7–12 months | 20 mcg |
| Children 1–3 years | 20 mcg |
| Children 4–8 years | 30 mcg |
| Children 9–13 years | 40 mcg |
| Teens 14–18 years | 55 mcg |
| Adults 19–50 years | 55 mcg |
| Adults 51–70 years | 55 mcg |

This chapter includes text excerpted from "Selenium," Office of Dietary Supplements (ODS), National Institutes of Health (NIH), February 17, 2016.

**Table 33.1.** Continued

| Life Stage | Recommended Amount |
|---|---|
| Adults 71 years and older | 55 mcg |
| Pregnant teens and women | 60 mcg |
| Breastfeeding teens and women | 70 mcg |

## Foods That Provide Selenium

Selenium is found naturally in many foods. The amount of selenium in plant foods depends on the amount of selenium in the soil where they were grown. The amount of selenium in animal products depends on the selenium content of the foods that the animals ate. You can get recommended amounts of selenium by eating a variety of foods, including the following:

- Seafood

- Meat, poultry, eggs, and dairy products

- Bread, cereals, and other grain products

## Selenium Dietary Supplements Available in the Market

Selenium is available in many multivitamin-mineral supplements and other dietary supplements. It can be present in several different forms, including selenomethionine and sodium selenite.

## Am I Getting Enough Selenium?

Most Americans get enough selenium from their diet because they eat food grown or raised in many different areas, including areas with soil that is rich in selenium. Certain groups of people are more likely than others to have trouble getting enough selenium:

- People undergoing kidney dialysis

- People living with human immunodeficiency virus (HIV)

- People who eat only local foods grown in soils that are low in selenium

## Health Risks of Selenium Deficiency

Selenium deficiency is very rare in the United States and Canada. Selenium deficiency can cause Keshan disease (a type of heart disease) and male infertility. It might also cause Kashin-Beck disease, a type of arthritis that produces pain, swelling, and loss of motion in your joints.

## Health Effects of Selenium

Scientists are studying selenium to understand how it affects health. Here are some examples of what the research has shown.

### Cancer

Studies suggest that people who consume lower amounts of selenium could have an increased risk of developing cancers of the colon and rectum, prostate, lung, bladder, skin, esophagus, and stomach. But whether selenium supplements reduce cancer risk is not clear. More research is needed to understand the effects of selenium from food and dietary supplements on cancer risk.

### Cardiovascular Disease

Scientists are studying whether selenium helps reduce the risk of cardiovascular disease. Some studies show that people with lower blood levels of selenium have a higher risk of heart disease, but other studies do not. More studies are needed to better understand how selenium in food and dietary supplements affects heart health.

### Cognitive Decline

Blood selenium levels decrease as people age, and scientists are studying whether low selenium levels contribute to a decline in brain function in the elderly. Some studies suggest that people with lower blood selenium levels are more likely to have a poorer mental function. But a study of elderly people in the United States found no link between selenium levels and memory. More research is needed to find out whether selenium dietary supplements might help reduce the risk of or treat cognitive decline in elderly people.

### Thyroid Disease

The thyroid gland has high amounts of selenium that play an important role in thyroid function. Studies suggest that people—especially women—who have low blood levels of selenium (and iodine) might develop problems with their thyroid. But whether selenium dietary supplements can help treat or reduce the risk of thyroid disease is not clear. More research is needed to understand the effects of selenium on thyroid disease.

## Can Selenium Be Harmful?

Yes, if you get too much. Brazil nuts, for example, contain very high amounts of selenium (68–91 mcg per nut) and can cause you to go over the upper limit if you eat too many. Getting too much selenium over time can cause the following:

- Garlic breath
- Nausea
- Diarrhea
- Skin Rashes
- Irritability
- Metallic taste in the mouth
- Brittle hair or nails
- Loss of hair or nails
- Discolored teeth
- Nervous system problems

Extremely high intakes of selenium can cause severe problems, including difficulty breathing, tremors, kidney failure, heart attacks, and heart failure.

The upper limits for selenium from foods and dietary supplements are listed below.

**Table 33.2.** Selenium Intake: Upper Limit

| Ages | Upper Limit |
|---|---|
| Birth to 6 months | 45 mcg |
| Infants 7–12 months | 60 mcg |
| Children 1–3 years | 90 mcg |
| Children 4–8 years | 150 mcg |
| Children 9–13 years | 280 mcg |
| Teens 14–18 years | 400 mcg |
| Adults | 400 mcg |

## Interactions of Medicines with Selenium

Some of the medications you take may interact with selenium. For example, cisplatin, a chemotherapy drug used to treat cancer, can lower selenium levels, but the effect this has on the body is not clear.

Tell your doctor, pharmacist, and other healthcare providers about any dietary supplements and prescription or over-the-counter (OTC) medicines you take. They can tell you if the dietary supplements might interact with your medicines or if the medicines might interfere with how your body absorbs, uses, or breaks down nutrients.

## Selenium and Healthful Eating

People should get most of their nutrients from food, advises the federal government's *Dietary Guidelines for Americans*. Foods contain vitamins, minerals, dietary fiber, and other substances that benefit health. In some cases, fortified foods and dietary supplements may provide nutrients that otherwise may be consumed in less-than-recommended amounts.

# Chapter 34

# *Bone and Joint Health Supplements*

## *Chapter Contents*

# Section 34.1

## *Calcium Supplements and Bone Health*

This section includes text excerpted from "Calcium,"
Office of Dietary Supplements (ODS), National
Institutes of Health (NIH), November 17, 2016.

Calcium is a mineral found in many foods. The body needs calcium to maintain strong bones and to carry out many important functions. Almost all calcium is stored in bones and teeth, where it supports their structure and hardness. The body also needs calcium for muscles to move and for nerves to carry messages between the brain and every body part. In addition, calcium is used to help blood vessels move blood throughout the body and to help release hormones and enzymes that affect almost every function in the human body.

### *How Much Calcium Do I Need?*

The amount of calcium you need each day depends on your age. Average daily recommended amounts are listed below in milligrams (mg):

**Table 34.1.** Calcium Intake: Recommended Amount

| Life Stage | Recommended Amount |
|---|---|
| Birth to 6 months | 200 mg |
| Infants 7–12 months | 260 mg |
| Children 1–3 years | 700 mg |
| Children 4–8 years | 1,000 mg |
| Children 9–13 years | 1,300 mg |
| Teens 14–18 years | 1,300 mg |
| Adults 19–50 years | 1,000 mg |
| Adult men 51–70 years | 1,000 mg |
| Adult women 51–70 years | 1,200 mg |
| Adults 71 years and older | 1,200 mg |

**Table 34.1.** Continued

| Life Stage | Recommended Amount |
|---|---|
| Pregnant and breastfeeding teens | 1,300 mg |
| Pregnant and breastfeeding adults | 1,000 mg |

## Foods That Provide Calcium

Calcium is found in many foods. You can get recommended amounts of calcium by eating a variety of foods, including the following:

- Milk, yogurt, and cheese are the main food sources of calcium for the majority of people in the United States.

- Kale, broccoli, and Chinese cabbage are fine vegetable sources of calcium.

- Fish with soft bones that you eat, such as canned sardines and salmon, are fine animal sources of calcium.

- Most grains (such as bread, pasta, and unfortified cereals), while not rich in calcium, add significant amounts of calcium to the diet because people eat them often or in large amounts.

- Calcium is added to some breakfast cereals, fruit juices, soy and rice beverages, and tofu. To find out whether these foods have calcium, check the product labels.

## Calcium Dietary Supplements

Calcium is found in many multivitamin-mineral supplements, though the amount varies by product. Dietary supplements that contain only calcium or calcium with other nutrients such as vitamin D are also available. Check the Supplement Facts label to determine the amount of calcium provided.

The two main forms of calcium dietary supplements are carbonate and citrate. Calcium carbonate is inexpensive but is absorbed best when taken with food. Some over-the-counter (OTC) antacid products, such as Tums® and Rolaids®, contain calcium carbonate. Each pill or chew provides 200–400 mg of calcium. Calcium citrate, a more expensive form of the supplement, is absorbed well on an empty or a full stomach. In addition, people with low levels of stomach acid (a condition more common in people older than 50) absorb calcium citrate more easily than calcium carbonate. Other forms of calcium in supplements and fortified foods include gluconate, lactate, and phosphate.

Calcium absorption is best when a person consumes no more than 500 mg at one time. So a person who takes 1,000 mg/day of calcium from supplements, for example, should split the dose rather than take it all at once.

Calcium supplements may cause gas, bloating, and constipation in some people. If any of these symptoms occur, try spreading out the calcium dose throughout the day, taking the supplement with meals, or changing the supplement brand or calcium form you take.

## Take Adequate Calcium

Many people don't get recommended amounts of calcium from the foods they eat, including:

- Boys aged 9–13 years

- Girls aged 9–18 years

- Women older than 50 years

- Men older than 70 years

When total intakes from both food and supplements are considered, many people—particularly adolescent girls—still fall short of getting enough calcium, while some older women likely get more than the upper limit.

Certain groups of people are more likely than others to have trouble getting enough calcium:

- Postmenopausal (PMS) women because they experience greater bone loss and do not absorb calcium as well. Sufficient calcium intake from food, and supplements if needed can slow the rate of bone loss.

- Women of childbearing age whose menstrual periods stop (amenorrhea) because they exercise heavily, eat too little, or both. They need sufficient calcium to cope with the resulting decreased calcium absorption, increased calcium losses in the urine, and slowdown in the formation of new bone.

- People with lactose intolerance cannot digest this natural sugar found in milk and experience symptoms like bloating, gas, and diarrhea when they drink more than small amounts at a time. They usually can eat other calcium-rich dairy products that are low in lactose, such as yogurt, and many cheeses, and drink lactose-reduced or lactose-free milk.

- Vegans (vegetarians who eat no animal products) and ovo-vegetarians (vegetarians who eat eggs but no dairy products), because they avoid the dairy products that are a major source of calcium in other people's diets.

Many factors can affect the amount of calcium absorbed from the digestive tract, including:

- Age. Efficiency of calcium absorption decreases as people age. Recommended calcium intakes are higher for people over age 70.

- Vitamin D intake. This vitamin, present in some foods and produced in the body when skin is exposed to sunlight, increases calcium absorption.

- Other components in food. Both oxalic acid (in some vegetables and beans) and phytic acid (in whole grains) can reduce calcium absorption. People who eat a variety of foods don't have to consider these factors. They are accounted for in the calcium recommended intakes, which take absorption into account.

Many factors can also affect how much calcium the body eliminates in urine, feces, and sweat. These include consumption of alcohol and caffeine-containing beverages as well as intake of other nutrients (protein, sodium, potassium, and phosphorus). In most people, these factors have little effect on calcium status.

## Risks of Calcium Deficiency

Insufficient intakes of calcium do not produce obvious symptoms in the short term because the body maintains calcium levels in the blood by taking it from bone. Over the long term, intakes of calcium below recommended levels have health consequences, such as causing low bone mass (osteopenia) and increasing the risks of osteoporosis and bone fractures.

Symptoms of serious calcium deficiency include numbness, and tingling in the fingers, convulsions, and abnormal heart rhythms that can lead to death if not corrected. These symptoms occur almost always in people with serious health problems or who are undergoing certain medical treatments.

## Health Effects of Calcium

Scientists are studying calcium to understand how it affects health. Here are several examples of what the research has shown:

## Bone Health and Osteoporosis

Bones need plenty of calcium and vitamin D throughout childhood and adolescence to reach their peak strength and calcium content by about age 30. After that, bones slowly lose calcium, but people can help reduce these losses by getting recommended amounts of calcium throughout adulthood and by having a healthy, active lifestyle that includes weight-bearing physical activity (such as walking and running).

Osteoporosis is a disease of the bones in older adults (especially women) in which the bones become porous, fragile, and more prone to fracture. Osteoporosis is a serious public health problem for more than 10 million adults over the age of 50 in the United States. Adequate calcium and vitamin D intakes, as well as regular exercise, are essential to keep bones healthy throughout life.

Taking calcium and vitamin D supplements reduce the risk of breaking a bone and the risk of falling in frail, elderly adults who live in nursing homes and similar facilities. But it's not clear if the supplements help prevent bone fractures and falls in older people who live at home.

## Cancer

Studies have examined whether calcium supplements or diets high in calcium might lower the risks of developing cancer of the colon or rectum or increase the risk of prostate cancer. The research to date provides no clear answers. Given that cancer develops over many years, longer-term studies are needed.

## Cardiovascular Disease

Some studies show that getting enough calcium might decrease the risk of heart disease and stroke. Other studies find that high amounts of calcium, particularly from supplements, might increase the risk of heart disease. But when all the studies are considered together, scientists have concluded that as long as intakes are not above the upper limit, calcium from food or supplements will not increase or decrease the risk of having a heart attack or stroke.

## High Blood Pressure

Some studies have found that getting recommended intakes of calcium can reduce the risk of developing high blood pressure (hypertension). One large study, in particular, found that eating a diet high in fat-free and low-fat dairy products, vegetables, and fruits lowered blood pressure.

### Preeclampsia

Preeclampsia is a serious medical condition in which a pregnant woman develops high blood pressure and kidney problems that cause protein to spill into the urine. It is a leading cause of sickness and death in pregnant women and their newborn babies. For women who get less than about 900 mg of calcium a day, taking calcium supplements during pregnancy (1,000 mg a day or more) reduces the risk of preeclampsia. But most women in the United States who become pregnant get enough calcium from their diets.

### Kidney Stones

Most kidney stones are rich in calcium oxalate. Some studies have found that higher intakes of calcium from dietary supplements are linked to a greater risk of kidney stones, especially among older adults. But calcium from foods does not appear to cause kidney stones. For most people, other factors (such as not drinking enough fluids) probably have a larger effect on the risk of kidney stones than calcium intake.

### Weight Loss

Although several studies have shown that getting more calcium helps lower body weight or reduce weight gain over time, most studies have found that calcium—from foods or dietary supplements—has little if any effect on body weight and amount of body fat.

## Risks Associated with Calcium Intake

Getting too much calcium can cause constipation. It might also interfere with the body's ability to absorb iron and zinc, but this effect is not well established. In adults, too much calcium (from dietary supplements but not food) might increase the risk of kidney stones. Some studies show that people who consume high amounts of calcium might have increased risks of prostate cancer and heart disease, but more research is needed to understand these possible links.

The upper limits for calcium are listed below. Most people do not get amounts above the upper limits from food alone; excess intakes usually come from the use of calcium supplements. Surveys show that

some older women in the United States probably get amounts somewhat above the upper limit since the use of calcium supplements is
common among these women.

**Table 34.2.** Calcium Intake: Upper Limit

| Life Stage | Upper Limit |
|---|---|
| Birth to 6 months | 1,000 mg |
| Infants 7–12 months | 1,500 mg |
| Children 1–8 years | 2,500 mg |
| Children 9–18 years | 3,000 mg |
| Adults 19–50 years | 2,500 mg |
| Adults 51 years and older | 2,000 mg |
| Pregnant and breastfeeding teens | 3,000 mg |
| Pregnant and breastfeeding adults | 2,500 mg |

## Interactions of Medicines with Calcium

Calcium dietary supplements can interact or interfere with certain
medicines that you take, and some medicines can lower or raise calcium levels in the body. Here are some examples:

- Calcium can reduce the absorption of these drugs when taken
  together:
    - Bisphosphonates (to treat osteoporosis)
    - Antibiotics of the fluoroquinolone and tetracycline families
    - Levothyroxine (to treat low thyroid activity)
    - Phenytoin (an anticonvulsant)
    - Tiludronate disodium (to treat Paget disease).
    - Diuretics differ in their effects. Thiazide-type diuretics
      (such as Diuril® and Lozol®) reduce calcium excretion by
      the kidneys which in turn can raise blood calcium levels
      too high. But loop diuretics (such as Lasix® and Bumex®)
      increase calcium excretion and thereby lower blood calcium
      levels.
    - Antacids containing aluminum or magnesium increase
      calcium loss in the urine.
    - Mineral oil and stimulant laxatives reduce calcium
      absorption.

- Glucocorticoids (such as prednisone) can cause calcium depletion and eventually osteoporosis when people use them for months at a time.

Tell your doctor, pharmacist, and other healthcare providers about any dietary supplements and medicines you take. They can tell you if those dietary supplements might interact or interfere with your prescription or OTC medicines or if the medicines might interfere with how your body absorbs, uses, or breaks down nutrients.

### *Calcium and Healthful Eating*

People should get most of their nutrients from food, advises the federal government's *Dietary Guidelines for Americans*. Foods contain vitamins, minerals, dietary fiber, and other substances that benefit health. In some cases, fortified foods and dietary supplements may provide nutrients that otherwise may be consumed in less-than-recommended amounts.

## Section 34.2

# *Glucosamine/Chondroitin Supplements and Joint Health*

This section includes text excerpted from "Glucosamine and Chondroitin for Osteoarthritis," National Center for Complementary and Integrative Health (NCCIH), November 2014. Reviewed May 2018.

Glucosamine and chondroitin are structural components of cartilage, the tissue that cushions the joints. Both are produced naturally in the body. They are also available as dietary supplements. Researchers have studied the effects of these supplements, individually or in combination, on osteoarthritis (OA), a common type of arthritis that destroys cartilage in the joints.

Cartilage is the connective tissue that cushions the ends of bones within the joints. In OA, the surface layer of cartilage between the bones of a joint wears down. This allows the bones to rub together, which can cause pain and swelling and make it difficult to move the joint. The knees, hips, spine, and hands are the parts of the body most likely to be affected by OA.

## What the Science Says about Glucosamine and Chondroitin for Osteoarthritis (OA)

Major studies of glucosamine for OA of the knee have had conflicting results.

- A large National Institutes of Health (NIH) study, called the Glucosamine/chondroitin Arthritis Intervention Trial (GAIT), compared glucosamine hydrochloride, chondroitin, both supplements together, celecoxib (a prescription drug used to manage OA pain), or a placebo (an inactive substance) in patients with knee OA. Most participants in the study had mild knee pain.

- Those who received the prescription drug had better short-term pain relief (at 6 months) than those who received a placebo.

- Overall, those who received the supplements had no significant improvement in knee pain or function, although the investigators saw evidence of improvement in a small subgroup of patients with moderate-to-severe pain who took glucosamine and chondroitin together.

- In several European studies, participants reported that their knees felt and functioned better after taking glucosamine. The study participants took a large, once-a-day dose of a preparation of glucosamine sulfate sold as a prescription drug in Europe.

- Researchers don't know why the results of these large, well-done studies differ. It may be because of differences in the types of glucosamine used (glucosamine hydrochloride in the National Institutes of Health (NIH) study versus glucosamine sulfate in the European studies), differences in the way they were administered (one large daily dose in the European studies versus three smaller ones in the NIH study), other differences in the way the studies were done, or chance.

### Chondroitin

In general, research on chondroitin has not shown it to be helpful for pain from knee or hip OA. More than 20 studies have looked at the effect of chondroitin on pain from knee or hip OA. The quality of the studies varied and so did the results. However, the largest and best studies showed that chondroitin doesn't lessen OA pain.

## Joint Structure

A few studies have looked at whether glucosamine or chondroitin can have beneficial effects on joint structure. Some but not all studies found evidence that chondroitin might help, but the improvements may be too small to make a difference to patients. There is little evidence that glucosamine has beneficial effects on joint structure.

## Experts' Recommendations

Experts disagree on whether glucosamine and chondroitin may help knee and hip OA. The American College of Rheumatology (ACR) has recommended that people with knee or hip OA not use glucosamine or chondroitin. But the recommendation was not a strong one, and the ACR acknowledged that it was controversial.

## For Other Parts of the Body

Only a small amount of research has been done on glucosamine and chondroitin for OA of joints other than the knee and hip. Because there have been only a few relatively small studies, no definite conclusions can be reached.

- Chondroitin for OA of the hand. A 6-month trial of chondroitin in 162 patients with severe OA of the hand showed that it may improve pain and function.

- Glucosamine for OA of the jaw. One study of 45 patients with OA of the jaw showed that those given glucosamine had less pain than those given ibuprofen. But another study, which included 59 patients with OA of the jaw, found that those taking glucosamine did no better than those taking a placebo (pills that don't contain the active ingredient).

- Glucosamine for chronic low-back pain and OA of the spine. A Norwegian trial involving 250 people with chronic low-back pain and OA of the lower spine found that participants who received glucosamine fared the same at 6 months as those who received placebo.

## What the Science Says about Safety and Side Effects

- No serious side effects have been reported in large, well-conducted studies of people taking glucosamine, chondroitin, or both for up to 3 years.

- Glucosamine or chondroitin may interact with the anticoagulant (blood-thinning) drug warfarin (Coumadin).

- A study in rats showed that long-term use of moderately large doses of glucosamine might damage the kidneys. Although results from animal studies don't always apply to people, this study does raise concern.

- Glucosamine might affect the way your body handles sugar, especially if you have diabetes or other blood sugar problems, such as insulin resistance or impaired glucose tolerance.

## Section 34.3

# *Vitamin A and Bone Health*

This section includes text excerpted from "Vitamin A and Bone Health," National Institutes of Health (NIH), May 2015.

Vitamin A is a family of compounds that play an important role in vision, bone growth, reproduction, cell division, and cell differentiation. We get vitamin A from a variety of sources. Two of the most common sources are retinol and beta carotene. Retinol is sometimes called "true" vitamin A because it is nearly ready for the body to use. Retinol is found in such animal foods as liver, eggs, and fatty fish. It also can be found in many fortified foods, such as breakfast cereals, and in dietary supplements.

Beta carotene is a precursor for vitamin A. The body needs to convert it to retinol or vitamin A for use. Beta carotene is found naturally in mostly orange and dark green plant foods, such as carrots, sweet potatoes, mangos, and kale. The body stores both retinol and beta-carotene in the liver, drawing on this store whenever more vitamin A is needed.

## How Much Vitamin A Do I Need?

The Institute of Medicine (IOM)developed the Recommended Dietary Allowance (RDA) for vitamin A (retinol). The recommended intakes are listed in International Units (IU) in the table, below:

**Table 34.3.** Vitamin A Intake: Upper Limit

| Life Stage | Upper Limit |
|---|---|
| Birth to 6 months | 1,000 mg |
| Infants 7–12 months | 1,500 mg |
| Children 1–8 years | 2,500 mg |
| Children 9–18 years | 3,000 mg |
| Adults 19–50 years | 2,500 mg |
| Adults 51 years and older | 2,000 mg |
| Pregnant and breastfeeding teens | 3,000 mg |
| Pregnant and breastfeeding adults | 2,500 mg |

The body can convert beta carotene into vitamin A to help meet these requirements. Although there is no RDA for beta carotene, the National Institutes of Health (NIH) Office of Dietary Supplements (ODS) recommends eating five or more servings of fruits and vegetables per day, including dark green and leafy vegetables and deep yellow or orange fruits to get appropriate amounts of beta carotene.

## Vitamin A Can Affect Your Bones

Vitamin A is a family of fat-soluble compounds that play an important role in vision, bone growth, reproduction, cell division, and cell differentiation. Vitamin A is important for healthy bones. However, too much vitamin A has been linked to bone loss and an increase in the risk of hip fracture. Scientists believe that excessive amounts of vitamin A trigger an increase in osteoclasts, the cells that break down bone. They also believe that too much vitamin A may interfere with vitamin D, which plays an important role in preserving bone.

Retinol is the form of vitamin A that causes concern. In addition to getting retinol from their diets, some people may be using synthetic retinoid preparations that are chemically similar to vitamin A to treat acne, psoriasis, and other skin conditions. These preparations have been shown to have the same negative impact on bone health as dietary retinol. Use of these medications in children and teens also has been linked to delays in growth.

Beta carotene, on the other hand, is largely considered to be safe and has not been linked to adverse effects in bone or elsewhere in the body.

## Making Sure That You Get the Right Amount of Vitamin

Surveys suggest that most Americans are getting adequate amounts of vitamin A. The IOM cautions against daily intakes of retinol above 10,000 IU. The table below identifies some common food sources of retinol. Most of the reported cases of vitamin A toxicity have been blamed on the use of supplements. Healthy individuals who eat a balanced diet generally do not need a vitamin A supplement.

Plant sources of beta carotene are not as well absorbed as the animal sources of vitamin A listed in the table, but they are still an important source of this vitamin. Dark orange and green vegetables and fruit, including carrots, sweet potatoes, spinach, cantaloupe, and kale are excellent sources of beta carotene. Because of concerns about the negative effects of too much retinol, some people prefer to eat more foods rich in beta carotene to satisfy their need for vitamin A.

## People at Special Risk of Getting Too Much Vitamin A

Older people who regularly take dietary supplements containing vitamin A may be at higher risk of getting too much vitamin A. Studies suggest that taking dietary supplements is a common practice among many older adults. However, the routine use of vitamin A supplements, as well as fortified foods, in older men and women are increasingly being questioned. Older adults are at significant risk for osteoporosis and related fractures, and their serum (blood) levels of retinol increase with age. As a result, fortified foods and supplements containing vitamin A in the form of beta carotene may be a better choice for bone health in this population.

The supplement label provides information about how much vitamin A is provided, in both International Units (IU) and as a percentage of the RDA. The list of ingredients will contain information about which forms of vitamin A are included. Other names for retinol include retinyl, palmitate, and retinyl acetate.

# Chapter 35

# *Immune System Support Supplements*

## *Chapter Contents*

Section 35.1

# *Astragalus*

This section includes text excerpted from "Astragalus,"
National Center for Complementary and Integrative
Health (NCCIH), September 2016.

Astragalus has been used for centuries in traditional Chinese medicine (TCM) in combination with other herbs, such as ginseng, dong quai, and licorice. There are more than 2,000 species of astragalus. It has been used as a dietary supplement for many conditions, including for diarrhea, fatigue, anorexia, upper respiratory infections, heart disease, hepatitis, fibromyalgia (FM), and as an adjunctive therapy for cancer. The root of the astragalus plant is put in soups, teas, extracts, or capsules.

## *How Much Do We Know?*

There are no high-quality studies in people of astragalus for any health conditions.

## *What Have We Learned?*

- Patients with nephrotic syndrome (health problems related to kidney damage) are susceptible to infections. A 2012 research review found that taking astragalus granules may be associated with a lower risk of infections in children with nephrotic syndrome. However, the review concluded that the studies were poor quality.

- People with diabetic nephropathy (a type of kidney disease) who received an intravenous (IV) drip of astragalus over a period of 2–6 weeks did better on some measures of kidney function, compared to people who didn't get astragalus, according to a 2011 analysis of 25 studies. However, most of the trials involved were poor quality.

- There's weak evidence that astragalus may help heart function in some patients with viral myocarditis (an infection of the heart), a 2013 research review showed.

- Because of limitations in the studies, a 2013 research review on the effects of astragalus on fatty liver disease, which causes fat to build up in liver cells, couldn't determine whether astragalus helps.

- An astragalus-based herbal formula didn't extend the life of patients with advanced lung cancer, a small trial reported. The study was supported in part by the National Center for Complementary and Integrative Health (NCCIH).

## What Do We Know about Safety?

- Astragalus is considered safe for many adults. The most commonly reported side effects are diarrhea and other mild gastrointestinal effects. However, it may affect blood sugar levels and blood pressure and be risky for people with certain health problems, such as blood disorders, diabetes, or hypertension.

- Astragalus may interact with medications that suppress the immune system, such as drugs taken by organ transplant recipients and some cancer patients.

- Some Astragalus species, usually not found in dietary supplements, can be toxic. Several species that grow in the United States contain the neurotoxin swainsonine and have caused "locoweed" poisoning in animals. Other species contain potentially toxic levels of selenium.

## Keep in Mind

Tell all your healthcare providers about any complementary or integrative health approaches you use. Give them a full picture of what you do to manage your health. This will help ensure coordinated and safe care.

## Section 35.2

# *Echinacea*

This section includes text excerpted from "Echinacea," National Center for Complementary and Integrative Health (NCCIH), September 2016.

There are nine known species of echinacea, all of which are native to North America They were used by Native Americans of the Great Plains region as traditional medicines. Echinacea is used as a dietary supplement for the common cold and other infections, based on the idea that it might stimulate the immune system to more effectively fight infection. Echinacea preparations have been used topically (applied to the skin) for wounds and skin problems. The roots and above-ground parts of the echinacea plant are used fresh or dried to make teas, squeezed (expressed) juice, extracts, capsules, and tablets, and preparations for external use. Several species of echinacea, most commonly *Echinacea purpurea* or *Echinacea Angustifolia*, may be included in dietary supplements.

## How Much Do We Know?

Many studies have been done on echinacea and the common cold. Much less research has been done on the use of echinacea for other health purposes.

## What Have We Learned?

- Taking echinacea after you catch a cold has not been shown to shorten the time that you'll be sick.

- Taking echinacea while you're well may slightly reduce your chances of catching a cold. However, the evidence on this point isn't completely certain.

## What Do We Know about Safety?

- There are many different echinacea products. They may contain different species of plants or different parts of the plant, be manufactured in different ways, and have other ingredients in addition to echinacea. Most of these products have not been tested in people.

- For most people, short-term oral (by mouth) use of echinacea is probably safe; the safety of long-term use is uncertain.

- The most common side effects of echinacea are digestive tract symptoms, such as nausea or stomach pain.

- Some people have allergic reactions to echinacea, which may be severe. Some children participating in a clinical trial of echinacea developed rashes, which may have been caused by an allergic reaction. People with atopy (a genetic tendency toward allergic reactions) may be more likely to have an allergic reaction when taking echinacea.

- Current evidence indicates that the risk of interactions between echinacea supplements and most medications is low.

### Keep in Mind

Tell all your healthcare providers about any complementary or integrative health approaches you use. Give them a full picture of what you do to manage your health. This will help ensure coordinated and safe care.

# Section 35.3

# *European Elder*

This section includes text excerpted from "European Elder,"
National Center for Complementary and Integrative
Health (NCCIH), September 2016.

European elder is a tree native to Europe and parts of Asia and Africa, and it also grows in the United States. The name "elder" comes from the Anglo-Saxon word "aeld," meaning fire. The terms "elderflower" and "elderberry" may refer to either European elder or a different herb called American elder. This section focuses only on

European elder. Various parts of the elder tree, including the bark, leaves, flowers, fruits, and roots, have long been used in traditional medicine. Currently, elderberry and elderflower are used as dietary supplements for flu, colds, constipation, and other conditions. The dried flowers (elderflower) and the dried ripe or fresh berries (elderberry) of the European elder tree are used in teas, extracts, and capsules.

## How Much Do We Know?

A small number of studies in people have evaluated European elder for various health conditions. Some of these studies used products that included several ingredients, so the actions of individual ingredients are unclear.

## What Have We Learned?

- Although some preliminary research indicates that elderberry may relieve flu symptoms, the evidence is not strong enough to support its use for this purpose.

- A few studies have suggested that combination products containing elderflower and other herbs might be helpful for sinusitis, but because the products contain multiple ingredients, it's unclear what role, if any, elderflower plays in their effects.

- There's not enough information to show whether elderflower and elderberry are helpful for any other purposes.

## What Do We Know about Safety?

The leaves, stems, raw, and unripe berries, and other plant parts of the elder tree contain a toxic substance and, if not properly prepared, may cause nausea, vomiting, and severe diarrhea. Because the substance may also be present in the flower, consuming large amounts of the flower might be harmful; however, no illnesses caused by elderflower have been reported.

## Keep in Mind

Tell all your healthcare providers about any complementary or integrative health approaches you use. Give them a full picture of what you do to manage your health. This helps to ensure coordinated and safe care.

# Section 35.4

# *Zinc*

This section includes text excerpted from "Zinc," Office
of Dietary Supplements (ODS), National Institutes of
Health (NIH), February 17, 2016.

Zinc is a nutrient that people need to stay healthy. Zinc is found in
cells throughout the body. It helps the immune system fight off invading bacteria and viruses. The body also needs zinc to make proteins and
deoxyribonucleic acid (DNA), the genetic material in all cells. During
pregnancy, infancy, and childhood, the body needs zinc to grow and
develop properly. Zinc also helps wounds heal and is important for
proper senses of taste and smell.

## *How Much Zinc Do I Need?*

The amount of zinc you need each day depends on your age. Average daily recommended amounts for different ages are listed below in
milligrams (mg):

**Table 35.1.** Zinc Intake: Recommended Amount

| Life Stage | Recommended Amount |
|---|---|
| Birth to 6 months | 2 mg |
| Infants 7–12 months | 3 mg |
| Children 1–3 years | 3 mg |
| Children 4–8 years | 5 mg |
| Children 9–13 years | 8 mg |
| Teens 14–18 years (boys) | 11 mg |
| Teens 14–18 years (girls) | 9 mg |
| Adults (men) | 11 mg |
| Adults (women) | 8 mg |
| Pregnant teens | 12 mg |
| Pregnant women | 11 mg |

**Table 35.1.** Continued

| Life Stage | Recommended Amount |
|---|---|
| Breastfeeding teens | 13 mg |
| Breastfeeding women | 12 mg |

## *Foods That Provide Zinc*

Zinc is found in a wide variety of foods. You can get recommended amounts of zinc by eating a variety of foods including the following:

- Oysters, which are the best source of zinc

- Red meat, poultry, seafood such as crab, and lobsters, and fortified breakfast cereals, which are also good sources of zinc

- Beans, nuts, whole grains, and dairy products, which provide some zinc

## *Zinc Dietary Supplements Available in Market*

Zinc is present in almost all multivitamin/mineral dietary supplements. It is also available alone or combined with calcium, magnesium, or other ingredients in dietary supplements. Dietary supplements can have several different forms of zinc including zinc gluconate, zinc sulfate, and zinc acetate. It is not clear whether one form is better than the others.

Zinc is also found in some oral over-the-counter (OTC) products, including those labeled as homeopathic medications for colds. Use of nasal sprays and gels that contain zinc has been associated with the loss of the sense of smell, in some cases long-lasting or permanent. Currently, these safety concerns have not been found to be associated with oral products containing zinc, such as cold lozenges.

Zinc is also present in some denture adhesive creams. Using large amounts of these products, well beyond recommended levels, could lead to excessive zinc intake and copper deficiency. This can cause neurological problems, including numbness and weakness in the arms and legs.

## *Intake Sufficient Zinc*

Most people in the United States get enough zinc from the foods they eat. However, certain groups of people are more likely than others to have trouble getting enough zinc:

- People who have had gastrointestinal surgery, such as weight loss surgery, or who have digestive disorders, such as ulcerative colitis (UC), or Crohn's disease. These conditions can both decrease the amount of zinc that the body absorbs and increase the amount lost in the urine.

- Vegetarians because they do not eat meat, which is a good source of zinc. Also, the beans and grains they typically eat have compounds that keep zinc from being fully absorbed by the body. For this reason, vegetarians might need to eat as much as 50 percent more zinc than the recommended amounts.

- Older infants who are breastfed because breast milk does not have enough zinc for infants over 6 months of age. Older infants who do not take formula should be given foods that have zinc such as pureed meats. Formula-fed infants get enough zinc from infant formula.

- Alcoholics because alcoholic beverages decrease the amount of zinc that the body absorbs and increase the amount lost in the urine. Also, many alcoholics eat a limited amount and variety of food, so they may not get enough zinc.

- People with sickle cell disease because they might need more zinc

## Risk of Zinc Deficiency

Zinc deficiency is rare in North America. It causes slow growth in infants and children, delayed sexual development in adolescents and impotence in men. Zinc deficiency also causes hair loss, diarrhea, eye, and skin sores, and loss of appetite. Weight loss, problems with wound healing, decreased ability to taste food, and lower alertness levels can also occur.

Many of these symptoms can be signs of problems other than zinc deficiency. If you have these symptoms, your doctor can help determine whether you might have a zinc deficiency.

## Health Effects of Zinc

Scientists are studying zinc to learn about its effects on the immune system (the body's defense system against bacteria, viruses, and other foreign invaders). Scientists are also researching possible connections between zinc and the health problems discussed below.

## Immune System and Wound Healing

The body's immune system needs zinc to do its job. Older people and children in developing countries who have low levels of zinc might have a higher risk of getting pneumonia and other infections. Zinc also helps the skin stay healthy. Some people who have skin ulcers might benefit from zinc dietary supplements, but only if they have low levels of zinc.

## Diarrhea

Children in developing countries often die from diarrhea. Studies show that zinc dietary supplements help reduce the symptoms and duration of diarrhea in these children, many of whom are zinc deficient or otherwise malnourished. The World Health Organization (WHO) and the United Nations International Children's Emergency Fund (UNICEF) recommend that children with diarrhea take zinc for 10–14 days (20 mg/day, or 10 mg/day for infants under 6 months). It is not clear whether zinc dietary supplements can help treat diarrhea in children who get enough zinc, such as most children in the United States.

## The Common Cold

Some studies suggest that zinc lozenges or syrup (but not zinc dietary supplements in pill form) help speed recovery from the common cold and reduce its symptoms if taken within 24 hours of coming down with a cold. However, more study is needed to determine the best dose and form of zinc, as well as how long it should be taken before zinc can be recommended as a treatment for the common cold.

## Age-Related Macular Degeneration (AMD)

AMD is an eye disease that gradually causes vision loss. Research suggests that zinc might help slow AMD progression. In a large study among older people with AMD who were at high risk of developing advanced AMD, those who took a daily dietary supplement with 80 mg zinc, 500 mg vitamin C, 400 IU vitamin E, 15 mg beta carotene, and 2 mg copper for about 6 years had a lower chance of developing advanced AMD and less vision loss than those who did not take the dietary supplement. In the same study, people at high risk of the disease who took dietary supplements containing only zinc also had a lower risk of getting advanced AMD than those who did not take zinc dietary supplements. People who have or are developing the disease might want to talk with their doctor about taking dietary supplements.

## Too Much of Zinc Can Be Harmful

Zinc can be harmful if you get too much. Signs of too much zinc include nausea, vomiting, loss of appetite, stomach cramps, diarrhea, and headaches. When people take too much zinc for a long time, they sometimes have problems such as low copper levels, lower immunity, and low levels of high-density lipoproteins (HDL) cholesterol (the "good" cholesterol).

The upper limits for zinc are listed below. These levels do not apply to people who are taking zinc for medical reasons under the care of a doctor:

**Table 35.2.** Zinc Intake: Upper Limit

| Life Stage | Upper Limit |
|---|---|
| Birth to 6 months | 4 mg |
| Infants 7–12 months | 5 mg |
| Children 1–3 years | 7 mg |
| Children 4–8 years | 12 mg |
| Children 9–13 years | 23 mg |
| Teens 14–18 years | 34 mg |
| Adults | 40 mg |

## Interactions of Medicines with Zinc

Zinc dietary supplements can interact or interfere with medicines that you take and, in some cases, medicines can lower zinc levels in the body. Here are several examples:

- Taking a zinc dietary supplement along with quinolone or tetracycline antibiotics (such as Cipro®, Achromycin®, and Sumycin®) reduces the amount of both zinc and the antibiotic that the body absorbs. Taking the antibiotic at least 2 hours before or 4–6 hours after taking a zinc dietary supplement helps minimize this effect.

- Zinc dietary supplements can reduce the amount of penicillamine (a drug used to treat rheumatoid arthritis (RA)) that the body absorbs. They also make penicillamine work less well. Taking zinc dietary supplements at least 2 hours before or after taking penicillamine helps minimize this effect.

- Thiazide diuretics, such as chlorthalidone (brand name Hygroton®) and hydrochlorothiazide (brand names Esidrix® and

HydroDIURIL®) increase the amount of zinc lost in the urine. Taking thiazide diuretics for a long time could decrease the amount of zinc in the body.

Tell your doctor, pharmacist, and other healthcare providers about any dietary supplements and medicines you take. They can tell you if those dietary supplements might interact or interfere with your prescription or over-the-counter medicines or if the medicines might interfere with how your body absorbs, uses, or breaks down nutrients.

## Zinc and Healthy Eating

People should get most of their nutrients from food, advises the federal government's *Dietary Guidelines for Americans*. Foods contain vitamins, minerals, dietary fiber, and other substances that benefit health. In some cases, fortified foods and dietary supplements may provide nutrients that otherwise may be consumed in less-than-recommended amounts.

Chapter 36

# *Mood and Brain Health Supplements*

## *Chapter Contents*

# Section 36.1

# *Ginkgo Biloba*

This section includes text excerpted from "Ginkgo,"
National Center for Complementary and Integrative
Health (NCCIH), September 2016.

## *Background*

- Ginkgo, one of the oldest living tree species in the world, has a long history in traditional Chinese medicine (TCM). Members of the royal court were given ginkgo nuts for senility. Other historical uses for ginkgo were for asthma, bronchitis, and kidney, and bladder disorders.

- Today, the extract from ginkgo leaves is used as a dietary supplement for many conditions, including dementia, eye problems, intermittent claudication (leg pain caused by narrowing arteries), tinnitus, and other health problems.

- Ginkgo is made into tablets, capsules, extracts, tea, and cosmetics.

## *How Much Do We Know?*

- There have been a lot of studies on the possible health effects and risks of people using ginkgo.

## *What Have We Learned?*

- There's no conclusive evidence that ginkgo is helpful for any health condition.

- Ginkgo doesn't help prevent or slow dementia or cognitive decline, according to studies, including the long-term Ginkgo Evaluation Memory Study, which enrolled more than 3,000 older adults and was funded in part by the National Center for Complementary and Integrative Health (NCCIH).

- There's no strong evidence that ginkgo helps with memory enhancement in healthy people, blood pressure, intermittent claudication, tinnitus, age-related macular degeneration, the risk of having a heart attack or stroke, or with other conditions.

- Ongoing NCCIH-funded research is looking at whether a compound in ginkgo may help with diabetes.

## What Do We Know about Safety?

- For many healthy adults, ginkgo appears to be safe when taken by mouth in moderate amounts.

- Side effects of ginkgo may include headache, stomach upset, and allergic skin reactions. If you're older, have a known bleeding risk, or are pregnant you should be cautious about ginkgo possibly increasing your risk of bleeding.

- In a 2013 research study, rodents given ginkgo had an increased risk of developing liver and thyroid cancer at the end of the 2-year tests.

- Ginkgo may interact with some conventional medications, including anticoagulants (blood thinners).

- Eating fresh (raw) or roasted ginkgo seeds can be poisonous and have serious side effects.

## Keep in Mind

- Tell all your healthcare providers about any complementary or integrative health approaches you use. Give them a full picture of what you do to manage your health. This will help ensure coordinated and safe care.

## Section 36.2

## *St. John's Wort*

This section includes text excerpted from "St. John's Wort,"
National Center for Complementary and Integrative
Health (NCCIH), September 2016.

### *Background*

- St. John's wort is a plant with yellow flowers that has been used
  in traditional European medicine as far back as the ancient
  Greeks. The name St. John's wort apparently refers to John the
  Baptist, as the plant blooms around the time of the feast of St.
  John the Baptist in late June.

- Historically, St. John's wort has been used for a variety of
  conditions, including kidney and lung ailments, insomnia, and
  depression, and to aid wound healing.

- Currently, St. John's wort is most often used as a dietary
  supplement for depression. People also use it as a dietary
  supplement for other conditions, including menopausal
  symptoms, attention deficit hyperactivity disorder (ADHD), and
  obsessive-compulsive disorder (OCD). It is used topically for
  wound healing.

- The flowering tops of St. John's wort are used to prepare teas,
  tablets, capsules, and liquid extracts. Topical preparations are
  also available.

### *How Much Do We Know?*

- There has been extensive research on St. John's wort,
  especially on its use for depression and on its interactions with
  medications. It has been clearly shown that St. John's wort can
  interact in dangerous, sometimes life-threatening ways with a
  variety of medicines.

## What Have We Learned?

- The results of studies on the effectiveness of St. John's wort for depression are mixed

- St. John's wort has also been studied for conditions other than depression. For some, such as ADHD, irritable bowel syndrome (IBS), and quitting smoking, current evidence indicates that St. John's wort is not helpful. For others, such as menopausal symptoms, premenstrual syndrome, and obsessive-compulsive disorder, the evidence is inconclusive.

## What Do We Know about Safety?

- St. John's wort can weaken the effects of many medicines, including crucially important medicines such as

- Antidepressants

- Birth control pills

- Cyclosporine, which prevents the body from rejecting transplanted organs

- Digoxin, a heart medication

- Some human immunodeficiency virus (HIV) drugs including indinavir

- Some cancer medications including irinotecan

- Warfarin, an anticoagulant (blood thinner).

- Taking St. John's wort with certain antidepressants or other drugs that affect serotonin, a substance produced by nerve cells, may lead to increased serotonin-related side effects, which may be potentially serious.

- St. John's wort may cause increased sensitivity to sunlight. Other side effects can include anxiety, dry mouth, dizziness, gastrointestinal symptoms, fatigue, headache, or sexual dysfunction.

## Keep in Mind

- Depression can be a serious illness. If you or someone in your family may have depression, consult a healthcare provider.

- Although it is important to tell all your healthcare providers about any complementary health approaches you use, this is especially crucial for St. John's wort because this herb interacts with so many medicines. Interactions with St. John's wort can weaken the effects of lifesaving medicines or cause dangerous side effects.

# Chapter 37

# *Probiotics: Supplements for Gastrointestinal Health*

## *About Probiotics*

Probiotics are live microorganisms that are intended to have health benefits. Products sold as probiotics include foods (such as yogurt), dietary supplements, and products that aren't used orally, such as skin creams.

Although people often think of bacteria and other microorganisms as harmful "germs," many microorganisms help our bodies function properly. For example, bacteria that are normally present in our intestines help digest food, destroy disease-causing microorganisms, and produce vitamins. Large numbers of microorganisms live on and in our bodies. In fact, microorganisms in the human body outnumber human cells by 10 to 1. Many of the microorganisms in probiotic products are the same as or similar to microorganisms that naturally live in our bodies.

### *The History of Probiotics*

The concept behind probiotics was introduced in the early 20th century, when Nobel laureate Elie Metchnikoff, known as the "father

---

This chapter includes text excerpted from "Probiotics: In Depth," National Center for Complementary and Integrative Health (NCCIH), October 2016.

of probiotics," proposed that consuming beneficial microorganisms could improve people's health. Researchers continued to investigate this idea, and the term "probiotics"—meaning "for life"—eventually came into use.

### What Kinds of Microorganisms Are in Probiotics?

Probiotics may contain a variety of microorganisms. The most common are bacteria that belong to groups called *Lactobacillus* and *Bifidobacterium*. Each of these two broad groups includes many types of bacteria. Other bacteria may also be used as probiotics, and so may yeasts such as *Saccharomyces boulardii*.

### Probiotics, Prebiotics, and Synbiotics

Prebiotics are not the same as probiotics. The term "prebiotics" refers to dietary substances that favor the growth of beneficial bacteria over harmful ones. The term "synbiotics" refers to products that combine probiotics and prebiotics.

### How Popular Are Probiotics?

Data from the 2012 National Health Interview Survey (NHIS) show that about 4 million (1.6 percent) U.S. adults had used probiotics or prebiotics. Among adults, probiotics or prebiotics were the third most commonly used dietary supplement other than vitamins and minerals, and the use of probiotics quadrupled between 2007–2012. The 2012 NHIS also showed that 300,000 children age 4–17 (0.5 percent) had used probiotics or prebiotics.

## What the Science Says about the Effectiveness of Probiotics

Researchers have studied probiotics to find out whether they might help prevent or treat a variety of health problems, including:

- Digestive disorders such as diarrhea caused by infections, antibiotic-associated diarrhea, irritable bowel syndrome (IBS), and inflammatory bowel disease (IBD)

- Allergic disorders such as atopic dermatitis (eczema) and allergic rhinitis (hay fever)

- Tooth decay, periodontal disease, and other oral health problems
- Colic in infants
- Liver disease
- Common cold
- Prevention of necrotizing enterocolitis in very low birth weight infants

There's preliminary evidence that some probiotics are helpful in preventing diarrhea caused by infections and antibiotics and in improving symptoms of IBS, but more needs to be learned. We still don't know which probiotics are helpful and which are not. We also don't know how much of the probiotic people would have to take or who would most likely benefit from taking probiotics. Even for the conditions that have been studied the most, researchers are still working toward finding the answers to these questions.

Probiotics are not all alike. For example, if a specific kind of Lactobacillus helps prevent an illness, that doesn't necessarily mean that another kind of Lactobacillus would have the same effect or that any of the Bifidobacterium probiotics would do the same thing.

Although some probiotics have shown promise in research studies, strong scientific evidence to support specific uses of probiotics for most health conditions is lacking. The U.S. Food and Drug Administration (FDA) has not approved any probiotics for preventing or treating any health problem. Some experts have cautioned that the rapid growth in marketing and use of probiotics may have outpaced scientific research for many of their proposed uses and benefits.

### How Might Probiotics Work?

Probiotics may have a variety of effects in the body, and different probiotics may act in different ways.

Probiotics might:

- Help to maintain a desirable community of microorganisms

- Stabilize the digestive tract's barriers against undesirable microorganisms or produce substances that inhibit their growth

- Help the community of microorganisms in the digestive tract return to normal after being disturbed (for example, by an antibiotic or a disease)

- Outcompete undesirable microorganisms

- Stimulate the immune response

### Government Regulation of Probiotics

Government regulation of probiotics in the United States is complex. Depending on a probiotic product's intended use, the FDA might regulate it as a dietary supplement, a food ingredient, or a drug.

Many probiotics are sold as dietary supplements, which do not require FDA approval before they are marketed. Dietary supplement labels may make claims about how the product affects the structure or function of the body without FDA approval, but they cannot make health claims (claims that the product reduces the risk of a disease) without the FDA's consent.

If a probiotic is marketed as a drug for specific treatment of a disease or disorder in the future, it will be required to meet more stringent requirements. It must be proven safe and effective for its intended use through clinical trials and be approved by the FDA before it can be sold.

## What the Science Says about the Safety and Side Effects of Probiotics

Whether probiotics are likely to be safe for you depends on the state of your health.

- In people who are generally healthy, probiotics have a good safety record. Side effects, if they occur at all, usually consist only of mild digestive symptoms such as gas.

- On the other hand, there have been reports linking probiotics to severe side effects, such as dangerous infections, in people with serious underlying medical problems. The people who are most at risk of severe side effects include critically ill patients, those who have had surgery, very sick infants, and people with weakened immune systems.

Even for healthy people, there are uncertainties about the safety of probiotics. Because many research studies on probiotics haven't looked closely at safety, there isn't enough information right now to answer some safety questions. Most of our knowledge about safety comes from studies of Lactobacillus and Bifidobacterium; less is known about other probiotics. Information on the long-term safety of probiotics is limited, and safety may differ from one type of probiotic to another. For example, even though a National Center for Complementary and Integrative Health (NCCIH)-funded study showed that a particular kind of Lactobacillus appears safe in healthy adults age 65 and older, this does not mean that all probiotics would necessarily be safe for people in this age group.

# Chapter 38

# *Sports and Energy Supplements*

## *Chapter Contents*

# Section 38.1

# *Sports Supplements*

This section includes text excerpted from "Dietary Supplements
for Exercise and Athletic Performance," Office of Dietary
Supplements (ODS), National Institutes of Health (NIH), June 30, 2017.

Dietary supplements to enhance exercise and athletic performance come in a variety of forms, including tablets, capsules, liquids, powders, and bars. Many of these products contain numerous ingredients in varied combinations and amounts. Among the more common ingredients are amino acids, protein, creatine, and caffeine. According to one estimate, retail sales of the category of "sports nutrition supplements" totaled $5.67 billion in 2016 or 13.8 percent of $41.16 billion total sales for dietary supplements and related nutrition products for that year.

It is difficult to make generalizations about the extent of dietary supplement use by athletes because the studies on this topic are heterogeneous. But the data suggest that:

- A larger proportion of athletes than the general U.S. population takes dietary supplements.

- Elite athletes (e.g., professional athletes and those who compete on a national or international level) use dietary supplements more often than their nonelite counterparts.

- The supplements used by male and female athletes are similar, except that a larger proportion of women use iron and a larger proportion of men take vitamin E, protein, and creatine.

For any individual to physically perform at his or her best, a nutritionally adequate diet and sufficient hydration are critical. The *Dietary Guidelines for Americans* and MyPlate recommend such an eating plan for everyone. Athletes require adequate daily amounts of calories, fluids, carbohydrates (to maintain blood glucose levels and replace muscle glycogen; typically 1.4 to 4.5 g/lb body weight [3 to 10 g/kg body weight]), protein (0.55 to 0.9 g/lb body weight [1.2 to 2.0 g/kg body weight]), fat (20% to 35% of total calories), and vitamins and minerals.

A few dietary supplements might enhance performance only when they add to, but do not substitute for, this dietary foundation. Athletes engaging in endurance activities lasting more than an hour or performed in extreme environments (e.g., hot temperatures or high altitudes) might need to replace lost fluids and electrolytes and consume additional carbohydrates for energy. Even with proper nutritional preparation, the results of taking any dietary supplement(s) for exercise and athletic performance vary by level of training; the nature, intensity, and duration of the activity; and the environmental conditions.

Most studies to assess the potential value and safety of supplements to enhance exercise and athletic performance include only conditioned athletes. Therefore, it is often not clear whether the supplements discussed in this chapter may be of value to recreational exercisers or individuals who engage in athletic activity only occasionally. In addition, much of the research on these supplements involves young adults (more often male than female), and not adolescents who may also use them against the advice of pediatric and high-school professional associations. The quality of many studies is limited by their small samples and short durations, use of performance tests that do not simulate real-world conditions or are unreliable or irrelevant, and poor control of confounding variables. Furthermore, the benefits and risks shown for the supplements might not apply to the supplement's use to enhance types of physical performance not assessed in the studies. In most cases, additional research is needed to fully understand the efficacy and safety of particular ingredients.

## Selected Ingredients in Dietary Supplements for Exercise and Athletic Performance

Many exercises and athletic-performance dietary supplements in the marketplace contain multiple ingredients (especially those marketed for muscle growth and strength). However, much of the research has focused only on single ingredients. One, therefore, cannot know or predict the effects and safety of combinations in these multi-ingredient products unless clinical trials have investigated that particular combination. Furthermore, the amounts of these ingredients vary widely among products. In some cases, the products contain proprietary blends of ingredients listed in order by weight, but labels do not provide the amount of each ingredient in the blend. Manufacturers and sellers of dietary supplements for exercise and athletic performance rarely fund or conduct scientific research on their proprietary products of a caliber that reputable biomedical journals require for publication.

301

## Antioxidants (Vitamin C, Vitamin E, and Coenzyme $Q_{10}$)

Exercise increases the body's consumption of oxidative stress, leading to the production of reactive oxygen and nitrogen species (i.e., free radicals) and the creation of more oxidized molecules in various tissues, including muscle. In theory, free radicals could impair exercise performance by impeding muscles' ability to produce force, thereby accelerating muscle damage and fatigue and producing inflammation and soreness. Some researchers have suggested that supplements containing antioxidants, such as vitamins C and E and coenzyme $Q_{10}$ ($CoQ_{10}$), could reduce this free-radical formation, thereby minimizing skeletal muscle damage and fatigue and promoting recovery.

### Arginine

L-arginine is an amino acid found in many protein-containing foods, especially animal products and nuts. The typical dietary intake is 4–5 grams/day. The body also synthesizes arginine (from citrulline), mainly in the kidneys.

Some experts suggest that taking arginine in supplement form enhances exercise and athletic performance in several ways. First, some arginine is converted to nitric oxide, a potent vasodilator that can increase blood flow and the delivery of oxygen and nutrients to skeletal muscle. Second, increased vasodilation can speed up the removal of metabolic waste products related to muscle fatigue, such as lactate, and ammonia, that the body produces during exercise. Third, arginine serves as a precursor for the synthesis of creatine, which helps supply muscle with energy for short-term, intense activity. Fourth, arginine may increase the secretion of human growth hormone (HGH), which in turn increases insulin-like growth factor-1 (IGF-1) levels, both of which stimulate muscle growth.

### Beetroot or Beet Juice

Beets are one of the richest food sources of inorganic nitrate. Ingested nitrate might enhance exercise and athletic performance in several ways, primarily through its conversion into nitric oxide in the body. Nitric acid is a potent vasodilator that can increase blood flow and the delivery of oxygen and nutrients to skeletal muscle. Ingested nitrate might also enhance performance by dilating blood vessels in exercising muscle when oxygen levels decline, thereby increasing oxygen and nutrient delivery, reducing the oxygen cost of submaximal exercise, attenuating the adenosine triphosphate (ATP)-creatine phosphate energy system's cost associated with skeletal muscle force production, and improving oxidative phosphorylation in mitochondria. Beetroot is available as a juice or juice concentrate and in powdered form; the amount of nitrate can vary considerably among products.

## Beta-Alanine

Beta-alanine, a type of amino acid that the body does not incorporate into proteins, is the rate-limiting precursor to the synthesis of carnosine—a dipeptide of histidine and beta-alanine—in skeletal muscle. Carnosine helps buffer changes in muscle pH from the anaerobic glycolysis that provides energy during high-intensity exercise but results in the buildup of hydrogen ions as lactic acid accumulates and dissociates to form lactate, leading to reduced force and to fatigue. More carnosine in muscle leads to greater potential attenuation of exercise-induced reductions in pH, which could enhance the performance of intense activities of short to moderate duration, such as rowing and swimming.

Beta-alanine is produced in the liver, and relatively small amounts are present in animal-based foods such as meat, poultry, and fish. Estimated dietary intakes range from none in vegans to about 1 g/day in heavy meat eaters. Carnosine is present in animal-based foods, such as beef and pork. However, oral consumption of carnosine is an inefficient method of increasing muscle carnosine concentrations because the dipeptide is digested into its constituent amino acids. Consumption of beta-alanine, in contrast, reliably increases the amount of carnosine in the body. Four to six grams of beta-alanine for 10 weeks, for example, can increase muscle carnosine levels by up to 80 percent, especially in trained athletes, although the magnitude of response differs widely. For example, in one study of young, physically active but untrained adult men who took 4.8 g/day beta-alanine for 5–6 weeks, the percent increase in muscle carnosine content after 9 weeks of follow-up ranged from 2 percent to 69 percent. Among the "low responders," the duration of the washout period when beta alanine concentrations returned to baseline values was less than half that for the "high responders" (6 weeks versus 15 weeks).

## Beta-Hydroxy-Beta-Methylbutyrate (HMB)

Beta-hydroxy-beta-methyl butyrate (HMB) is a metabolite of the branched-chain amino acid leucine. About 5 percent of the body's leucine is converted into HMB, which is then converted in the liver to a precursor (known as beta-hydroxy-beta-methyl glutaryl coenzyme A) needed for cholesterol biosynthesis. Some experts hypothesize that skeletal muscle cells that become stressed and damaged from exercise require an exogenous source of the coenzyme for synthesis of cholesterol in their cellular membranes to restore structure and function. Experts also believe that the conversion of leucine to HMB activates muscle protein synthesis and reduces protein breakdown. Supplementation is the only practical way to obtain 3 g/day HMB because one would otherwise need to consume over 600 g/day of high-quality protein (from 5 lb of beef tenderloin, for example) to obtain enough leucine (60 g) for conversion into HMB.

## Betaine

Betaine, also known as trimethylglycine, is found in foods such as beets, spinach, and whole-grain bread. Average daily intakes of betaine range from 100 to 300 mg/day. The mechanisms by which betaine might enhance exercise and athletic performance are not known, but many are hypothesized. For example, betaine might increase the biosynthesis of creatine, levels of blood nitric acid, and/or the water retention of cells.

## Branched-Chain Amino Acids (BCAA)

Three essential amino acids—leucine, isoleucine, and valine—are the branched-chain amino acids (BCAAs), whose name reflects their chemical structure. BCAAs make up approximately 25 percent of the amino acids in foods containing complete proteins (including all essential amino acids); most of these foods are animal products, such as meat, poultry, fish, eggs, and milk. BCAAs comprise about 14 percent–18 percent of the amino acids in human skeletal muscle proteins. Unlike other essential amino acids, the BCAAs can be metabolized by mitochondria in skeletal muscle to provide energy during exercise. The BCAAs, especially leucine, might also stimulate protein synthesis in exercised muscle.

## Caffeine

Caffeine is a methylated xanthine naturally found in variable amounts in coffee; tea; cacao pods (the source of chocolate); and other herbal/botanical sources, such as guarana, kola (or cola) nut, and yerba mate. Caffeine stimulates the central nervous system (CNS), muscles, and other organs, such as the heart, by binding to adenosine receptors on cells, thereby blocking the activity of adenosine, a neuromodulator with sedative-like properties. In this way, caffeine enhances arousal, increases vigor, and reduces fatigue. Caffeine also appears to reduce perceived pain and exertion. During the early stages of endurance exercise, caffeine might mobilize free fatty acids as a source of energy and spare muscle glycogen.

Caffeine is commonly used in energy drinks and "shots" touted for their performance-enhancement effects. It is also found in energy gels containing carbohydrates and electrolytes as well as in anhydrous caffeine-only pills.

### Citrulline

L-citrulline is a nonessential amino acid produced in the body, mainly from glutamine, and obtained from the diet. Watermelon is the best-known source; 1 cup diced seedless watermelon has about 365 mg citrulline. About 80 percent of the body's citrulline is converted in the kidneys into arginine, another amino acid. The subsequent conversion of arginine to nitric oxide, a potent dilator of blood vessels, might be the mechanism by which citrulline could serve as an ergogenic aid. In fact, consumption of citrulline might be a more efficient way to raise blood arginine levels than consumption of arginine because more citrulline is absorbed from the gut than arginine.

Most studies have used citrulline malate, a combination of citrulline with malic acid (a constituent in many fruits that is also produced endogenously), because malate, an intermediate in the Krebs cycle, might enhance energy production.

### Creatine

Creatine is one of the most thoroughly studied and widely used dietary supplements to enhance exercise and sports performance. Creatine is produced endogenously and obtained from the diet in small amounts. It helps generate adenosine triphosphate (ATP) and thereby supplies the muscles with energy, particularly for short-term events. Creatine might improve muscle performance in four ways: by increasing stores of phosphocreatine used to generate ATP at the beginning of the intense exercise, accelerating the resynthesis of phosphocreatine after exercise, depressing the degradation of adenine nucleotides and the accumulation of lactate, and/or enhancing glycogen storage in skeletal muscles.

The liver and kidneys synthesize about 1 g/day creatine from the amino acids glycine, arginine, and methionine. Animal-based foods, such as beef (2 g/lb), pork (2.3 g/lb), and salmon (2 g/lb), also contain creatine. A person weighing 154 pounds has about 120 g creatine and phosphocreatine in his or her body, almost all in the skeletal and cardiac muscles. However, it is only when users consume much greater amounts of creatine over time as a dietary supplement that it could have ergogenic effects. Metabolized creatine is converted into the waste product creatinine, which is eliminated from the body through the kidneys.

### Deer Antler Velvet

Deer antler velvet consists of cartilage and epidermis from growing deer or elk antlers before ossification. It is used as a general health aid in traditional Chinese medicine. Several growth factors have been detected in deer antler velvet, such as IGF-1, that could promote muscle tissue growth in a similar way to the quick growth of deer antlers.

### Dehydroepiandrosterone

Dehydroepiandrosterone (DHEA) is a steroid hormone secreted by the adrenal cortex. The body can convert DHEA to the male hormone testosterone; testosterone's intermediary, androstenedione; and the female hormone estradiol. Testosterone is an anabolic steroid that promotes gains in muscle mass and strength when combined with resistance training.

### Ginseng

Ginseng is a generic term for botanicals from the genus Panax. Some popular varieties are known as Chinese, Korean, American, and Japanese ginseng. Preparations made from ginseng roots have been used in traditional Chinese medicine for millennia as a tonic to improve stamina and vitality. So-called Siberian or Russian ginseng (*Eleutherococcus senticosus*), although unrelated to *Panax ginseng*, has also been used in traditional Chinese medicine to combat fatigue and strengthen the immune system.

### Glutamine

Glutamine is the most abundant amino acid in muscle, blood, and the body's free-amino-acid pool. It is synthesized in the body primarily from the BCAAs, and an adult consumes about 3–6 g/day in protein-containing foods. Glutamine is a key molecule in metabolism and energy production, and it contributes nitrogen for many critical biochemical reactions. It is an essential amino acid for critically ill patients when the body's need for glutamine exceeds its capacity to produce sufficient amounts.

## *Iron*

Iron is an essential mineral and a structural component of hemoglobin, an erythrocyte protein that transfers oxygen from the lungs to the tissues, and myoglobin, a protein in muscles that provides them with oxygen. Iron is also necessary to metabolize substrates for energy as a component of cytochromes and to dehydrogenase enzymes involved in substrate oxidation. Iron deficiency impairs oxygen-carrying capacity and muscle function, and it limits people's ability to exercise and be active. Its detrimental effects can include fatigue and lethargy, lower aerobic capacity, and slower times in performance trials.

Iron balance is an important consideration for athletes who must pay attention to both iron intakes and iron losses. Teenage girls and premenopausal women are at increased risk of obtaining insufficient amounts of iron from their diets. They require more iron than teenage boys and men because they lose considerable iron due to menstruation, and they might not eat sufficient amounts of iron-containing foods.

Athletes of both sexes lose additional iron for several reasons. Physical activity produces acute inflammation that reduces iron absorption from the gut and iron use via a peptide, hepcidin, that regulates iron homeostasis. Iron is also lost in sweat. The destruction of erythrocytes in the feet because of frequent striking on hard surfaces leads to foot-strike hemolysis. Also, use of anti-inflammatories and pain medications can lead to some blood loss from the gastrointestinal tract, thereby decreasing iron stores.

The richest dietary sources of heme iron (which is highly bioavailable) include lean meats and seafood. Plant-based foods—such as nuts, beans, vegetables, and fortified grain products—contain non-heme iron, which is less bioavailable than heme iron.

## *Protein*

Protein is necessary to build, maintain, and repair muscle. Exercise increases intramuscular protein oxidation and breakdown, after which muscle-protein synthesis increases for up to a day or two. Regular resistance exercise results in the accretion of myofibrillar protein (the predominant proteins in skeletal muscle) and an increase in skeletal muscle fiber size. Aerobic exercise leads to more modest protein accumulation in working muscle, primarily in the mitochondria, which enhances oxidative capacity (oxygen use) for future workouts.

Athletes must consider both protein quality and quantity to meet their needs for the nutrient. They must obtain essential amino acids (EAAs) from the diet or from supplementation to support muscle growth, maintenance, and repair. The nine EAAs are histidine, isoleucine, leucine, lysine, methionine, phenylalanine, threonine, tryptophan, and valine. Most complete proteins (those that contain all EAAs) are composed of about 40 percent EAAs, so a meal or snack with 25 g total protein provides about 10 g EAAs.

### Ribose

Ribose, a naturally occurring 5-carbon sugar synthesized by cells and found in some foods, is involved in the production of ATP. The amount of ATP in muscle is limited, and it must continually be resynthesized. Therefore, theoretically, the more ribose in the body, the more potential ATP production.

### Sodium Bicarbonate

Sodium bicarbonate is commonly known as baking soda. The consumption of several teaspoons of sodium bicarbonate over a short time temporarily increases blood pH by acting as a buffering agent. The precise mechanism by which this induced alkalosis leads to an ergogenic response to exercise is unclear. It is thought that "bicarbonate loading" enhances disposal of hydrogen ions that accumulate and efflux from working muscles as they generate energy in the form of ATP via anaerobic glycolysis from high-intensity exercise, thereby reducing the metabolic acidosis that contributes to fatigue. As a result, supplementation with sodium bicarbonate might improve performance in short-term, intense exercises (e.g., sprinting and swimming) and in intermittently intense sports (e.g., boxing and tennis).

### Tart or Sour Cherry

The Montmorency variety of tart or sour cherry (*Prunus cerasus*) contains anthocyanins and other polyphenolic phytochemicals, such as quercetin. Researchers hypothesize that these compounds have anti-inflammatory and antioxidant effects that might facilitate exercise recovery by reducing pain and inflammation, strength loss and muscle damage from intense activity, and hyperventilation trauma from endurance activities. The labels on tart-cherry juice and concentrate products do not usually indicate that they are dietary supplements, although the labels on products containing encapsulated tart-cherry powder do.

## *Tribulus Terrestris*

*Tribulus Terrestris* (common names include bindii, goat's-head, bullhead, and tackweed), is a fruit-bearing plant that is most common in Africa, Asia, Australia, and Europe. It has been used since ancient times in Greece, China, and Asia to treat low libido and infertility. *Tribulus Terrestris* extracts contain many compounds, including steroidal saponins. Some marketers claim that *Tribulus Terrestris* enhances exercise and athletic performance by increasing serum concentrations of testosterone and luteinizing hormone, but studies have not adequately determined its potential mechanisms of action.

## Ingredients Banned from Dietary Supplements

This chapter provides examples of ingredients that the FDA currently prohibits in dietary supplements and that some consumers have used in the past as ergogenic aids, despite the lack of evidence supporting their use.

### *Androstenedione*

Androstenedione is an anabolic steroid precursor, or prohormone, that the body converts to testosterone (which induces muscle growth) and estrogen. Major League Baseball slugger Mark McGwire popularized androstenedione as an ergogenic aid in 1998. However, two randomized clinical trials found no performance benefits from androstenedione supplements. In one study, 10 healthy young men (ages 19–29 years) took a single 100-mg dose of androstenedione. Another 20 were randomized to receive either 300 mg/day androstenedione or a placebo for 6 or 8 weeks while undergoing resistance-training and muscle-strengthening exercises. The short-term or longer-term use of the supplement did not affect serum testosterone concentrations, nor did it produce any significantly greater gains in resistance-training performance, muscle strength, or lean body mass. However, participants who took androstenedione for the 6 weeks experienced significant declines in their high-density lipoprotein (HDL) cholesterol levels and significant increases in serum estrogens. A similar study randomized 50 men (ages 35–65 years) to take 200 mg/day androstenedione, 200 mg/day of the related androstenediol, or a placebo for 12 weeks while participating in a high-intensity resistance training program. The supplements did not improve participants' muscular strength or lean body mass compared with placebo, but they significantly decreased HDL cholesterol levels and raised levels of serum estrogens. Among participants taking the androstenedione, testosterone levels increased significantly by 16 percent after 1 month of use but declined to pre-treatment levels by 12 weeks, in part due to downregulation of endogenous testosterone synthesis.

### Dimethylamylamine

Dimethylamylamine (DMAA) is a stimulant formerly included in some preworkout and other dietary supplements claimed to enhance exercise performance and build muscle. Studies have not evaluated DMAA in humans as a potential ergogenic aid. In 2013, FDA declared products containing this ingredient to be illegal after it received 86 reports of deaths and illnesses associated with dietary supplements containing DMAA. These reports described heart problems as well as nervous system and psychiatric disorders. Furthermore, FDA had never approved DMAA as a new dietary ingredient that would reasonably be expected to be safe. Although products marketed as dietary supplements containing DMAA are illegal in the United States, discontinued, reformulated, or even new products containing DMAA might still be found in the U.S. marketplace. The Department of Defense's (DoD) Human Performance Resource Center (HPRC) maintains a list of currently available products that contain DMAA or are labeled as containing DMAA, 1-3-dimethylamylamine, or an equivalent chemical or marketing name (e.g., methylhexanamine or geranium extract).

The FDA also determined that dietary supplements containing 1,3-dimethylbutylamine (DMBA), a stimulant chemically related to DMAA, are adulterated. As with DMAA, FDA had never approved this stimulant as a new dietary ingredient. The FDA contended that there is no history of use or data offering sufficient assurance that this compound is not associated with "a significant or unreasonable risk of illness or injury."

### Ephedra

Ephedra (also known as ma huang), a plant native to China, contains ephedrine alkaloids, which are stimulant compounds; the primary alkaloid is ephedrine. In the 1990s, ephedra—frequently combined with caffeine—was a popular ingredient in dietary supplements sold to enhance exercise and athletic performance and to promote weight loss.

No studies have evaluated the use of ephedra dietary supplements, with or without caffeine, as ergogenic aids. Instead, available studies have used the related synthetic compound ephedrine together with caffeine and typically measured the effects 1–2 hours after a single dose. These studies showed that the ephedrine-caffeine combination produced a 20–30 percent increase in power and endurance, but ephedrine alone had no significant effects on exercise-performance parameters, such as oxygen consumption or time to exhaustion. No data show any sustained improvement in athletic performance over time with continued dosing of ephedrine with caffeine.

Ephedra use has been associated with death and serious adverse effects, including nausea, vomiting, psychiatric symptoms (such as anxiety and mood change), hypertension, palpitations, stroke, seizures, and heart attack. In 2004, FDA banned the sale of dietary supplements containing ephedrine alkaloids in the United States because they are associated with "an unreasonable risk of illness or injury." The World Anti-Doping Agency prohibits the use of ephedrine in amounts that lead to urine concentrations of ephedrine (or the related methylephedrine) exceeding 10 mcg/ml.

## Regulation of Dietary Supplements to Enhance Exercise and Athletic Performance

The FDA regulates dietary supplements for exercise and athletic performance in accordance with the Dietary Supplement Health and Education (DSHE) Act of 1994. Like other dietary supplements, exercise and athletic-performance supplements differ from over-the-counter (OTC) or prescription medications in that they do not require premarket review or approval by FDA. Supplement manufacturers are responsible for determining that their products are safe and their label claims are truthful and not misleading, although they are not required to provide this evidence to FDA before marketing their products. If FDA finds a supplement to be unsafe, it may remove the product from the market or ask the manufacturer to voluntarily recall the product. The FDA and Federal Trade Commission (FTC) may also take regulatory actions against manufacturers that make unsubstantiated physical-performance or other claims about their products.

The FDA permits dietary supplements to contain only "dietary ingredients," such as vitamins, minerals, amino acids, herbs, and other botanicals. It does not permit these products to contain pharmaceutical ingredients, and manufacturers may not promote them to diagnose, treat, cure, or prevent any disease.

## Safety Considerations

Like all dietary supplements, supplements used to enhance exercise and athletic performance can have side effects and might interact with prescription and over-the-counter medications. In some cases, the active constituents of botanical or other ingredients promoted as ergogenic aids are unknown or uncharacterized. Furthermore, many such products contain multiple ingredients that have not been adequately tested in combination with one another. People interested in taking dietary supplements to enhance their exercise and athletic performance should talk with their healthcare providers about the use of these products.

The Uniformed Services University of the Health Sciences (USUHS) and the U.S. Anti-Doping Agency (ADA) maintain a list of products marketed as dietary supplements that contain stimulants, steroids, hormone-like ingredients, controlled substances, or unapproved drugs and that can have health risks for warfighters and others who take them for bodybuilding or other forms of physical performance.

### *Fraudulent and Adulterated Products*

The FDA requires the manufacture of dietary supplements to comply with quality standards that ensure that these products contain only the labeled ingredients and amounts and are free of undeclared substances and unsafe levels of contaminants. However, FDA notes that products marketed as dietary supplements for bodybuilding are among those most often adulterated with undeclared or deceptively labeled ingredients, such as synthetic anabolic steroids or prescription medications. As one example, some products sold for bodybuilding are adulterated with selective androgen receptor modulators (SARMs); these synthetic drugs are designed to mimic the effects of testosterone. Using such tainted products can cause health problems and lead to disqualification of athletes from competition if a drug test shows that they have consumed prohibited substances, even if they have done so unknowingly. FDA has warned against the use of any body- building products that claim to contain steroids or steroid-like substances. It recommends that a user contact their healthcare provider if they experience symptoms possibly related to these products, especially nausea, weakness, fatigue, fever, abdominal pain, chest pain, shortness of breath, jaundice (yellowing of skin or whites of eyes), or brown or discolored urine.

Some dietary-supplement firms have hired third-party certification companies to verify the identity and content of their supplements to enhance exercise and athletic performance, thus providing some extra, independent assurance that the products contain the labeled amounts of ingredients and are free of any banned substances and drugs. The major companies providing this certification service are the National Science Foundation NSF (nsf.org) through its Certified for Sport® program, Informed-Choice (informed-choice.org), and the Banned Substances Control Group (bscg.org). The products that meet the requirements of these companies may carry the certifier's official logo and are listed on the certifier's website.

### Interactions with Medications

Some ingredients in dietary supplements used to enhance exercise and athletic performance can interact with certain medications. For example, intakes of large doses of antioxidant supplements, such as vitamins C and E, during cancer chemotherapy or radiotherapy could reduce the effectiveness of these therapies by inhibiting cellular oxidative damage in cancerous cells. Ginseng can reduce the anticoagulant effects of the blood thinner warfarin (Coumadin or Jantoven). Iron supplements can reduce the bioavailability of levodopa (used to treat Parkinson disease) and levothyroxine (Levothroid, Levoxyl, Synthroid, and others, for hypothyroidism and goiter), so users should take iron supplements at a different time of the day than these two drugs. Cimetidine (Tagamet HB, used to treat duodenal ulcers) can slow the rate of caffeine clearance from the body and thereby increase the risk of adverse effects from caffeine consumption.

Individuals taking dietary supplements and medications on a regular basis should discuss the use of these products with their healthcare providers.

## Choosing a Sensible Approach to Enhance Exercise and Athletic Performance

According to Academy of Nutrition and Dietetics (AND), Dietitians of Canada (DoC), and American College of Sports Medicine (ACSM), sound science supports the use of only a few dietary supplements whose labels claim ergogenic benefits. These organizations add that the best way to use supplements is as additions to a carefully chosen diet, that dietary supplements rarely have ergogenic benefits when not used in these conditions, and that there is no justification for their use by young athletes. The National Federation of State High School Associations (NHFS) also expresses strong opposition to the use of supplements to enhance athletic performance by high school students. The American Academy of Pediatrics (AAP) adds that performance-enhancing substances do not result in significant improvements in most teen-aged athletes beyond those that can result from proper nutrition and training basics.

Elite and recreational athletes perform at their best and recover most quickly when they consume a nutritionally adequate diet with sufficient fluids and when they have appropriate physical conditioning and proper training.

## Section 38.2

## *Energy Drinks*

This section includes text excerpted from "Energy Drinks,"
National Center for Complementary and Integrative
Health (NCCIH), October 4, 2017.

Energy drinks are widely promoted as products that increase alertness and enhance physical and mental performance. Marketing targeted at young people has been quite effective. Next to multivitamins, energy drinks are the most popular dietary supplement consumed by American teens and young adults. Males between the ages of 18 and 34 years consume the most energy drinks, and almost one-third of teens between 12 and 17 years drink them regularly.

Caffeine is the major ingredient in most energy drinks—a 24-ounce (oz) energy drink may contain as much as 500 mg of caffeine (similar to that in four or five cups of coffee). Energy drinks also may contain guarana (another source of caffeine sometimes called Brazilian cocoa), sugars, taurine, ginseng, B vitamins, glucuronolactone, Yohimbe, carnitine, and bitter orange.

Consuming energy drinks also increases important safety concerns. Between 2007 and 2011, the overall number of energy-drink-related visits to emergency departments doubled, with the most significant increase (279 percent) in people aged 40 and older. A growing trend among young adults and teens is mixing energy drinks with alcohol. About 25 percent of college students consume alcohol with energy drinks, and they binge-drink significantly more often than students who don't mix them. In 2011, 42 percent of all energy-drink-related emergency department visits involved combining these beverages with alcohol or drugs (including illicit drugs, like marijuana, as well as central nervous systems (CNS) stimulants, like Ritalin, or Adderall).

## Bottom Line

- Although there's very limited data that caffeine-containing energy drinks may temporarily improve alertness and physical endurance, evidence that they enhance strength or power is lacking. More important, they can be dangerous because large amounts of caffeine may cause serious heart rhythm, blood flow, and blood pressure problems.

- There's not enough evidence to determine the effects of additives other than caffeine in energy drinks.

- The amounts of caffeine in energy drinks vary widely, and the actual caffeine content may not be identified easily.

## Safety

- Large amounts of caffeine may cause serious heart and blood vessel problems such as heart rhythm disturbances and increases in heart rate and blood pressure. Caffeine also may harm children's still-developing cardiovascular and nervous systems.

- Caffeine use may be associated with palpitations, anxiety, sleep problems, digestive problems, elevated blood pressure, and dehydration.

- Guarana, commonly added to energy drinks, contains caffeine. Therefore, the addition of guarana increases the drink's total caffeine content.

- Young adults who combine caffeinated drinks with alcohol may not be able to tell how intoxicated they are.

- Excessive energy drink consumption may disrupt teens' sleep patterns and may fuel risk-taking behavior.

- Many energy drinks contain as much as 25–50 g of simple sugars; this may be problematic for people who are diabetic or prediabetic.

# Chapter 39

# Supplements Used for Weight Loss

## Chapter Contents

## Section 39.1

# *Green Tea*

This section includes text excerpted from "Green Tea,"
National Center for Complementary and Integrative
Health (NCCIH), September 2016.

Green, black, and oolong teas all come from the same plant, Camellia sinensis, but are prepared using different methods. To produce green tea, fresh leaves from the plant are lightly steamed. Tea has been used for medicinal purposes in China and Japan for thousands of years. Current uses of green tea as a beverage or dietary supplement include improving mental alertness, relieving digestive symptoms and headaches, and promoting weight loss. Green tea and its extracts, such as one of its components, epigallocatechin gallate (EGCG), have been studied for their possible protective effects against heart disease and cancer.

Green tea is consumed as a beverage. It is also sold in liquid extracts, capsules, and tablets, and is sometimes used in topical products (intended to be applied to the skin).

## *How Much Do We Know?*

Although many studies have been done on green tea and its extracts, definite conclusions cannot yet be reached on whether green tea is helpful for most of the purposes for which it is used.

## *What Have We Learned?*

There's evidence that green tea enhances mental alertness, as would be expected because of its caffeine content. The U.S. Food and Drug Administration (FDA) has approved a specific green tea extract ointment as a prescription drug for treating genital warts. Studies of green tea and cancer in people have had inconsistent results. The National Cancer Institute (NCI) does not recommend for or against using green tea to reduce the risk of any type of cancer. Very few long-term studies have investigated the effects of tea on heart disease risk.

However, the limited evidence currently available suggests that both green and black tea might have beneficial effects on some heart disease risk factors, including blood pressure and cholesterol.

Green tea extracts haven't been shown to produce a meaningful weight loss in overweight or obese adults. They also haven't been shown to help people maintain a weight loss. The National Center for Complementary and Integrative Health (NCCIH) is funding research on green tea and its extracts, including studies of the effects of high doses of tea components on the liver, whether substances in green tea can be helpful for iron overload disease, and the safety of a component of green tea in people who are human immunodeficiency virus (HIV)-positive.

## What Do We Know about Safety?

Green tea, when consumed as a beverage, is believed to be safe when used in moderate amounts. Liver problems have been reported in a small number of people who took concentrated green tea extracts. Although the evidence that the green tea products caused the liver problems is not conclusive, experts suggest that concentrated green tea extracts be taken with food and that people discontinue use and consult a healthcare provider if they have a liver disorder or develop symptoms of liver trouble, such as abdominal pain, dark urine, or jaundice. Except for decaffeinated green tea products, green tea, and green tea extracts contain substantial amounts of caffeine. Too much caffeine can make people feel jittery and shaky; interfere with sleep, and cause headaches.

Green tea has been shown to reduce blood levels (and, therefore, the effectiveness) of the drug nadolol, a beta blocker used for high blood pressure and heart problems. It may also interact with other medicines.

## Keep in Mind

Tell all your healthcare providers about any complementary or integrative health approaches you use. Give them a full picture of what you do to manage your health. This will help ensure coordinated and safe care.

Section 39.2

# *Hoodia*

This section includes text excerpted from "Hoodia," National
Center for Complementary and Integrative
Health (NCCIH), September 2016.

Hoodia is a flowering, cactus-like plant that grows in the Kalahari
Desert in Africa. Historically, the San Bushmen used Hoodia to suppress appetite. Hoodia dietary supplements are used as an appetite
suppressant for weight loss. It is available as liquids, powders, tablets,
and capsules. Some hoodia products also contain other herbs or minerals, such as green tea, or chromium.

## *How Much Do We Know and What Have We Learned?*

We know very little about hoodia because only one study of this herb
has been done in people. In the one small study of hoodia in people,
overweight women who took hoodia for 15 days didn't lose more weight
than those who took a placebo.

## *What Do We Know about Safety?*

Little is known about the safety of hoodia. However, the one completed study in people raises concerns. In that study, participants taking hoodia had more side effects than those taking placebos, including
nausea, vomiting, dizziness, and odd skin sensations; they also had
increases in blood pressure and undesirable changes in some blood
tests. Whether hoodia interacts with medicines or other supplements
is not known.

## *Keep in Mind*

Tell all your healthcare providers about any complementary or
integrative health approaches you use. Give them a full picture of
what you do to manage your health. This will help ensure coordinated
and safe care.

# Chapter 40

# *Using Dietary Supplements Wisely*

Like many Americans, you may take dietary supplements in an effort to stay healthy. With so many dietary supplements available and so many claims made about their health benefits, how can you decide whether a supplement is safe or useful? This chapter provides a general overview of dietary supplements, discusses safety considerations, and suggests sources for additional information.

- Dietary supplements contain a variety of ingredients, such as vitamins, minerals, amino acids, and herbs or other botanicals. Research has confirmed health benefits of some dietary supplements but not others.

- To use dietary supplements safely, read and follow the label instructions, and recognize that "natural" does not always mean "safe." Be aware that an herbal supplement may contain dozens of compounds and that all of its ingredients may not be known.

- Some dietary supplements may interact with medications or pose risks if you have medical problems or are going to have surgery. Most dietary supplements have not been tested in pregnant women, nursing mothers, or children.

---

This chapter includes text excerpted from "Using Dietary Supplements Wisely," National Center for Complementary and Integrative Health (NCCIH), June 2014. Reviewed May 2018.

- The U.S. Food and Drug Administration (FDA) regulates dietary supplements, but the regulations for dietary supplements are different and less strict than those for prescription or over-the-counter (OTC) drugs.

- Tell all your healthcare providers about any complementary health approaches you use. Give them a full picture of what you do to manage your health. This will help ensure coordinated and safe care.

## About Dietary Supplements

Dietary supplements were defined in a law passed by Congress in 1994 called the Dietary Supplement Health and Education Act (DSHEA). According to DSHEA, a dietary supplement is a product that:

- Is intended to supplement the diet

- Contains one or more dietary ingredients (including vitamins, minerals, herbs or other botanicals, amino acids, and certain other substances) or their constituents

- Is intended to be taken by mouth, in forms such as tablet, capsule, powder, softgel, gelcap, or liquid

- Is labeled as being a dietary supplement

Herbal supplements are one type of dietary supplement. An herb is a plant or plant part (such as leaves, flowers, or seeds) that is used for its flavor, scent, and/or potential health-related properties. "Botanical" is often used as a synonym for "herb." An herbal supplement may contain a single herb or mixtures of herbs. The law requires that all of the herbs be listed on the product label.

Research has shown that some uses of dietary supplements are beneficial to health. For example, scientists have found that folic acid (a vitamin) prevents certain birth defects. Other research on dietary supplements has failed to show benefit; for example, several major studies of the herbal supplement echinacea did not find evidence of benefit against the common cold.

## Federal Regulation of Dietary Supplements

The federal government regulates dietary supplements through the FDA. The regulations for dietary supplements are not the same as those for prescription or OTC drugs.

- Manufacturers of dietary supplements are responsible for ensuring that their products are safe and that the label information is truthful and not misleading. However, a manufacturer of a dietary supplement does not have to provide the FDA with data that demonstrate the safety of the product before it is marketed. In contrast, manufacturers of drugs have to provide the FDA with evidence that their products are both safe and effective before the drugs can be sold.

- Manufacturers may make three types of claims for their dietary supplements: health claims, structure/function claims, and nutrient content claims. Some of these claims describe the link between a food substance and a disease or health-related condition; the intended benefits of using the product; or the amount of a nutrient or dietary substance in a product. Different requirements apply to each type of claim. If a dietary supplement manufacturer makes a claim about a product's effects, the manufacturer must have data to support the claim. Claims about how a supplement affects the structure or function of the body must be followed by the words "This statement has not been evaluated by the U.S. Food and Drug Administration (FDA). This product is not intended to diagnose, treat, cure, or prevent any disease."

- Manufacturers must follow "current good manufacturing practices" for dietary supplements to ensure that these products are processed, labeled, and packaged consistently and meet quality standards.

- Once a dietary supplement is on the market, the FDA evaluates safety by doing research and keeping track of any side effects reported by consumers, healthcare providers, and supplement companies. If the FDA finds a product to be unsafe, it can take action against the manufacturer and/or distributor, and may issue a warning or require that the product is removed from the marketplace.

Also, once a dietary supplement is on the market, the FDA monitors product information, such as label claims and package inserts. The Federal Trade Commission (FTC) is responsible for regulating product advertising; it requires that all information be truthful and not misleading. The federal government has taken legal action against dietary supplement promoters or websites that promote or sell dietary supplements for making false or deceptive statements about their products or because marketed products have proven to be unsafe. In 2010, an investigation by the U.S. Government Accountability Office found instances in which written sales materials for herbal dietary supplements sold through online retailers included illegal claims that the products could treat, prevent, or cure diseases such as diabetes, cancer, or cardiovascular disease.

According to the 2007 National Health Interview Survey (NHIS), which included questions on Americans' use of natural products (not including vitamins and minerals), 17.7 percent of American adults had used these types of products in the past 12 months. The most popular of these products used by adults in the past 30 days were fish oil/ omega 3/docosahexaenoic acid (DHA) (37.4 percent), glucosamine (19.9 percent), echinacea (19.8 percent), flaxseed oil, or pills (15.9 percent), and ginseng (14.1 percent). National Health and Nutrition Examination Survey (NHANES) data collected from 2003 to 2006 that covered all types of dietary supplements indicate that 53 percent of American adults took at least one dietary supplement, most commonly multivitamin/multimineral supplements (taken by 39 percent of all adults). Women were more likely than men to take dietary supplements.

## Sources of Science-Based Information

It's important to look for reliable sources of information on dietary supplements so you can evaluate the claims that are made about them. The most reliable information on dietary supplements is based on the results of rigorous scientific testing.

To get reliable information on a particular dietary supplement:

- Ask your healthcare providers. Even if they don't know about a specific dietary supplement, they may be able to access the latest medical guidance about its uses and risks.

- Look for scientific research findings on the dietary supplement. The National Center for Complementary and Integrative Health (NCCIH) and the National Institutes of Health (NIH) Office of Dietary Supplements (ODS), as well as other federal agencies, have free publications, clearinghouses, and information on their websites.

## Safety Considerations

If you're thinking about or currently using a dietary supplement, here are some points to keep in mind.

- Tell all your healthcare providers about any complementary health approaches you use. Give them a full picture of what you do to manage your health. This will help ensure coordinated and safe care.

- It's especially important to talk to your healthcare providers if you:

  - Take any medications (whether prescription or over-the-counter). Some dietary supplements have been found to interact with medications. For example, the herbal supplement St. John's wort interacts with many medications, making them less effective.

  - Are thinking about replacing your regular medication with one or more dietary supplements

  - Expect to have surgery. Certain dietary supplements may increase the risk of bleeding or affect the response to anesthesia.

  - Are pregnant, nursing a baby, attempting to become pregnant, or considering giving a child a dietary supplement. Most dietary supplements have not been tested in pregnant women, nursing mothers, or children.

  - Have any medical conditions. Some dietary supplements may harm you if you have particular medical conditions. For example, by taking supplements that contain iron, people with hemochromatosis, a hereditary disease in which too much iron accumulates in the body, could further increase their iron levels and, therefore, their risk of complications such as liver disease.

- If you're taking a dietary supplement, follow the label instructions. Talk to your healthcare provider if you have any questions, particularly about the best dosage for you to take. If you experience any side effects that concern you, stop taking the dietary supplement, and contact your healthcare provider. You can report serious problems suspected with dietary supplements to the FDA and the NIH through the Safety Reporting Portal.

- Keep in mind that although many dietary supplements (and some prescription drugs) come from natural sources, "natural" does not always mean "safe." For example, the herbs comfrey and kava can cause serious harm to the liver. Also, a manufacturer's use of the term "standardized" (or "verified" or "certified") does not necessarily guarantee product quality or consistency.

- Be aware that an herbal supplement may contain dozens of compounds and that all of its ingredients may not be known. Researchers are studying many of these products in an effort to identify what ingredients may be active and understand their effects on the body. Also, consider the possibility that what's on the label may not be what's in the bottle. Analyses of dietary supplements sometimes find differences between labeled and actual ingredients. For example:

  - An herbal supplement may not contain the correct plant species.

  - The amounts of the ingredients may be lower or higher than the label states. That means you may be taking less—or more—of the dietary supplement than you realize.

  - The dietary supplement may be contaminated with other herbs, pesticides, or metals, or even adulterated with unlabeled, illegal ingredients such as prescription drugs.

# Chapter 41

# *Beware of Fraudulent Dietary Supplements*

Federal regulators continue to warn consumers about tainted, dangerous products that are marketed as dietary supplements. These fraudulent products can cause serious injury or even death.

The U.S. Food and Drug Administration (FDA) has found nearly 300 fraudulent products—promoted mainly for weight loss, sexual enhancement, and bodybuilding—that contain hidden or deceptively labeled ingredients, such as:

- The active ingredients in the FDA-approved drugs or their analogs (closely-related drugs)

- Other compounds, such as novel synthetic steroids, that do not qualify as dietary ingredients

"These products are masquerading as dietary supplements—they may look like dietary supplements but they are not legal dietary supplements," says Michael Levy, director of the FDA's Division of New Drugs and Labeling Compliance (DNDLC). "Some of these products contain hidden prescription ingredients at levels much higher than those found in an approved drug product and are dangerous."

---

This chapter includes text excerpted from "Consumer Updates—Beware of Fraudulent Dietary Supplements," U.S. Food and Drug Administration (FDA), January 23, 2018.

The FDA has received numerous reports of harm associated with the use of these products, including stroke, liver injury, kidney failure, heart palpitations, and death.

## *Advice for Consumers*

"We need consumers to be aware of these dangerous products and to learn how to identify and avoid them," says Levy. Consumers should look for potential warning signs of tainted products marketed as dietary supplements, such as:

- Products claiming to be alternatives to the FDA-approved drugs or to have effects similar to prescription drugs

- Products claiming to be a legal alternative to anabolic steroids

- Products that are marketed primarily in a foreign language or those that are marketed through mass Emails

- Sexual enhancement products promising rapid effects, such as working in minutes to hours, or long-lasting effects, such as working for 24–72 hours

- Product labels warning that you may test positive in performance enhancement drug tests

Generally, if you are using or considering using any product marketed as a dietary supplement, the FDA suggests that you:

- Check with your healthcare professional or a registered dietician about any nutrients you may need in addition to your regular diet.

- Ask your healthcare professional for help distinguishing between reliable and questionable information.

- Ask yourself if it sounds too good to be true.

- Be cautious if the claims for the product seem exaggerated or unrealistic.

- Watch out for extreme claims—for example, "quick and effective," "cure-all," "can treat or cure diseases," or "totally safe."

- Be skeptical about anecdotal information from personal "testimonials" about incredible benefits or results obtained from using a product.

- See the FDA's website to help recognize fraudulent weight-loss products and claims.

If you suspect a dietary supplement sold online may be illegal, the FDA urges you to report that information online. In addition, you or your healthcare professional can also report an illness or injury you believe to be related to the use of a dietary supplement by phone at 1-800-FDA-1088 or online.

## Dietary Supplements and the U.S. Food and Drug Administration (FDA)

Dietary supplements, in general, are not the FDA-approved. Under the law (Dietary Supplement Health and Education Act (DSHEA) of 1994), dietary supplement firms do not need the FDA's approval prior to marketing their products. It is the company's responsibility to make sure its products are safe and that any claims are true.

Just because you see a supplement product on a store shelf does NOT mean it is safe or effective. When safety issues are suspected, the FDA must investigate and, when warranted, take steps to have the product removed from the market. However, it is much easier for a firm to get a product on the market than it is for the FDA to take a product off the market.

The FDA has worked with industry to recall numerous products with potentially harmful ingredients including:

- More than 40 products marketed for weight loss

- More than 70 products marketed for sexual enhancement

- More than 80 products marketed for bodybuilding

The FDA last alerted the public to tainted products in December 2010, and will continue to issue consumer alerts and press announcements about these products. The FDA has issued warning letters, seized products, and conducted criminal prosecutions. In December 2010, a woman pleaded guilty to an 18-count indictment charging her with the illegal importation and distribution of more than four million diet pills that contained a controlled substance, unapproved drugs, and a possible cancer-causing agent.

Remember, the FDA cannot test all products on the market to identify those that contain potentially harmful hidden ingredients. Consumers must also be aware of these dangerous products and learn how to identify and avoid them using the warning signs described above.

## Keep Up-to-Date on Tainted Products

Get the latest news on tainted products by using the FDA's "widget" and "RSS (Really Simple Syndication) feed." Both of these online tools contain alerts, health information, and the FDA actions on tainted products marketed as dietary supplements.

A widget is a portable application that displays featured content directly on a webpage. Bloggers or owners of websites can embed this content into their sites. Once the FDA's widget is added, there's no technical maintenance—the FDA will automatically provide updates to content displayed on the widget.

The RSS feed, like the widget, includes updated content published on the FDA's website. RSS is usually used for news and blog websites and requires an RSS news reader (a special software program) to pick up the content in the feed. Organizations and bloggers can subscribe to the RSS feed to receive updates automatically and put together their own customized lists of news and information.

# Part Four


# Biologically Based Therapies

# Chapter 42

# *Biologically Based Therapies: An Overview*

## Chapter Contents

## Section 42.1

# *Aromatherapy and Essential Oils*

This section includes text excerpted from "Aromatherapy and
Essential Oils (PDQ®)—Patient Version," National
Cancer Institute (NCI), February 23, 2018.

### *About Aromatherapy*

Aromatherapy is the use of essential oils from plants to improve
the mind, body, and spirit. It is used by patients with cancer to
improve quality of life and reduce stress, anxiety, nausea, and vomiting caused by cancer and its treatment. Aromatherapy may be
used with other complementary treatments like massage therapy,
and acupuncture, as well as with standard treatments, for symptom
management.

### *About Essential Oils*

Essential oils (also known as volatile oils) are the fragrant (aro-
matic) part found in many plants, often under the surface of leaves,
bark, or peel. The fragrance is released if the plant is crushed or a
special steam process is used. There are many essential oils used in
aromatherapy, including those from Roman chamomile, geranium,
lavender, tea tree, lemon, ginger, cedarwood, and bergamot. Each
plant's essential oil has a different chemical makeup that affects how
it smells, how it is absorbed, and how it affects the body.

Essential oils are very concentrated. For example, it takes about
220 pounds of lavender flowers to make about 1 pound of essential oil.
The aroma of essential oils fades away quickly when left open to air.

### *How Is Aromatherapy Given or Taken?*

Aromatherapy is used in several ways. It includes:

- Indirect inhalation. The patient breathes in an essential oil by
  using a room diffuser, which spreads the essential oil through
  the air, or by placing drops nearby.

- Direct inhalation. The patient breathes in an essential oil by using an individual inhaler made by floating essential oil drops on top of hot water.

- Massage. In aromatherapy massage, one or more essential oils are diluted into a carrier oil and massaged into the skin.

Essential oils may also be mixed with bath salts and lotions, or applied to bandages.

There are some essential oils used to treat specific conditions. However, the types of essential oils used and the ways they are combined may vary, depending on the experience and training of the aromatherapist.

## Preclinical (Laboratory or Animal) Studies on Using Aromatherapy

In laboratory studies, tumor cells are used to test a substance to find out if it is likely to have any anticancer effects. In animal studies, tests are done to see if a drug, procedure, or treatment is safe and effective in animals. Laboratory and animal studies are done before a substance is tested in people. Laboratory and animal studies have tested the effects of essential oils.

## Clinical Trials (Research Studies with People) on Using Aromatherapy

Clinical trials of aromatherapy have studied its use in the treatment of anxiety, nausea, vomiting, and other health-related conditions in cancer patients. No studies of aromatherapy used to treat cancer have been published in a peer-reviewed scientific journal. Studies of aromatherapy massage or inhalation have had mixed results. There have been some reports of improved mood, anxiety, sleep, nausea, and pain. Other studies reported that aromatherapy showed no change in symptoms.

A trial of 103 cancer patients studied the effects of massage compared to massage with Roman chamomile essential oil. A decrease in anxiety and improved symptoms were noted in the group that had massage with essential oil. The group that had massage only did not have the same benefit.

A study of inhaled ginger essential oil in women receiving chemotherapy for breast cancer showed improvements in acute nausea, but no improvement in vomiting or chronic nausea.

A study of inhaled bergamot essential oil in children and adolescents at the time of stem cell infusion reported an increase in anxiety and nausea and no effect on pain. In a study of adult patients at the time of stem cell infusion, tasting, or sniffing sliced oranges was more effective at reducing nausea, retching, and coughing than inhaling an orange essential oil.

A study of tea tree essential oil as a topical treatment to clear antibiotic-resistant methicillin-resistant *Staphylococcus aureus* (MRSA) bacteria from the skin of hospital patients found that it was as effective as the standard ointment.

## Side Effects or Risks from Aromatherapy

Safety testing on essential oils shows very few side effects or risks when they are used as directed. Most essential oils have been approved as ingredients in food and fragrances and are labeled as GRAS (generally recognized as safe) by the U.S. Food and Drug Administration (FDA). Swallowing large amounts of essential oils is not recommended.

Allergic reactions and skin irritation may occur when essential oils are in contact with the skin for long periods of time. Sun sensitivity may occur when citrus or other essential oils are applied to the skin before going out in the sun.

Lavender and tea tree essential oils have been found to have effects similar to estrogen (female sex hormone) and also block or decrease the effect of androgens (male sex hormones). Applying lavender and tea tree essential oils to the skin over a long period of time was linked in one study to breast growth in boys who had not yet reached puberty.

## Status of Aromatherapy Approved for Use as a Cancer Treatment in the United States

Aromatherapy products do not need FDA approval. Aromatherapy is not regulated by state law, and there is no licensing required to practice aromatherapy in the United States. Practitioners often combine aromatherapy training with another field in which they are licensed, for example, massage therapy, nursing, acupuncture, or naturopathy.

# Section 42.2

# *Oxygen Therapy*

This section contains text excerpted from the following sources: Text beginning with the heading "Oxygen" is excerpted from "Oxygen Therapy," MedlinePlus, National Institutes of Health (NIH), November 14, 2016; Text beginning with the heading "How Is Oxygen Therapy Administered?" is excerpted from "Oxygen Therapy," National Heart, Lung, and Blood Institute (NHLBI), December 26, 2012. Reviewed May 2018.

## *Oxygen*

Oxygen is a gas that your body needs to function. Normally, your lungs absorb oxygen from the air you breathe. But some conditions can prevent you from getting enough oxygen. You may need oxygen if you have:

- Chronic obstructive pulmonary disease (COPD)

- Pneumonia

- A severe asthma attack

- Late-stage heart failure

- Cystic fibrosis (CF)

- Sleep apnea

## *What Is Oxygen Therapy?*

Oxygen therapy is a treatment that provides you with extra oxygen. A different kind of oxygen therapy is called hyperbaric oxygen therapy. It uses oxygen at high pressure to treat wounds and serious infections.

## *How Is Oxygen Therapy Administered?*

You can receive oxygen therapy from tubes resting in your nose, a face mask, or a tube placed in your trachea, or windpipe. This treatment increases the amount of oxygen your lungs receive and deliver to your blood. Oxygen therapy may be prescribed for you when you have a condition that causes your blood oxygen levels to be too low. Low blood oxygen may make you feel short of breath, tired, or confused, and can damage your body.

Oxygen therapy can be given for a short or long period of time in the hospital, another medical setting, or at home. Oxygen is stored as a gas or liquid in special tanks. These tanks can be delivered to your home and contain a certain amount of oxygen that will require refills. Another device for use at home is an oxygen concentrator, which pulls oxygen out of the air for immediate use. Because oxygen concentrators do not require refills, they won't run out of oxygen. Portable tanks and oxygen concentrators may make it easier for you to move around while using your therapy.

### Are There Any Risks?

Oxygen poses a fire risk, so you should never smoke or use flammable materials when using oxygen. You may experience side effects from this treatment, such as a dry or bloody nose, tiredness, and morning headaches. Oxygen therapy is generally safe.

## Section 42.3

## *Hyperbaric Oxygen Therapy: Don't Be Misled*

This section includes text excerpted from "For Consumers—Hyperbaric Oxygen Therapy: Don't Be Misled," U.S. Food and Drug Administration (FDA), January 4, 2018.

Hyperbaric oxygen therapy (HBOT) has not been clinically proven to cure or be effective in the treatment of cancer, autism, or diabetes. But do a quick search on the Internet, and you'll see all kinds of claims for these and other diseases for which the device has not been cleared or approved by the U.S. Food and Drug Administration (FDA). HBOT involves breathing oxygen in a pressurized chamber. The FDA has cleared hyperbaric chambers for certain medical uses, such as treating decompression sickness suffered by divers.

HBOT has not, however, been proven to be the kind of universal treatment it has been touted to be on some Internet sites. The FDA is concerned that some claims made by treatment centers using HBOT may give consumers a wrong impression that could ultimately endanger their health. "Patients may incorrectly believe that these devices have been proven safe and effective for uses not cleared by the FDA, which may cause them to delay or forgo proven medical therapies," says Nayan Patel, a biomedical engineer in the FDA's Anesthesiology Devices Branch (ADB). "In doing so, they may experience a lack of improvement and/or worsening of their existing condition(s)."

Patients may be unaware that the safety and effectiveness of HBOT has not been established for these diseases and conditions, including:

- Acquired immunodeficiency syndrome (AIDS)/ human immunodeficiency virus (HIV)

- Alzheimer disease (AD)

- Asthma

- Bell palsy

- Brain injury

- Cerebral palsy (CP)

- Depression

- Heart disease

- Hepatitis

- Migraine

- Multiple sclerosis (MS)

- Parkinson disease (PD0

- Spinal cord injury (SCI)

- Sport's injury

- Stroke

Patel says that the FDA has received 27 complaints from consumers and healthcare professionals over the past three years about treatment centers promoting the hyperbaric chamber for uses not cleared by the FDA.

## How HBOT Works

HBOT involves breathing oxygen in a pressurized chamber in which the atmospheric pressure is raised up to three times higher than normal. Under these conditions, your lungs can gather up to three times more oxygen than would be possible breathing oxygen at normal air pressure. Patel explains that your body's tissues need an adequate supply of oxygen to function. When tissue is injured, it may require more oxygen to heal. "HBOT increases the amount of oxygen dissolved in your blood," says Patel. An increase in blood oxygen may improve oxygen delivery for vital tissue function to help fight infection or minimize injury.

Hyperbaric chambers are medical devices that require the FDA clearance. FDA clearance of a device for a specific use means the FDA has reviewed valid scientific evidence supporting that use and determined that the device is at least as safe and effective as another legally U.S.-marketed device. Thirteen uses of a hyperbaric chamber for HBOT have been cleared by the FDA. They include treatment of air or gas embolism (dangerous "bubbles" in the bloodstream that obstruct circulation), carbon monoxide poisoning, decompression sickness (often known by divers as "the bends"), and thermal burns (caused by heat or fire).

## What Are the Risks?

Patients receiving HBOT are at risk of suffering an injury that can be mild (such as sinus pain, ear pressure, painful joints) or serious (such as paralysis, air embolism). Since hyperbaric chambers are oxygen-rich environments, there is also a risk of fire. "If you're considering using HBOT, it's essential that you first discuss all possible options with your healthcare professional," Patel says. "Whatever treatment you're getting, you need to understand its benefits and risks. Your healthcare professional can help you determine which treatment is your best option."

# Chapter 43

# *Apitherapy*

Modern medicine is increasingly focusing on the use of natural and biological products in clinical practice. Apitherapy is one example. Described as a traditional medicine that uses products from the honeybee hive—honey, bee pollen, propolis, royal jelly, and bee venom—apitherapy has been in use for centuries and may be as old as human medicine itself. Beehive products have been used for prophylaxis treatment and to treat various conditions.

The immune-boosting properties of honey are believed to make it an excellent tonic for maintaining general health and well-being. The earliest reference to the use of apitherapy can be traced to the thirty-first century, in ancient Egypt. Ancient Greeks and Romans also believed in the curative properties of honey and other hive products. Prescriptions dating back to the third century establish the use of honey in traditional Chinese medicine, and various civilizations around the world have used bee-sting therapy to treat several diseases. Hippocrates, a Greek physician and father of modern medicine, also described the nutritional and therapeutic uses of beehive products.

## *Bee Products in Traditional Medicine*

Folk medicine has used bee products to treat a multitude of medical conditions, including neurological disorders (multiple sclerosis, Lou Gehrig disease, and shingles) and immune system dysfunction

"Apitherapy," © 2018 Omnigraphics. Reviewed May 2018.

(rheumatoid arthritis, gout, and allergies). Beehive products have also been used widely to treat musculoskeletal diseases (such as bursitis or tendinitis). Respiratory illnesses (such as a recalcitrant cough, cold, and tuberculosis) have been traditionally treated using apitherapy. In addition, gastrointestinal disorders, infections, cancer, tumors, pain, burns, and trauma have all been treated with alternative practices involving beehive products.

Hive product preparations are available over the counter (OTC) and typically combine two or more hive products, depending on the condition being treated. They are usually prepared as a dietary supplement and come in the form of liquids, tablets, liniment, sprays, and suppositories. Some formulations also contain essential oils, herbs, or other natural ingredients or biologicals.

## Some Important Products of the Hive

### Honey

Honey is a sweet, viscous liquid regurgitated by bees and a few other insects. It contains the floral nectar of plants. Stored in waxy colony cells called honeycombs, raw honey—particularly the type secreted by a member of the genus *Apis*—has been widely used as a potent internal and topical medicine for thousands of years by various cultures.

Honey is orally ingested to relieve dyspepsia, insomnia, anorexia, constipation, osteoporosis, cholesterolemia, and laryngitis. Its hydrophilic nature attracts water molecules and makes it unavailable for microbial growth. This may explain the antimicrobial properties attributed to honey.

When externally applied, honey is believed to help treat athlete's foot, eczema, wounds, and abscesses. Honey is also an excellent source of readily digestible sugars (fructose and glucose) and can serve as a quick source of energy. It is also rich in a variety of important vitamins, minerals, and antioxidants, which makes it a valuable nutritional supplement.

Some studies show synergy between honey and certain beneficial bacteria in the colon. It has been suggested that short-chain carbohydrate compounds in honey stimulate the growth of useful gut flora, help to maintain the health of the gastrointestinal tract, and confer prebiotic effects—making honey a popular functional food with physiological benefits.

### Bee Pollen

Often called "bee bread," pollen is the male germ cells of seed plants and a major protein source for bees. It is a rich source of enzymes, phytochemicals, and antioxidants and has been used in traditional medicine for its anti-inflammatory, anti-arthritic, and anti-cancer properties. Reportedly, bee pollen has been used to treat a variety of other medical conditions, including varicose veins, hypercholesterolemia, fatigue, infertility, anorexia, obesity, hypertension, gastrointestinal disturbances, prostatitis, and depression. Pollen is also recommended for reducing scar formation and hastening recovery from surgery.

### *Propolis*

Also called "bee glue," propolis is made by bees from a plant or tree resins and serves as an anti-infective agent to protect the colony from harmful microorganisms. Propolis has been used in folk medicine as a detoxifying agent. The flavonoid compounds present in propolis are known for their antioxidant activity and anti-inflammatory properties. Some studies have also attributed propolis with some tissue regenerative/anti-aging effects.

Before the advent of antibiotics, propolis was used as an anti-infective salve to prevent infection of wounds, burns, and other skin lesions. It also finds use as a mouthwash to treat halitosis (bad breath), gingivitis, or tooth decay. Propolis can help with the symptoms associated with arthritis, boils, acne, asthma, dermatitis, ulcers, and inflammatory bowel diseases as well. Some herbalists also recommend propolis for its antimutagenic effects and possible role in cancer prevention. In conjunction with royal jelly, propolis is used to ameliorate the side effects of chemo and radiation therapies.

### *Bee Venom*

Secreted from glands associated with the sting apparatus of worker bees, bee venom is believed to have beneficial effects in treating a large number of ailments and has been used by many ancient civilizations. Comprising a complex mixture of proteins, bee venom is reported to possess antibacterial and antiviral, antithrombotic, and anti-inflammatory effects. Bee venom is also used in alternative medicine to ameliorate conditions such as fibromyalgia, rheumatoid arthritis, and irritable bowel syndrome. While there are various claims on the efficacy of bee venom in treating a variety of conditions, most are considered unsubstantiated because of a lack of sufficient research.

Bee venom immunotherapy is the only FDA-approved apitherapy and is used for desensitization in persons with allergic reactions to a bee sting. A subcutaneous injection of purified bee venom provides nearly 99 percent protection from adverse reactions to bee stings.

## Royal Jelly

A milky substance produced by nurse bees to initially feed bee larvae, and later to feed only the queen bee-designated larva, royal jelly has played a significant role in traditional Chinese medicine and continues to be widely used as a therapeutic agent for a variety of conditions, including anxiety, depression, arthritis, arteriosclerosis, asthma, impaired libido, hair loss, and insomnia. Folk medicine also prescribes royal jelly for varicose veins, weakened immune systems, abnormal blood pressure, and menopausal symptoms. Rich in B vitamins, royal jelly is considered to enhance metabolism, and its antioxidant qualities are believed to have an inhibitory effect on free radical formation, one of the major risk factors for carcinogenicity. Royal jelly is also an ingredient in several dermatologic products because of its perceived ability to promote synthesis of collagen, the main structural protein in skin.

## Apitherapy in Modern Medicine

Studies in modern medicine have attributed certain anti-inflammatory and antimicrobial characteristics to honey. Bee honey as well as other hive products, including royal jelly, propolis, and venom have been shown to play a role as immune system stimulants. Controlled clinical trials have also shown honey to be a promising treatment in chronic wound healing. While proponents of apitherapy have attributed a multitude of health benefits to beehive products, these claims, for the most part, remain unsubstantiated by evidence-based medicine and require high-quality research to confirm the efficacy and safety of apitherapy in clinical practice.

## Who Practices Apitherapy

Apitherapy is typically practiced by beekeepers who can offer advice on the science and art of beekeeping, provide people with beehive product, and instruct them on how to use beehive products for therapeutic purposes. Trained practitioners, such as physicians, nurses, acupuncturists, or naturopaths may also provide apitherapy.

## Health Risks Associated with Apitherapy

Adverse events related to bee venom therapy have been reported, making it an unsafe alternative medicine to treat conditions such as multiple sclerosis. Contact with venom is also known to set off allergic reactions ranging from local swelling to life-threatening anaphylactic shock, multiple organ failures, or even death.

## References

1.  "Bee Venom an Effective Potential for Bacteria," U.S. National Library of Medicine (NLM), September 19, 2016.

2.  "Apitherapy," American Apitherapy Society, September 15, 2011.

# Chapter 44

# *Diet-Based Therapies*

## *Chapter Contents*

# Section 44.1

# *Popular Fad Diets*

"Popular Fad Diets,"
© 2015 Omnigraphics. Reviewed May 2018.

## Introduction to Popular Fad Diets

The many popular diets and diet plans on the market today can be confusing and overwhelming for consumers to navigate. People who want to lose weight are bombarded with advertisements for various diets all claiming to provide the secret to rapid weight loss with little or no effort. Some of these diets eliminate or restrict various foods, while others focus on including only certain foods. A diet can be considered a fad if it promises to deliver drastic weight loss in a short amount of time, without exercise, and if it is based on an unbalanced approach to nutrition. Many popular fad diets can be organized by type: high protein, low carbohydrate, fasting, food-specific, liquid only, and so on.

## High-Protein Diets

High-protein diets promote an eating plan based largely on foods containing protein, usually meat, eggs, cheese, and other dairy products. The theory behind high-protein diets is that the body must work harder to digest protein, and in doing so, more calories are burned. Studies have found that diets high in protein can cause certain health problems, as the body works to process excess protein. High-protein diets can cause rapid initial weight loss as the body eliminates water while processing extra protein. Typically, any weight lost on a high-protein diet will be regained.

## Low-Carbohydrate Diets

The main premise of low-carbohydrate diets is the severe restriction of calories from carbohydrates (sugar). Most low-carbohydrate diets suggest replacing foods high in carbohydrates with foods high in protein. In this way, low-carbohydrate diets are similar to high-protein diets. A low-carbohydrate diet is often high in fat. A high-fat diet causes a condition known as ketosis, which can act as an appetite suppressant. The theory of low-carbohydrate diets is that the suppressed appetite will result in the dieter consuming fewer calories overall. Studies of low-carbohydrate diets have shown that dieters are at risk for health problems including kidney malfunction and heart disease. Many people who follow a low-carbohydrate diet report feeling sluggish and tired, and typically any weight that is lost will be regained.

## Detoxifying Diets

Detoxifying diets are often high-fiber diets, and sometimes include increased consumption of fats and oils. The theory of this type of detoxification is that the fiber helps the dieter to feel full, thereby consuming fewer calories throughout the day. It is also believed that a high-fiber diet will cleanse the digestive system through the elimination of more solid waste. Side effects of a high-fiber detoxifying diet often include gastrointestinal distress, bloating, cramps, and dehydration. Studies have shown no permanent weight loss from this type of detoxifying diet.

## Fasting Diets

Fasting diets require dieters to consume nothing but clear liquids for a short period of time, typically one to five days. This is believed to help rid the body of toxins. Fasting can result in temporary weight loss due to consuming far fewer calories than normal, though the weight generally returns once the fast is ended. Fasting produces a host of side effects, including dizziness, lethargy, and feeling weak or tired.

## Food-Specific Diets

Food-specific diets recommend consumption of a single type of food, such as grapefruit, cabbage, or protein shakes. These diets are based on the theory that certain foods have special properties that promote weight-loss. Food-specific diets do not provide the range of vitamins, minerals, and other nutrients needed to support bodily functions. If maintained over an extended period of time, the side effects of food-specific diets can be serious.

## Popular Diet Plans

### The Atkins Diet

The Atkins Diet is a low-carbohydrate, high-protein diet created by Dr. Robert Atkins, an American cardiologist. The main premise of the Atkins Diet is that eating too many carbohydrates causes obesity and other health problems. A diet that is low in carbohydrates produces metabolic activity that results in less hunger and also in weight loss. The Atkins Diet is structured in four phases: induction; weight loss; premaintenance; lifetime maintenance. Dieters move through the four phases at their own pace. Early phases of the Atkins Diet allow consumption of seafood, poultry, meat, eggs, cheese, salad vegetables, oils, butter, and cream. Later phases allow consumption of foods such as nuts, fruits, wine, beans, whole grains, and other vegetables. The Atkins Diet recommends avoidance of certain foods such as fruit, bread, most grains, starchy vegetables, and dairy products other than cheese, cream, and butter. The Atkins Diet may help people feel full longer, and may result in weight loss as long as the diet is continued. Side effects may result from consuming low amounts of fiber and certain vitamins and minerals, while consuming larger amounts of saturated fat, cholesterol, and red meat.

### The Zone Diet

The Zone Diet was created by Dr. Barry Spears and is based on the genetic evolution of humans. The main premise of the Zone Diet is that humans should maintain a diet similar to that of our ancient hunter-gatherer ancestors. The Zone Diet focuses on lean protein, natural carbohydrates (fruit) and natural fiber (vegetables) while avoiding or eliminating processed carbohydrates such as grains and products made from grains. The Zone Diet recommends a food plan that is made up of 40 percent natural carbohydrates. 30 percent fat, and 30 percent protein. The emphasis is on food choices, not amount of calories. This percentage should apply to every meal and snack that is eaten. Close evaluation of the Zone Diet has revealed that at its core, the Zone Diet is a very low-calorie eating plan that is lacking in certain nutrients, vitamins, and minerals.

### Weight Watchers

Weight Watchers was founded by Jean Nidetch in 1963. The Weight Watchers program focuses on weight loss through diet, exercise, and the use of support networks. Members are given the option of joining a group or following the program online. In either case, educational materials and support are available to assist members. The Weight Watchers support network is considered a critical aspect of the program, as it is believed that dieters need constant positive reinforcement in order to achieve and maintain long-term weight loss. The Weight Watchers program is structured in two phases: weight loss and maintenance. During weight loss, dieters work to lose weight slowly, with the goal of one to two pounds per week. Once the goal weight has been attained, dieters move into the maintenance phase, during which they gradually adjust their food intake until they are neither losing nor gaining weight. In general, Weight Watchers is viewed as providing a healthy approach to dieting.

## Ornish Lifestyle Medicine

The Ornish Lifestyle Medicine program was created by Dr. Dean Ornish. The main premise of the program is that foods are neither good nor bad, but some are healthier than others. The Ornish diet focuses on fruits, vegetables, whole grains, legumes, soy products, nonfat dairy, natural egg whites, and fats that contain omega three fatty acids. The Ornish diet is plant-based; meat, poultry, and fish are excluded. Portion control is recommended, but caloric intake is not restricted unless a person is trying to lose weight. The program recommends small, frequent meals spread out throughout the day to support constant energy and avoid hunger. The consumption of caffeine is discouraged though allowed in small amounts. The Ornish program recommends exercise and low-dose multivitamin supplements. In general, the Ornish program is viewed as a healthy diet.

## Diet Safety

Fad diets may produce initial weight loss results, but the potential for undesirable side effects should not be ignored. The human body needs simple carbohydrates (glucose) for energy and brain function. Low-carbohydrate and high-protein diets are not nutritionally balanced enough to meet the needs of children and some adults, particularly women who are pregnant, plan to become pregnant, or are nursing a baby. If maintained for an extended period of time, high-protein, low-carbohydrate diets can result in health problems such as heart disease, kidney problems, and certain cancers.

351

Weight loss is achieved by eating fewer calories than are consumed by physical activity. Because most fad diets require people to consume very few calories, these diets can result in weight loss. However, because most fad diets are not nutritionally balanced and cannot be maintained for long periods of time, people usually find that any weight lost is regained once they stop following the diet and return to their old eating habits. The most effective weight-loss strategies are those that include a healthy, balanced diet combined with exercise.

### References

1. "Diet Fads vs. Diet Truths," January 2004.

2. Nordqvist, Christian. "The Eight Most Popular Diets Today," Medical News Today, October 1, 2015.

3. "Nutrition Fact Sheet," Alaska Department of State Health Services, Nutrition Services Section, 2005.

## Section 44.2

# *Detoxification Diets*

Detoxification is concerned with identifying and eliminating toxic substances that may accumulate in the human body. It is a common technique used in alternative medicine for the purpose of curing disease and improving general health. Detoxification has been used for centuries by practitioners of the Ayurvedic and Chinese medical systems, who have taught that eating certain types of food can help eliminate toxins from the body and restore good health. Complementary and alternative medicine (CAM) practitioners often recommend detoxification therapies for people with allergies, anxiety, asthma, cancer, depression, diabetes, headaches, heart disease, obesity, and other chronic conditions. People who are exposed to high levels of toxic substances in the environment due to industrial accidents or pollution may also benefit from detoxification therapy.

Detoxification programs have increased in popularity in recent years. The trend may have started with celebrities touting the benefits of various regimens designed to cleanse the body of chemicals and impurities, cure chronic illnesses, promote weight loss, or end addictions. Such programs have quickly gained adherents among ordinary people hoping to reverse the ill effects of fast food, sugar, caffeine, and other dietary excesses. Detoxification has emerged as a major nutrition and health industry worldwide, with hundreds of different diets, supplements, and holiday retreats promising to help people cleanse their bodies of toxins. The options range from simple diets based on cucumber or grapefruit juice to elaborate vacation packages offering fasts, mud baths, and colonic irrigation. Many people sign up for detoxification therapies as inpatients in order to speed up the process and gain the reassurance of having a practitioner monitor their treatment.

## The Idea behind Detoxification

From pollution in the air to pesticides on crops and growth hormones in meat, people are exposed to a wide variety of organic pollutants and chemical contaminants every day. While the human body naturally eliminates many harmful substances in wastes, some toxic substances can build up in fat cells and other living tissues. Heavy metals, persistent organic pollutants, and fat-soluble chemicals, for instance, tend to bioaccumulate and remain in the body's cells for a long time. The buildup of toxins can contribute to serious physiological problems, including cancer and diseases of the kidneys, liver, lungs, and heart. Detoxification programs attempt to address these problems by ridding the body of toxins that pose health risks. Detoxification thus holds an obvious appeal for many people. They like the idea that following a special diet can remove harmful substances from the body and eliminate the health risks associated with them.

## The Science behind Detoxification

The mainstream medical community, however, tends to regard detoxification as a myth. Although toxins are undoubtedly present in the environment, they argue that the body is capable of eliminating those encountered by a typical person through natural mechanisms involving the skin, lungs, liver, and kidneys. If a person is exposed to such high levels of toxic substances that their bodily systems cannot process and eliminate them, then they are likely to require medical attention. Critics say that there is no scientific evidence to substantiate the lofty claims made by promoters of various detoxification programs. They argue that no special diet, supplement, or regimen can eliminate all toxins from the body, and that most of these programs are unlikely to lead to significant improvements in health. Critics point out that the makers of detoxification products—ranging from smoothies to shampoos—do not specify exactly what toxins the products purportedly eliminate. As a result, a patient's bodily levels of these toxins cannot be measured before and after they undergo treatment in order to prove the products' efficacy. The only kind of medically validated detoxification programs are those intended to help people overcome alcohol or drug addictions.

## Types of Detoxification Programs

Although there are many different detoxification diets and programs available, most are based on the same principles. They encourage people to restrict their exposure to chemicals for a specific period of time (usually 5–7 days) while also consuming foods or supplements that are believed to stimulate the release of stored toxins from the body. Many detoxification diets begin with a period of fasting, which is intended to rest the organs and reset the digestive system. Ancient Chinese and Ayurvedic medical traditions claim that regular fasting cleanses the digestive tract and enhances health and longevity.

Rather than restricting food intake in general, other detoxification diets focus on eliminating certain foods that are believed to increase the toxin load in the body—such alcohol, caffeine, refined sugar, saturated fats, and processed grains. Along the same lines, some detoxification programs recommend minimizing exposure to household cleaners, personal care products, lawn treatments, and other common environmental sources of toxic chemicals, and replacing them with natural alternatives when possible.

After reducing the exposure to toxins, the next step in many detoxification programs involves stimulating the body to eliminate built-up toxins from the organs and tissues. Common strategies for achieving this goal include drinking lots of water to improve kidney function, eating foods high in fiber to improve colon function, exercising to increase blood circulation, sitting in a sauna to excrete toxins through sweating, getting a massage to release toxins in muscles and fat tissues, and exfoliating to remove dead skin.

Finally, many detoxification programs recommend refueling the body with healthy nutrients. Although countless detox diet plans exist, most tend to emphasize a high-fiber diet full of organic fruits and vegetables and lots of water. Some programs promote the use of dietary supplements to aid in the detoxification process. Many of these supplements are diuretics or laxatives made from herbal extracts. They should be used with care, as diuretics can cause dehydration and fatigue, while laxatives can lead to frequent bowel movements and malabsorption of nutrients.

## The Pros and Cons of Detoxification

Despite the disapproval of the mainstream medical community, millions of people try detoxification programs each year, and some of them swear that they lose weight, feel better, or experience other health benefits. Some aspects of the typical detox diet can lead to healthier food choices and more mindful eating. Many people abstain from alcohol, tobacco, and caffeine during detoxification, for instance, and increase their consumption of fruits, vegetables, whole grains, and water. Completing a detoxification program can help people break bad eating habits by retraining the palate to enjoy whole foods and reject processed foods. It can also help people recover from disorders like emotional eating or binge eating.

By temporarily limiting food choices, detox diets can also help people consume fewer calories and lose weight. In many cases, though, the weight loss takes the form of water and stored glycogen, and people will typically regain the pounds once they resume a normal eating pattern. The restrictions in some detoxification plans can also create nutritional deficiencies, especially for teenagers, pregnant or lactating women, or people with health conditions like diabetes or cardiovascular disease. Doctors warn that detox diets—and especially those that involve fasting—can be harmful to the health and well-being of these groups of people. Finally, detoxification programs and supplements can be very expensive.

### References

1. Smith, Deborahann. "10 Ways to Detoxify Your Body," *Gaiam Life*, 2014.

2. Torrens, Kerry. "What Is a Detox Diet?" *BBC GoodFood*, n.d.

# Section 44.3

# *Gerson Therapy*

This section includes text excerpted from "Gerson Therapy (PDQ®)—
Patient Version," National Cancer Institute (NCI), January 7, 2015.

The Gerson therapy has been used by some people to treat cancer
and other diseases. It is based on the role of minerals, enzymes, and
other dietary factors.

There are 3 key parts to the Gerson therapy:

- **Diet.** Organic fruits, vegetables, and whole grains to give the
  body plenty of vitamins, minerals, enzymes, and other nutrients.
  The fruits and vegetables are low in sodium (salt) and high in
  potassium.

- **Supplementation.** The addition of certain substances to the
  diet to help correct cell metabolism (the chemical changes that
  take place in a cell to make energy and basic materials needed
  for the body's life processes).

- **Detoxification.** It involves treatments, including enemas, to
  remove toxic (harmful) substances from the body.

## *Gerson Therapy as a Complementary or Alternative Treatment for Cancer*

The Gerson therapy was named after Dr. Max B. Gerson (1881–
1959), who first used it to treat his migraine headaches. In the 1930's,
Dr. Gerson's therapy became known to the public as a treatment for a
type of tuberculosis (TB). The Gerson therapy was later used to treat
other conditions, including cancer.

## *Theory behind the Claim That the Gerson Therapy Is Useful in Treating Cancer*

The Gerson therapy is based on the idea that cancer develops when
there are changes in cell metabolism because of the buildup of toxic

substances in the body. Dr. Gerson said the disease process makes more toxins and the liver becomes overworked. According to Dr. Gerson, people with cancer also have too much sodium and too little potassium in the cells in their bodies, which causes tissue damage and weakened organs.

The goal of the Gerson therapy is to restore the body to health by repairing the liver and returning the metabolism to its normal state. According to Dr. Gerson, this can be done by removing toxins from the body and building up the immune system with diet and supplements. The enemas are said to widen the bile ducts of the liver so toxins can be released. According to Dr. Gerson, the liver is further overworked as the treatment regimen breaks down cancer cells and rids the body of toxins. Pancreatic enzymes are given to decrease the demands on the weakened liver and pancreas to make enzymes for digestion. An organic diet and nutritional supplements are used to boost the immune system and support the body as the regimen cleans the body of toxins. Foods low in sodium and high in potassium are said to help correct the tissue damage caused by having too much sodium in the cells.

## How Gerson Therapy Is Administered

The Gerson therapy requires that the many details of its treatment plan be followed exactly. Some key parts of the regimen include the following:

- Drinking 13 glasses of juice a day. The juice must be freshly made from organic fruits and vegetables and be taken once every hour.

- Eating vegetarian meals of organically grown fruits, vegetables, and whole grains

- Taking a number of supplements, including:

    - Potassium

    - Lugol's Solution (potassium iodide, iodine, and water)

    - Coenzyme $Q_{10}$ injected with vitamin $B_{12}$ (The original regimen used crude liver extract instead of coenzyme $Q_{10}$)

    - Vitamins A, C, and $B_3$ (niacin)

    - Flaxseed oil

    - Pancreatic enzymes

- Pepsin (a stomach enzyme)

- Taking coffee or chamomile enemas regularly to remove toxins from the body

- Preparing food without salt, spices, or oils, and without using aluminum cookware or utensils

## Preclinical (Laboratory or Animal) Studies and Clinical Trials on Gerson Therapy

No results of laboratory or animal studies have been published in scientific journals. Most of the published information on the use of the Gerson therapy reports on retrospective studies (reviews of past cases). Dr. Gerson published case histories (detailed reports of the diagnosis, treatment, and follow-up of individual patients) of 50 of his patients. He treated several different types of cancer in his practice. The reports include Dr. Gerson's notes, with some X-rays of the patients over time. The follow-up was contact with patients by mail or phone and included anecdotal reports (incomplete descriptions of the medical and treatment histories of one or more patients).

The National Cancer Institute (NCI) reviewed the cases of a total of 60 patients treated by Dr. Gerson. The NCI found that the available information did not prove the regimen had benefit.

The following studies of the Gerson therapy were published:

- A retrospective study of 38 patients treated with the Gerson therapy was done. Medical records were not available to the authors of the study; information came from patient interviews. These case reviews did not provide information that supports the usefulness of the Gerson therapy for treating cancer.

- A study of a diet regimen similar to the Gerson therapy was done in Austria. The patients received standard treatment along with the special diet. The authors of the study reported that the diet appeared to help patients live longer than usual and have fewer side effects. The authors said it needed further study.

- The Gerson Research Organization did a retrospective study of their melanoma patients who were treated with the Gerson therapy. The study reported that patients who had stage III or stage IV melanoma lived longer than usual for patients with these stages of melanoma. There have been no clinical trials that support the findings of this retrospective study.

- A case review of 6 patients with metastatic cancer who used the Gerson therapy reported that the regimen helped patients in some ways, both physically and psychologically. Based on these results, the reviewers recommended that clinical trials of the Gerson therapy be conducted.

### Side Effects or Risks Reported from Use of the Gerson Therapy

Reports of three deaths that may be related to coffee enemas have been published. Taking too many enemas of any kind can cause changes in normal blood chemistry, chemicals that occur naturally in the body and keep the muscles, heart, and other organs working properly.

### Gerson Therapy Approval Status

The Gerson therapy has not been approved by the U.S. Food and Drug Administration (FDA) for use as a treatment for cancer or any other disease.

# Section 44.4

# *Vegetarianism*

This section contains text excerpted from the following sources:
Text in this section begins with excerpts from "Vegetarian Diet,"
MedlinePlus, National Institutes of Health (NIH), April 2, 2015;
Text beginning with the heading "Ten Tips: Healthy Eating for
Vegetarians" is excerpted from "10 Tips: Healthy Eating for
Vegetarians," ChooseMyPlate.gov, U.S. Department
of Agriculture (USDA), July 25, 2017.

A vegetarian diet focuses on plants for food. These include fruits, vegetables, dried beans and peas, grains, seeds, and nuts. There is no single type of vegetarian diet. Instead, vegetarian eating patterns usually fall into the following groups:

- The vegan diet, which excludes all meat and animal products

- The lacto vegetarian diet, which includes plant foods plus dairy products

- The lacto-ovo vegetarian diet, which includes both dairy products and eggs

People who follow vegetarian diets can get all the nutrients they need. However, they must be careful to eat a wide variety of foods to meet their nutritional needs. Nutrients vegetarians may need to focus on include protein, iron, calcium, zinc, and vitamin $B_{12}$.

## Ten Tips: Healthy Eating for Vegetarians

A vegetarian eating pattern can be a healthy option. The key is to consume a variety of foods and the right amount of foods to meet your calorie and nutrient needs.

1. **Think about protein.** Your protein needs can easily be met by eating a variety of plant foods. Sources of protein for vegetarians include beans and peas, nuts, and soy products (such as tofu, tempeh). Lacto-ovo vegetarians also get protein from eggs and dairy foods.

2. **Bone up on sources of calcium.** Calcium is used for building bones and teeth. Some vegetarians consume dairy products, which are excellent sources of calcium. Other sources of calcium for vegetarians include calcium-fortified soymilk (soy beverage), tofu made with calcium sulfate, calcium-fortified breakfast cereals and orange juice, and some dark-green leafy vegetables (collard, turnip, and mustard greens; and bok choy).

3. **Make simple changes.** Many popular main dishes are or can be vegetarian—such as pasta primavera, pasta with marinara or pesto sauce, veggie pizza, vegetable lasagna, tofu-vegetable stir-fry, and bean burritos.

4. **Enjoy a cookout.** For barbecues, try veggie or soy burgers, soy hot dogs, marinated tofu, or tempeh, and fruit kabobs. Grilled veggies are great, too!

5. **Include beans and peas.** Because of their high nutrient content, consuming beans and peas is recommended for everyone, vegetarians and nonvegetarians alike. Enjoy some vegetarian chili, three bean salad, or split pea soup. Make a hummus-filled pita sandwich.

6. **Try different veggie versions.** A variety of vegetarian products look—and may taste—like their nonvegetarian counterparts but are usually lower in saturated fat and contain no cholesterol. For breakfast, try soy-based sausage patties or links. For dinner, rather than hamburgers, try bean burgers, or falafel (chickpea patties).

7. **Make some small changes at restaurants.** Most restaurants can make vegetarian modifications to menu items by substituting meatless sauces or nonmeat items, such as tofu and beans for meat, and adding vegetables or pasta in place of meat. Ask about available vegetarian options.

8. **Nuts make great snacks.** Choose unsalted nuts as a snack and use them in salads or main dishes. Add almonds, walnuts, or pecans instead of cheese or meat to a green salad.

9. **Get your vitamin B$_{12}$.** Vitamin B$_{12}$ is naturally found only in animal products. Vegetarians should choose fortified foods such as cereals or soy products, or take a vitamin B$_{12}$ supplement if they do not consume any animal products. Check the Nutrition Facts label for vitamin B$_{12}$ in fortified products.

10. **Find a vegetarian pattern for you.** The *Dietary Guidelines for Americans, 2015* (www.health.gov/dietaryguidelines/2015/guidelines) can help you in finding a vegetarian pattern for you.

# Part Five


# Mind-Body Medicine

# Chapter 45

# *Mind-Body Medicine: An Overview*

Mind and body practices are a large and diverse group of techniques that are administered or taught to others by a trained practitioner or teacher. Examples include acupuncture, massage therapy, meditation, relaxation techniques, spinal manipulation, and yoga.

## Mind and Body Approaches

Several mind and body approaches, including relaxation techniques, yoga, tai chi, and meditation may be useful for managing symptoms of stress in patients. For some stress-related conditions, mind and body approaches are used as an adjunct to other forms of treatment.

### *Relaxation Techniques*

Relaxation techniques may be helpful in managing a variety of stress-related health conditions, including anxiety associated with

This chapter contains text excerpted from the following sources: Text in this chapter begins with excerpts from "Mind and Body Practices," National Center for Complementary and Integrative Health (NCCIH), September 24, 2017; Text under the heading "Mind and Body Approaches" is excerpted from "Mind and Body Approaches for Stress: What the Science Says," National Center for Complementary and Integrative Health (NCCIH), January 2016.

ongoing health problems and in those who are having medical procedures. Evidence suggests that relaxation techniques may also provide some benefit on symptoms of posttraumatic stress disorder (PTSD), and may help reduce occupational stress in healthcare workers. For some of these conditions, relaxation techniques are used as an adjunct to other forms of treatment.

Relaxation techniques are generally considered safe for healthy people. However, occasionally, people report unpleasant experiences such as increased anxiety, intrusive thoughts, or fear of losing control. There have been rare reports that certain relaxation techniques might cause or worsen symptoms in people with epilepsy or certain psychiatric conditions, or with a history of abuse or trauma.

### *Yoga, Tai Chi, and Qi Gong*

A range of research has examined the relationship between exercise and depression. Results from a much smaller body of research suggest that exercise may also affect stress and anxiety symptoms. Even less certain is the role of yoga, tai chi, and qi gong—for these and other psychological factors.

The clinical trial data suggest yoga, as taught and practiced in these research studies under the guidance of a skilled teacher, has a low rate of minor side effects. It is not uncommon for practitioners to have some minor, transient discomfort, as with most physical activity programs. However, injuries from yoga, some of them serious, have been reported in the popular press.

People with health conditions should work with an experienced yoga instructor who can help modify or avoid some yoga poses to prevent side effects.

Tai chi appears to be a safe practice. Complaints of musculoskeletal pain after starting tai chi may occur but have been found to improve with continued practice. Women who are pregnant and those with heart conditions should talk with their healthcare providers before beginning yoga, tai chi, or any other exercise program.

### *Meditation and Mindfulness-Based Stress Reduction*

The scientific evidence to date suggests that mindfulness meditation—a mind-body practice which cultivates abilities to maintain focused and clear attention and develop an increased awareness of the present—may help reduce symptoms of stress, including anxiety and depression.

Meditation is considered to be safe for healthy people. There have been rare reports that meditation could cause or worsen symptoms in people who have certain psychiatric problems, but this question has not been fully researched.

# Chapter 46

# *Art Therapy*

## *What Is Art Therapy?*

Art therapy is based on the idea that the creative process of art making is healing and life-enhancing, and is a form of nonverbal communication of thoughts and feelings. Art therapy encourages personal growth, increases self-understanding and assists in emotional reparation. Participation in this treatment modality does not require any artistic training. The therapists involved in providing this treatment are all trained registered/licensed art therapists.

This chapter contains text excerpted from the following sources: This chapter contains text excerpted from the following sources: Text under the heading "What Is Art Therapy?" is excerpted from "VA Palo Alto Health Care System—What Is Art Therapy?" U.S. Department of Veterans Affairs (VA), April 11, 2017; Text under the heading "Creative Art Therapy and the Integrated Healthcare Model" is excerpted from "Creative Arts Therapy a Useful Tool for Military Patients," National Endowment for the Arts (NEA), November 12, 2015; Text under the heading "Historical Context of Research into the Arts and Health" is excerpted from "The National Endowment for the Arts Guide to Community-Engaged Research in the Arts and Health," National Endowment for the Arts (NEA), December 2016; Text under the heading "How Arts Can Aid Trauma Recovery" is excerpted from "Calm through Creativity: How Arts Can Aid Trauma Recovery," Administration for Children and Families (ACF), U.S. Department of Health and Human Services (HHS), December 18, 2013. Reviewed May 2018; Text under the heading "Creative Art Therapists" is excerpted from "Art Therapist," U.S. Bureau of Labor Statistics (BLS), U.S. Department of Labor (DOL), April 2015.

Art therapy helps individuals to:

- Create meaning
- Achieve insight
- Find relief from overwhelming emotions or trauma and posttraumatic stress disorder (PTSD)
- Resolve conflicts and problems, enrich daily life
- Achieve an increased sense of well-being

## Creative Art Therapy and the Integrated Healthcare Model

Creative arts therapy is a noninvasive and cost-effective medical treatment in which certified creative arts therapists work closely with other health professionals to create individual treatment plans with measurable outcomes. Patients may receive therapies such as painting, ceramics, music therapy, and therapeutic writing to improve health conditions for a wide range of medical, physical, neurological, and psychological health issues, such as depression, anxiety, cognitive function, memory, and impaired motor skills. Patients have described how art therapy activities have improved their cognitive skills and ability to process trauma and confront issues relating to frustrations, transitions, and grief.

## Historical Context of Research into the Arts and Health

Therapeutic uses of the arts have been documented since antiquity. For centuries, artists, philosophers, physicians, and others have proposed specific benefits of the arts for health and well-being. For instance, early examples about the therapeutic value of music date back at least to the 18th century, when references to music appeared in medical texts and references to medicine in music treatises. An interest in using the arts to influence health developed substantially in the 20th century when arts professionals formalized distinct arts therapies by founding professional organizations and creating educational training programs. Among these interventions are music therapy, visual art therapy, dance/movement therapy, drama therapy, and several other genre-based forms of creative arts therapy.

## How Arts Can Aid Trauma Recovery

It takes a lot of effort for the brain to deal with trauma. Whether because of posttraumatic stress disorder (PTSD) or the many adaptive behaviors that victims use instinctively in threatening situations, the traumatized brain is constantly on high-alert, particularly its lower regions, where survival instincts originate. Simple artistic activities like drawing or sculpting clay can soothe those lower regions, which is why arts therapists argue that their methods can help trauma victims calm down and release some of that mental tension. These evidence-informed therapies use creativity to raise victims' awareness of their physical and mental states and build resilience and a sense of safety. Counselor and author Cathy Malchiodi, who has pioneered trauma-informed art therapy and trauma-informed expressive arts therapy, claims that the use of music, art, and other creative activities grant victims a means of expressing the effects of trauma even after therapy ends.

When the lower brain's instincts are over-activated, they can inhibit people's ability to perform higher cognitive functions until they have started healing from trauma. "Teens who are stressed may have diffi-culty answering questions about their drug use, or about making goals and plans for the future," Malchiodi says. However, as she and other researchers have found, these effects can be reversed with therapies that rebuild the brain from the ground up.

Nancy Gerber, Director of the Ph.D. Program in Creative Arts Therapies at Drexel University, explains that expressive arts support trauma recovery, especially for those victims who were traumatized or seek treatment at a young age, because they engage the regions of the brain that develop earlier in life. "A lot of kids in adolescence strug-gle with language," she says. "They know how to talk but they don't always know how to talk with emotional intelligence. The idea (of art therapy) is that images are a form of cognition, a way of knowing. They develop very early in our lives: little kids point at things before they have a word for them. These images provide a history of the early life, and when we grow up we don't have a word for that." Simply put, art therapy helps trauma victims reconnect with that image-based part of the brain, a process which calms the parts of the brain that have been overworked by trauma.

Here's how it works.

### Step 1. Getting in Touch with the "Lower Brain"

Traumatic stress manifests differently for different people; victims may be withdrawn and uncommunicative, or wild and confrontational.

371

(In therapeutic terms, this is referred to as "internalizing" or "externalizing" one's feelings.) In her previous work at an inpatient psychiatric hospital, mostly focused on adolescents, Gerber included drawing in every young patient's intake process. She would then share the drawings with staff when they met to decide on a treatment plan. It was particularly useful for those young people who couldn't easily express their experiences verbally.

"The art provides a different dimension that most of us don't know how to say," Gerber says. "A picture can tell a story about our internal life that isn't accessible in words."

"Malchiodi begins her therapy by observing her clients infer what kind of activities would help them best. Some may benefit from therapies that help them loosen up, such as movement activities with music. Others need to do something that will help calm them down and focus, such as drawing or painting.

In one treatment, she gives individuals a rubber duck and asks them to build a safe place for it using feathers, paper plates, leaves, fabric and other materials.

"This highly sensory experience, where you can actually feel the nest, pond, or whatever you build, engages the lower parts of your brain, whereas simply drawing a safe place or depicting goals require higher cognitive areas," Malchiodi explains.

### Step 2. Becoming More Expressive

For young and older people alike, the experience of traumatic events can be difficult to express in words. So Malchiodi uses the first step to get them feeling calmer and more creatively expressive. Then she engages them in storytelling activities that use higher cognitive areas. For example, she might ask, "If you could draw a bridge that starts in the past and goes into the future, show me where you are on the bridge," or to depict one's family in any way they choose to depict it.

Gerber says that expressive arts therapy allows victims to deal with trauma in the same deeply emotional way that they experience it, which in turn prepares them to address it more fully. "They no longer had to act out," she says of her clients. "They could have conversations about how they saw themselves and the world."

Malchiodi saw similar results in her young people. "Trauma memories are sensory memories," she says, "meaning that people feel them in their bodies and react with their bodies." Creativity can help them make that leap to full understanding and expression.

## Creative Art Therapists

### *What They Do*

Art therapists work in different settings with different types of clients. Some are in schools, where they work with students of all ages and meet with them in groups or one-on-one. Many others work in medical settings, such as community clinics and psychiatric hospitals, where they may help people who have a physical or mental illness. Still, others have their own practice, serving clients with various needs.

But no matter where they work or who their clients are, art therapists use art and psychology on the job.

**Art.** Every client has different needs, but for some, the process of creating may be valuable on its own. For example, people who have trouble focusing may become more grounded when working with clay. Using paints, in contrast, can help people release emotion.

Art therapists design projects using their understanding of how art media and techniques can influence people. For example, a therapist may ask students to create an image showing parts of their past that they would like to leave behind. Then, he or she may have them create an image that depicts their future and shows the positive elements they hope to build on. This helps them think about what they want to change about themselves, what they want to be.

**Psychology.** Knowledge of psychology allows an art therapist to help clients understand themselves and work toward specific goals. The art therapist engages clients in reflection about the art that they have created. It's all about exploring things they're trying to process that they can't verbally communicate. Sometimes they're not ready to talk, but just having a person there helps. When clients are ready to process their thoughts, the art therapist might discuss ways to help them deal with whatever they're facing. For example, an art therapist might work with clients to develop coping skills or strategies for changing behavior.

# Chapter 47

# *Biofeedback*

## *What Is Biofeedback?*

Biofeedback is a type of therapy that helps people control certain body functions that otherwise take place involuntarily, such as blood pressure, heart rate, skin temperature, and muscle tension. The biofeedback technique works on the principle that by harnessing the power of one's mind, a person can be aware of the processes taking place inside their body, and this can give them more control over their health. With biofeedback, electrodes or sensors are attached to the skin. These help receive information about the body, measure processes, and display the results on a monitor. Using this information, a biofeedback therapist can help a person learn how the heart rate or blood pressure can be controlled. The individual then uses the monitor to see his or her progress and eventually will be able to achieve success without it. The therapy is said to prevent or treat conditions such as high blood pressure, chronic pain, migraine headaches, and urinary incontinence.

## *Biofeedback Methods*

Depending on the individual's need, a biofeedback therapist recommends the appropriate course of action.

---

"Biofeedback," © 2018 Omnigraphics. Reviewed May 2018.

Some biofeedback therapies include:

- **Brainwave.** This method uses scalp sensors attached to an electroencephalograph (EEG) to monitor brain waves.

- **Breathing.** Breathing patterns and respiration rate are observed by placing bands around the abdomen and chest during respiration.

- **Muscle.** Electromyography (EMG) is used to measure muscle tension. This involves placing sensors over skeletal muscles to monitor electrical activity.

- **Heart rate.** An electrocardiograph (ECG) measures the heart rate and its variability. This method of feedback uses sensors placed on the chest, wrist, or lower torso.

- **Temperature.** Blood flow to the skin is measured using sensors attached to the fingers or feet.

- **Sweat glands.** Sweat gland activity and skin perspiration are measured by an electrodermograph (EDG) by attaching sensors to the fingers, palm, or wrist.

## How Does Biofeedback Work?

Biofeedback is known to promote relaxation and help relieve stress. Researchers are not sure how the method works; however, people who have undergone treatment report benefiting greatly from biofeedback therapy. When the body is under stress, certain internal processes, like blood pressure and heart rate, tend to become overactive. Biofeedback promotes relaxation, and many scientists believe that this is the key to stress reduction and other health benefits. A biofeedback therapist can help an individual learn to reduce stress through mental exercises and physical relaxation techniques.

## A Biofeedback Session

A typical biofeedback session involves attaching electrodes to an individual's skin. The electrodes send signals to a monitor that displays the current heart rate, breathing rate, skin temperature, blood pressure, muscle activity, and perspiration. If the individual is under stress, muscles tighten, heart rate becomes faster, blood pressure rises, sweating increases, and breathing quickens. When the monitor displays variation from normal rates, the biofeedback therapist trains the individual to manage these functions through various mental and physical relaxation techniques. This eventually helps the individual bring involuntary internal body functions under his or her control outside of the therapy session.

The following are some of the types of relaxation techniques used in biofeedback therapy:

- **Progressive muscle relaxation.** Tightening and relaxing different muscle groups.

- **Mindfulness meditation.** Negative emotions are purged by refocusing thought processes.

- **Guided imagery.** Focusing on a specific calming image makes one feel more relaxed.

- **Deep breathing.** A breathing exercise intended to promote a sense of well-being.

## Benefits of Biofeedback

Proponents of biofeedback cite many of its benefits that can be used to manage both physical and mental issues. Biofeedback therapy is found to be most effective for conditions influenced by stress, such as eating and learning disorders, bedwetting, and muscle spasms. Other problems that can be helped by biofeedback include asthma, incontinence, irritable bowel syndrome (IBS), constipation, high blood pressure, chronic pain, anxiety, depression, diabetes, headaches, and the effects of chemotherapy. Researchers have found that biofeedback has also helped improve intelligence and behavior in children, reportedly including attention deficit hyperactivity disorder (ADHD) and autism. Some people prefer biofeedback to other types of therapy since it is noninvasive and reduces the need for medication.

Biofeedback method is more useful and effective in children. For instance, EEG neurofeedback (especially when combined with cognitive therapy) has been found to improve behavior and intelligence scores in children with attention deficit hyperactivity disorder (ADHD) and autism. Abdominal pain can be relieved by biofeedback combined with a fiber-rich diet. Migraine and chronic tension headaches among children and teens can be relieved or controlled by thermal biofeedback.

## Risks of Biofeedback

Biofeedback is generally considered safe, and research has not revealed any side effects. A consultation with a primary healthcare provider is a good idea before beginning therapy since biofeedback may not be for everyone. For example, some people with existing serious mental health issues might not find this form of treatment to be beneficial.

### References

1. "Biofeedback," Mayo Clinic, January 3, 2018.

2. Kiefer, David, MD. "Overview of Biofeedback," WebMD, August 1, 2016.

3. Ehrlich, D. Steven, NMD. "Biofeedback," University of Maryland Medical Center (UMMC), November 6, 2015.

4. "Biofeedback," Healthline, January 11, 2016.

5. Nordqvist, Joseph. "Biofeedback," Medical News Today, January 10, 2017.

# Chapter 48

# *Deep Breathing Exercises*

## *What Is Deep Breathing?*

Deep breathing is a good way to relax. We don't always remember to breathe deeply. Most adults breathe from the chest, which is known as shallow breathing. When you breathe deeply, your body takes in more oxygen. You exhale more carbon dioxide. Your body naturally "resets" itself to a more relaxed and calm state.

## *Who Needs Deep Breathing Exercise?*

Deep breathing can be useful for anyone who has stress. You can practice deep breathing during your workday when you're feeling stressed or anxious. And you can choose to take a couple minutes and breathe deeply each day, or just use it when you need it.

## *What Are the Benefits of Deep Breathing?*

Deep breathing doesn't just work for handling day-to-day stress. It can be especially helpful to veterans and civilians who've experienced

This chapter contains text excerpted from the following sources: Text beginning with the heading "What Is Deep Breathing?" is excerpted from "Relaxation Exercise: Deep Breathing," U.S. Department of Veterans Affairs (VA), September 2, 2015; Text under the heading "How Is Deep Breathing Exercise Done?" is excerpted from "Practice It: Deep Conscious Breathing Exercise," Smokefree Women, U.S. Department of Health and Human Services (HHS), November 30, 2012. Reviewed May 2018.

traumatic events (such as military combat or a civilian assault). Deep breathing can help you cope with the stress from these events. Symptoms such as anxiety, "panic" or feeling "stuck in alarm mode" often respond well to deep breathing.

This exercise only takes a few minutes and can be performed anywhere. Nobody has to know you're doing it. You may do this exercise with your eyes open or closed. If you've gone through traumatic stress you may find that keeping eyes open helps you to stay "grounded" in the "here and now." Do what's most comfortable for you.

## How Is Deep Breathing Exercise Done?

You can do deep breathing exercise in the following way:

1.  Find a comfortable and quiet place to sit or lie down. If this is not possible, close your eyes and imagine yourself somewhere relaxing such as lying on the beach listening to ocean waves.

2.  Close and relax your eyes and relax your facial muscles, jaw, neck, and shoulders. Gently place one hand on your chest and the other hand on your belly button.

3.  As you breathe in, allow the breath to expand the body including the belly, chest, and lungs. As you breathe out, gently press your hands against the chest and belly a bit more to encourage full release of the breath.

4.  Focus on developing a steady breathing rhythm by making the inhale and exhale equal in length. Silently repeat to yourself, "Breathing in" while inhaling and "Breathing out" while exhaling.

5.  Be patient with the process. With practice, you can do this more easily and might not even need to place your hands on your belly and chest.

No time to sit and breathe? No problem; take your breathing practice with you! Deep conscious breathing can also be done with the eyes open wherever you happen to be—simply pause and take two to three full deep breaths (inhale deeply and exhale completely). Taking a few moments when you start to feel stressed can keep stress in check.

# Chapter 49

# *Guided Imagery*

## *What Is Visualization/Guided Imagery?*

Imagery or visualization involves using your imagination to help put your body in a more relaxed state. Just as your body can become tense and stressed in response to thoughts that make us angry or anxious, it can also become more calm and relaxed in response to calming, peaceful, and pleasant thoughts.

One of the most basic ways to use imagery to relax is to close your eyes and imagine being in a place that is peaceful and relaxing to you. It may be a place you have actually been in the past, or it may be a place created in your imagination. It might be a quiet beach; a cool, shady spot in the woods; snuggled in front of a fireplace; fishing; or any place else that is peaceful and soothing to you. Use all of your senses in your imagination. For example, see the waves gently lapping on the shore or the light filtering through the leaves of the trees. Hear the birds singing or the leaves rustling. Smell the flowers, the grass, or the salt air. Feel the sun or gentle breeze on your skin. Feel that you are actually there. Smile and let your body relax. Enjoy being there for a few minutes. You can use this as a regular relaxation exercise or in times of stress when you need to relax. Following is a scripted example of a visualization exercise.

Text in this chapter is excerpted from "Visualization/Guided Imagery," U.S. Department of Veterans Affairs (VA), July 2013. Reviewed May 2018.

## *Visualization Exercise*

Close your eyes. Allow yourself to get comfortable. Begin with a few slow deep breaths in through your nose and out through your mouth, letting your body get relaxed. Let the chair fully support your body as you continue to breath and relax.

Now, use your imagination to picture yourself walking slowly along a path. It's a pleasant path, any kind that you wish. It's a beautiful day, and you feel relaxed and happy. You can feel the warmth and energy of the sunlight on your skin. Soon you come to a gate. You know this gate leads to a special place where you feel welcomed, safe, and comfortable. Push the gate open and allow yourself to enter your very own private garden.

Your garden is filled with your favorite things. Whatever is pleasing to you can be found in this place. Perhaps there are flowers, trees, animals, birds, water, or even music. Look around and notice what is in your garden. See all the colors and objects that are in this place. Notice how beautiful they are. Look at the various shapes and see how varied they are. Look at the ground, look at the sky, and see where they meet. Your garden is calm and tranquil. Everything peacefully coexists in the garden. As you are looking, become aware of how things might feel in this private place of yours. Begin to explore this place with your sense of touch. Perhaps some things are soft and warm, and others are smooth and cool. Simply spend some time exploring, using your sense of touch as you continue to feel at peace and comfortable. Notice what the air feels like; is it cool or warm? Is there a breeze or is it still? Take the time to feel the peace and serenity in this private place. As you continue to explore your garden by seeing and feeling, become aware of the sounds that you hear in your garden. The sounds in your garden are pleasing to the ear and very comforting. Perhaps it is quiet in your garden, or maybe there are a number of sounds. Some of the sounds may be very soft, while others may be louder. Relax and listen for a while and see if you can identify the different sounds in your garden. As you're listening to the sounds in your garden, become aware of what smells you might smell. Take a deep breath in, and notice the fragrances that are present. Some of them may be famil-iar, while others may be unfamiliar. The fragrances are pleasant and soothing. Take your time and enjoy your visit to the garden, using it in whatever way that you wish. Spend the time that is necessary for you to rejuvenate and to care for yourself.

When you are ready to leave, slowly walk back towards the gate of your garden. You have enjoyed your visit to the garden and feel relaxed and content. This good feeling will remain with you throughout the day. Push the gate open and return to the path that led you to the garden. As you make your way back up the path to the here and now, remember that you can use your imagination to return to your private garden at any time you wish. Visit your garden any time you would like to relax, to be comforted, or just to enjoy its beauty. You are now ready to resume your day. Stretch gently and open your eyes, feeling refreshed and alert.

# Chapter 50

# *Hypnotherapy*

That time you were totally absorbed, whether you were sinking every jump shot or flying around Hogwarts? Well, you just might have been under hypnosis. Researchers believe that super-focused trance-like states can be harnessed to treat medical problems—to reduce pain or control neuromuscular disorders, for instance.

"Hypnosis is the oldest Western conception of a psychotherapy," said National Institute of Health (NIH) grantee Dr. David Spiegel in a National Center for Complementary and Integrative Health (NCCIH) Integrative Medicine Research Lecture. "It's the first time a talking interaction was thought to have therapeutic potential. It's useful as a model system for understanding how brain-body interactions work."

Spiegel is medical director of the Center for Integrative Medicine at Stanford University School of Medicine. His research—with funding over the years from the NIH, the National Cancer Institute (NCI), the National Institute of Mental Health (NIMH) and the NCCIH—spans

Text in this chapter begins with excerpts from "How Can Hypnosis Treat Medical Problems?" National Institutes of Health (NIH), June 19, 2015; Text under the heading "How Can Hypnosis Treat Medical Problems?" is excerpted from "Hypnosis," National Center for Complementary and Integrative Health (NCCIH), September 24, 2017; Text under the heading "Hypnotherapy and Irritable Bowel Syndrome (IBS)" is excerpted from "6 Tips: IBS and Complementary Health Practices," National Center for Complementary and Integrative Health (NCCIH), September 24, 2015; Text under the heading "Hypnotherapy and Smoking Cessation" is excerpted from "Complementary Health Approaches for Smoking Cessation: What the Science Says," National Center for Complementary and Integrative Health (NCCIH), November 13, 2017.

four decades in such areas as psycho-oncology, stress and health, pain control, and clinical applications of hypnosis.

## History of Hypnosis

Viennese physician Franz Anton Mesmer founded the field. In the 18th century, "he theorized that magnetic fields flow through the body. When people got sick, something went wrong with their magnetic fields. [Mesmer believed] if he put his magnetic field next to their magnetic field, theirs would get better." Mesmer moved to France, where his practice flourished. Not really surprising, Spiegel said. Compare hypnosis with what French doctors were using back then—bloodletting. Patients under the care of French physicians were more prone to die.

Mesmer's success did not endear him to the French medical establishment, which begged King Louis to investigate the Viennese doctor. A panel that included Benjamin Franklin and "pain-control expert" Dr. Joseph-Ignace Guillotin, inventor of the execution device that bears his name, concluded Mesmer's method was "nothing but heated imagination."

That episode ended Mesmer's career and recorded perhaps the first doubt about trances as medicine. It did not prevent further pursuit of hypnosis' potential healing powers nor further skepticism. Hypnosis, Spiegel quipped, "has been something like the oldest profession—everybody's interested in it, but no one wants to be seen in public with it. It was at the foundation of many very important movements, including psychoanalysis."

Sigmund Freud began psychoanalysis by using hypnosis as "a royal road to the unconscious," Spiegel said. When Freud found some patients formed irrational feelings for their physicians during hypnosis, he stopped the practice. Instead of entering trance-like states, patients were urged to free associate. At the end of his career, however, Freud returned to an interest in hypnosis.

## You Are Not Getting Very Sleepy

Defining hypnosis as a "state of aroused, attentive, focused concentration with diminished peripheral awareness," Spiegel also refuted a common misconception. "You don't go to sleep," he said. "Hypnosis is not sleep. It's a narrowing of the focus of attention. Hypnosis is to consciousness what a telephoto lens is to a camera: What you see you see with great detail, but you're less aware of the context."

So, can hypnosis make folks flap their arms and squawk like a chicken? No, usually not. Some vulnerability does come with the practice, though. "People in hypnosis are less likely to critically judge what you say to them," noted Spiegel, explaining suggestibility. "You've got to be careful what you say to them, because they're less likely to correct your mistakes. It makes people nervous, because we are all social creatures. We all respond to social cues and sometimes we do so irrationally. Hypnosis is an example of how much we can allow input from other people—even people we don't know very well—to control our perception, judgment and behavior."

## *In the Zone?*

We use hypnotic-like states in normal activities, Spiegel said. "Self-hypnosis is what people do when they want to enhance performance." Top athletes commonly describe their training techniques for competing at their highest levels as involving intensely focused imagination. They visualize their best performance to the exclusion of all else around them. Spiegel said that type of laser-focused attention is a form of self-hypnosis.

"People who are more highly hypnotizable have more self-altering states of attention—total absorption—in everyday life all the time," Spiegel noted. "They get lost in a sunset or a movie or reading a novel."

Studies indicate that hypnotizability cannot be taught. In fact, Spiegel said, it's a more stable trait over the lifespan than Intelligence quotient (IQ). Researchers estimate that about one-third of people cannot be hypnotized, while 15 percent of the population is considered highly hypnotizable. The rest of us have varying degrees of hypnotizability that we can be trained to use.

In terms of neurophysiology, Spiegel said researchers see brain differences between people who are high and low in hypnotizability. The brain's anterior cingulate cortex (ACC) region—where tasks such as attention, monitoring and pain management are located—seems to play a significant role in hypnotic experience.

Scientists have collected "data showing how if you change how distressing pain is—not the sensation itself, but how much it bothers you—then you reduce activity in the (ACC) as well," he explained.

Highly hypnotizable individuals have more functional connectivity—a functional magnetic resonance imaging (fMRI) term for neurons that fire together—between the dorsal ACC and portions of the executive control network in the dorsolateral prefrontal cortex, Spiegel pointed out. This means that paying attention and carrying out a task are highly coordinated among high hypnotizables, he said.

Researchers conducted brain scans of study participants while they were under hypnosis. Scientists examined which brain regions turn on and off and which areas work together. These studies helped clarify how dissociation occurs, Spiegel said. "When you're engaged in hypnosis, you're not ruminating about yourself," he noted. "People will engage in hypnotic experiences and they often won't remember what they did. We think it has to do with an inverse relationship between being hypnotized and functioning of the (brain's) default mode network. We're beginning to understand what goes on in the brain when people enter these altered states."

## Change Your Mind

Spiegel showed videos of some of his clinical work. In one clip, a patient with Parkinson disease (PD) who experienced near-constant involuntary tremors in his hand was able, under self-hypnosis, to rest his hand. He imagined himself in his happy place—Hawaii, in this case—and the tremors stopped.

Spiegel shared results from some of his group's other studies:

- One out of four patients under hypnosis can permanently quit smoking.

- Self-hypnotized metastatic breast cancer patients were able to cut their pain levels in half.

- Children taught to imagine themselves elsewhere better tolerated a painful invasive medical exam; procedure time was reduced by 17 minutes.

"In hypnosis, you actually use words to transform perception," Spiegel concluded. "So some of our ability to manipulate experience is not just from speech and motor activity but also from the ability to control our own perceptual processes. We have an amazing ability in our brain to alter not just how we react to perception but also what it is that we perceive. If you think it is taking away control, it isn't. Hypnosis is teaching people control."

## How Can Hypnosis Treat Medical Problems?

Hypnosis (also called hypnotherapy) has been studied for a number of conditions, including state anxiety (e.g., before medical procedures or surgeries), headaches, smoking cessation, pain control, hot flashes in breast cancer survivors, and irritable bowel syndrome (IBS).

## *Hypnotherapy and Irritable Bowel Syndrome (IBS)*

This practice involves the power of suggestion by a trained hypnotist or hypnotherapist during a state of deep relaxation, and is the most widely used mind and body intervention for IBS. According to reviews of the scientific literature, hypnotherapy may be a helpful treatment for managing IBS symptoms. Several studies of hypnotherapy for IBS have shown substantial long-term improvement of gastrointestinal symptoms as well as anxiety, depression, disability, and quality of life.

## *Hypnotherapy and Smoking Cessation*

There is some evidence to suggest that hypnotherapy may improve smoking cessation, but data are not definitive.

### *What Does the Research Show?*

- A 2014 randomized controlled trial of 164 patients hospitalized with cardiac or pulmonary illness compared the efficacy of hypnotherapy alone, as well as hypnotherapy with nicotine replacement therapy, to conventional nicotine replacement therapy alone. The study found that hypnotherapy patients were more likely than nicotine replacement therapy patients to be nonsmokers at 12 weeks and 26 weeks after hospitalization.

- A Cochrane review of eleven studies compared hypnotherapy with 18 different control interventions. The authors found that hypnotherapy did not have a greater effect on 6-month quit rates than other interventions or no treatment. They concluded that there is not enough evidence to show whether hypnotherapy could be as effective as counseling treatment.

- A 2012 meta-analysis of randomized controlled trials found that acupuncture, hypnotherapy, and aversive smoking increased smoking abstinence, but the patient population in the analysis was small and reports of smoking cessation were not validated by biochemical means.

### *Safety Considerations of Hypnotherapy*

Hypnosis is considered safe when performed by a health professional trained in hypnotherapy. Self-hypnosis also appears to be safe for most people. There are no reported cases of injury resulting from self-hypnosis.

# Chapter 51

# *Meditation*

Meditation is a mind and body practice that has a long history of use for increasing calmness and physical relaxation, improving psychological balance, coping with illness, and enhancing overall health and well-being. Mind and body practices focus on the interactions among the brain, mind, body, and behavior.

There are many types of meditation, but most have four elements in common:

1. a quiet location with as few distractions as possible;

2. a specific, comfortable posture (sitting, lying down, walking, or in other positions);

3. a focus of attention (a specially chosen word or set of words, an object, or the sensations of the breath); and

4. an open attitude (letting distractions come and go naturally without judging them).

## What the Science Says about the Effectiveness of Meditation

Many studies have investigated meditation for different conditions, and there's evidence that it may reduce blood pressure as well as symptoms of irritable bowel syndrome (IBS) and flare-ups in people who have had ulcerative colitis (UC). It may ease symptoms of anxiety and depression and may help people with insomnia.

Text in this chapter is excerpted from "Meditation: In Depth," National Center for Complementary and Integrative Health (NCCIH), September 7, 2017.

## Meditation for Pain

Research about meditation's ability to reduce pain has produced mixed results. However, in some studies, scientists suggest that meditation activates certain areas of the brain in response to pain. A small 2016 study funded in part by the National Center for Complementary and Integrative Health (NCCIH) found that mindfulness meditation does help to control pain and doesn't use the brain's naturally occurring opiates to do so. This suggests that combining mindfulness with pain medications and other approaches that rely on the brain's opioid activity may be particularly effective for reducing pain. In another 2016 NCCIH-funded study, adults aged 20–70 who had chronic low-back pain received either mindfulness-based stress reduction (MBSR) training, cognitive-behavioral therapy (CBT), or usual care. The MBSR and CBT participants had a similar level of improvement, and it was greater than those who got usual care, including long after the training ended. The researchers found that participants in the MBSR and CBT groups had greater improvement in functional limitation and back pain at 26 and 52 weeks compared with those who had usual care. There were no significant differences in outcomes between MBSR and CBT.

## Meditation for High Blood Pressure

The results of an NCCIH-funded trial involving 298 university students suggest that practicing Transcendental Meditation (TM) may lower the blood pressure of people at increased risk of developing high blood pressure. The findings also suggested that practicing meditation can help with psychological distress, anxiety, depression, anger/hostility, and coping ability.

A literature review and scientific statement from the American Heart Association (AHA) suggest that evidence supports the use of TM to lower blood pressure. However, the review indicates that it's uncertain whether TM is truly superior to other meditation techniques in terms of blood-pressure-lowering because there are few head-to-head studies.

## Meditation for Irritable Bowel Syndrome (IBS)

The few studies that have looked at mindfulness meditation training for IBS found no clear effects, the American College of Gastroenterology (ACG) stated in a 2014 report. But the authors noted that given the limited number of studies, they can't be sure that IBS doesn't help.

Results of an NCCIH-funded trial that enrolled 75 women suggest that practicing mindfulness meditation for 8 weeks reduces the severity of IBS symptoms. A review concluded that mindfulness training improved IBS patients' pain and quality of life but not their depression or anxiety. The amount of improvement was small.

## Meditation for Ulcerative Colitis (UC)

In a 2014 pilot study, 55 adults with UC in remission were divided into two groups. For 8 weeks, one group learned and practiced mindfulness-based stress reduction (MBSR) while the other group practiced a placebo procedure. Six and twelve months later, there were no significant differences between the two groups in the course of the disease, markers of inflammation, or any psychological measure except perceived stress during flare-ups. The researchers concluded that MBSR might help people in remission from moderate to moderately severe disease—and maybe reduce rates of a flare-up from stress.

## Meditation for Anxiety, Depression, and Insomnia

A 2014 literature review of 47 trials in 3,515 participants suggests that mindfulness meditation programs show moderate evidence of improving anxiety and depression. But the researchers found no evidence that meditation changed health-related behaviors affected by stress, such as substance abuse and sleep. A review of 36 trials found that 25 of them reported better outcomes for symptoms of anxiety in the meditation groups compared to control groups. In a small, NCCIH-funded study, 54 adults with chronic insomnia learned mindfulness-based stress reduction (MBSR), a form of MBSR specially adapted to deal with insomnia (mindfulness-based therapy for insomnia, or MBTI), or a self-monitoring program. Both meditation-based programs aided sleep, with MBTI providing a significantly greater reduction in insomnia severity compared with MBSR.

## Meditation for Smoking Cessation

The results of 13 studies of mindfulness-based interventions for stopping smoking had promising results regarding craving, smoking cessation, and relapse prevention, a 2015 research review found. However, the studies had many limitations. The findings from a review suggest that meditation-based therapies may help people quit smoking;

however, the small number of available studies is insufficient to determine rigorously if meditation is effective for this.

A trial comparing mindfulness training with a standard behavioral smoking cessation treatment found that individuals who received mindfulness training showed a greater rate of reduction in cigarette use immediately after treatment and at 17-week follow-up. The results of a brain imaging study suggest that mindful attention reduced the craving to smoke, and also that it reduced activity in a craving-related region of the brain. However, in a second brain imaging study, researchers observed that a 2-week course of meditation (5 hours total) significantly reduced smoking, compared with relaxation training, and that it increased activity in brain areas associated with craving.

## *Meditation for Other Conditions*

The results from an NCCIH-funded study of 279 adults who participated in an 8-week Mindfulness-Based Stress Reduction (MBSR) program found that changes in spirituality were associated with better mental health and quality of life. The guidelines from the American College of Chest Physicians suggest that MBSR and meditation may help to reduce stress, anxiety, pain, and depression while enhancing mood and self-esteem in people with lung cancer.

The clinical practice guidelines issued in 2014 by the Society for Integrative Oncology (SIC) recommend meditation as supportive care to reduce stress, anxiety, depression, and fatigue in patients treated for breast cancer. The SIC also recommends its use to improve quality of life in these people.

Meditation-based programs may be helpful in reducing common menopausal symptoms, including the frequency and intensity of hot flashes, sleep and mood disturbances, stress, and muscle and joint pain. However, differences in study designs mean that no firm conclusions can be drawn. Because only a few studies have been conducted on the effects of meditation for attention deficit hyperactivity disorder (ADHD), there isn't sufficient evidence to support its use for this condition.

A 2014 research review suggested that mind and body practices, including meditation, reduce chemical identifiers of inflammation and show promise in helping to regulate the immune system. The Results from an NCCIH-supported study involving 49 adults suggest that 8 weeks of mindfulness training may reduce stress-induced inflammation better than a health program that includes physical activity, education about diet, and music therapy.

## Meditation and the Brain

Some research suggests that meditation may physically change the brain and body and could potentially help to improve many health problems and promote healthy behaviors. In a study, researchers compared brain images from 50 adults who meditate and 50 adults who don't meditate. Results suggested that people who practiced meditation for many years have more folds in the outer layer of the brain. This process (called gyrification) may increase the brain's ability to process information.

A review of three studies suggests that meditation may slow, stall, or even reverse changes that take place in the brain due to normal aging. Results from an NCCIH-funded study suggest that meditation can affect activity in the amygdala (a part of the brain involved in processing emotions) and that different types of meditation can affect the amygdala differently even when the person is not meditating. Research about meditation's ability to reduce pain has produced mixed results. However, in some studies, scientists suggest that meditation activates certain areas of the brain in response to pain.

## What the Science Says about Safety and Side Effects of Meditation

Meditation is generally considered to be safe for healthy people. People with physical limitations may not be able to participate in certain meditative practices involving movement. People with physical health conditions should speak with their healthcare providers before starting a meditative practice, and make their meditation instructor aware of their condition.

There have been rare reports that meditation could cause or worsen symptoms in people with certain psychiatric problems like anxiety and depression. People with existing mental health conditions should speak with their healthcare providers before starting a meditative practice, and make their meditation instructor aware of their condition.

## More to Consider

If you are considering to try meditation then consider the following:

- Don't use meditation to replace conventional care or as a reason to postpone seeing a healthcare provider about a medical problem.

- Ask about the training and experience of the meditation instructor you are considering.

- Tell all your healthcare providers about any complementary or integrative health approaches you use. Give them a full picture of what you do to manage your health. This will help ensure coordinated and safe care.

Chapter 52

# *Music Therapy*

Music has been around since ancient times. It is part of every known culture. It can get your foot tapping, lift your mood, and even help you recall a distant memory. Did you know that music can bring other health benefits? Scientists are exploring the different ways music stimulates healthier bodies and minds.

"When you listen to or create music, it affects how you think, feel, move, and more," says neuroscientist Dr. Robert Finkelstein, who coleads National Institutes of Health's (NIH) music and health initiative. "Today, modern technologies are helping researchers learn more about how the brain works, what parts of the brain respond to music, and how music might help ease symptoms of certain diseases and conditions," he explains.

## *Your Brain on Music*

The brain is a complex processing hub. It's the control center of your nervous system, the network of nerve cells that carry messages to and from your body and the brain. A healthy brain tries to make sense of the world around you and the constant information it receives, including sound and music.

"Sound is an important and profound force in our lives," explains Northwestern University neuroscientist Dr. Nina Kraus. "The more we exercise our sound processing in the brain, the better the brain

Text in this chapter is excerpted from "Sound Health," *NIH News in Health*, National Institutes of Health (NIH), January 2018.

becomes at making sense of sound and the world around us. Music does this more than any other sound."

Music and other sounds enter the ear as sound waves. These create vibrations on our eardrum that are transformed into electrical signals. The electrical signals travel up the auditory nerve to the brain's auditory cortex. This brain area interprets the sound into something we recognize and understand.

But music affects more than the brain areas that process sound. Using techniques that take pictures of the brain, like functional magnetic resonance imaging or functional MRI (fMRI), scientists have found that music affects other brain areas. When music stimulates the brain, it shows up on brain images as flickers of bright light. Studies have shown that music "lights up" brain areas involved in emotion, memory, and even physical movement.

"Music can help facilitate movement," Finkelstein explains. NIH-funded scientists are investigating whether music can help patients with movement disorders, like Parkinson disease (PD). Patients with this condition slowly lose their ability to walk and move over time. "Studies show that when a certain beat is embedded in music, it can help people with PD walk," Finkelstein says. Another study is looking at how dance compares to other types of exercise in people with PD.

There's also evidence that music may be helpful for people with other health conditions, including Alzheimer disease (AD), dementia, traumatic brain injury (TBI), stroke, aphasia, autism, and hearing loss.

## Building Strong Minds

Playing a musical instrument engages many parts of the brain at once. This can especially benefit children and teens, whose brains are still developing. Introducing music to young kids can positively influence their ability to focus, how they act, and language development. Kraus's research team at Northwestern studies how musical training influences brain development. They found that music has positive effects on kids' learning abilities, even when the training starts as late as high school.

"The teens in our study showed biological changes in the brain after two years of participating in consistent music-making activities in school," she explains. Kraus says that these changes affect learning ability and can help improve skills like reading and writing. These benefits can be long-lasting, too. "Once you teach your brain how to respond to sound effectively it continues to do that well beyond when the music lessons stop," Kraus explains. "A little music goes a long way, but the longer you play, the stronger your brain becomes."

Being musical may also protect you from hearing loss as you age. We naturally lose our hearing ability over time. In particular, it becomes harder to hear conversations in a loud environment. But researchers have found that musicians are better at picking out a person's voice in a noisy background.

## Music Therapy Interventions

Listening to and making music on your own can bring health benefits. But some people may also benefit from the help of a board-certified music therapist. Music therapists are trained in how to use music to meet the mental, social, and physical needs of people with different health conditions. "Music therapy can take many forms that go beyond listening to music," explains Dr. Sheri Robb, a music therapist and behavioral intervention researcher at Indiana University.

Music therapists can use certain parts of music, like the rhythm or melody, to help people regain abilities they've lost from a brain injury or developmental disability. For example, a person who's had a stroke may be able to sing words, but not speak them. Music therapists also rely on the social qualities of music. Shared musical experiences can help a family member connect with a loved one who has dementia. Music can also be used to help young people with behavior disorders learn ways to manage their emotions.

Robb's research focuses on developing and testing music therapy interventions for children and teens with cancer and their families. In one study, music therapists helped young people undergoing high-risk cancer treatments to write song lyrics and create music videos about what was most important to them. "With the help of music therapists, these teenagers were able to identify their strengths and positive ways to cope, remain connected with family and friends, and improve communication during a challenging time," Robb explains.

## Music in Your Life

Music can offer many health benefits, but it may not be helpful for everyone. Traumatic injuries and brain conditions can change the way a person perceives and responds to music. Some people may find some types of music overstimulating. Others may find that certain music brings up emotional or traumatic memories.

"It's important for healthcare providers to identify and understand when music isn't helpful and may be harmful," Robb says. "And this is an area where music therapists can be helpful."

As scientists continue to learn more about music and the brain, try striking a chord for your health. Whether you're looking to boost your mood, stay connected to others, or improve symptoms of a health condition, add a little music to your life. "Think of music like physical fitness or what you eat," Kraus says. "To see the most health benefits, try to include music as a regular, consistent part of your life. It's never too late to add music to your life."

## Live with Music

- Listen to music during the day, like on your way to work or during exercise.
- Sing and dance while you're doing chores or cooking meals.
- Play a musical instrument. Consider taking lessons or joining friends to make music.
- Attend concerts, plays, and other community music activities in your area.
- Encourage your kids to listen to music, sing, play an instrument or participate in music programs at the school.
- Ask your doctor if music therapy is right for you. Consider working with a board-certified music therapist to improve your health.

# Chapter 53

# *Prayer and Spirituality*

## *Chapter Contents*

# Section 53.1

# *What Is Spirituality?*

This section includes text excerpted from "Spirituality and
Trauma: Professionals Working Together," National
Center for Posttraumatic Stress Disorder (NCPTSD), U.S.
Department of Veterans Affairs (VA), May 26, 2016.

Spirituality is a personal experience with many definitions. Spirituality might be defined as "an inner belief system providing an individual with meaning and purpose in life, a sense of the sacredness of life, and a vision for the betterment of the world." Other definitions emphasize "a connection to that which transcends the self." The connection might be to God, a higher power, a universal energy, the sacred, or to nature.

## *Three Dimensions of Spirituality*

Researchers in the field of spirituality have suggested three useful dimensions for thinking about one's spirituality:

1.  Beliefs

2.  Spiritual practices

3.  Spiritual Experiences

## *Spirituality in the United States*

Currently, in the United States, opinion surveys consistently find that most people endorse a belief in God or higher power. In a Gallup Poll, 86 percent of respondents indicated a belief in God, while only 6 percent stated they did not believe in God. Many of these individuals would describe religion or spirituality as the most important source of strength and direction for their lives. Because spirituality plays such a significant and central role in the lives of many people, it is likely to be affected by trauma, and in turn to affect the survivor's reaction to the trauma.

## Spirituality and Healthcare

Historically, there have been differences between the beliefs of scientists and healthcare practitioners and those of the general population. For example, one study indicated that only 66 percent of psychologists report a "belief in God." These differences in viewpoint may contribute to the lack of research on spirituality. The beliefs and training experiences of practitioners may also influence whether and how spirituality is incorporated into therapy.

## Section 53.2

# *Types of Spirituality*

This section includes text excerpted from "Three Types of Spirituality," U.S. Department of Veterans Affairs (VA), January 12, 2016.

We can live on junk food, at least for a while. However, junk food is not for healthy eating. Junk food is for pleasure. In time, we pay the price of our food choice. We have poorer health. In a like way, if we feed our inner spirit with pleasing but not healthy matter, over time we become poorer in spirit.

There are three types of spirituality, namely:

1. Religious spirituality

2. Nonreligious spirituality

3. Toxic spirituality

## *Religious Spirituality*

Most of us know religious spirituality. It involves belief in a being greater than oneself, church, and prayer. Some people try to be like the masters of spirituality in their church. Other people find their spirituality in the books of religions. It does not matter where or how they find their spirituality. For many people, their religious beliefs shape and define their spiritual lives. They are inseparable.

403

## Nonreligious Spirituality

The second type of spirituality is nonreligious spirituality. It centers on doing something positive. This gives a sense of peace in one's spirit. Nonreligious spiritual acts often mean creating things or making something by hand. This act gives a sense of satisfaction. Fans of the television show NCIS may recall a scene. After Agent Gibbs solves a disturbing crime, he retreats to his basement. There he quietly, carefully works on his hand-made boat. The message is simple. The act of creating something fed his soul. The acts of destruction he saw took away his sense of peace. Building something of beauty gives back his inner peace. His spirit is nourished back to health. Making the boat gives meaning and purpose to his life. This is an example of nonreligious spirituality.

## Toxic Spirituality

The third kind of spirituality is toxic, or pseudo-spirituality. More often than not, this involves an action or the use of a substance. At first, this causes a good feeling, a rush. Too much use of drugs, alcohol, gambling, food, and the like all provide the person with a rush or feeling high. Even exercise, when done in excess, can make us feel good at first.

The action is repeated often to try to get back that good feeling. After all, it is only natural to seek things that make us feel good about ourselves. People want to believe that their lives have meaning. The problem comes up when such actions take over our lives. The action becomes meaning itself for us.

## Choose Life

Once we see these different types of spirituality, we can make a choice. I doubt that any of us would choose a spirituality that kills. That is what toxins do. Toxins kill. We would choose a spirituality that brings growth and life. Religious and nonreligious spirituality bring growth and life. Toxic spirituality brings death. Sadly, the choice is not always easy to make. The task for you is simple, yet most important: Choose life!

# Section 53.3

# *Spirituality and Trauma*

This section includes text excerpted from "Spirituality and Trauma: Professionals Working Together," National Center for Posttraumatic Stress Disorder (NCPTSD), U.S. Department of Veterans Affairs (VA), May 26, 2016.

## *Relationship of Trauma to Spirituality*

Evidence suggests that trauma can produce both positive and negative effects on the spiritual experiences and perceptions of individuals. For example, depression and loneliness can lead to feelings of abandonment and loss of faith in God. These effects may change as time passes and a person moves further away from the acute phase of trauma recovery. On the positive side, some individuals experience increased appreciation of life, greater perceived closeness to God, increased sense of purpose in life, and enhanced spiritual well-being even following devastating events such as disasters and rape. For others, trauma can be associated with loss of faith, diminished participation in religious or spiritual activities, changes in belief, feelings of being abandoned or punished by God, and loss of meaning and purpose for living.

Aspects of spirituality are associated with positive outcomes, even when trauma survivors develop psychiatric difficulties such as posttraumatic stress disorder (PTSD) or depression. Research also indicates that healthy spirituality is often associated with lower levels of symptoms and clinical problems in some trauma populations. For example, anger, rage, and a desire for revenge following trauma may be tempered by forgiveness, spiritual beliefs, or spiritual practices.

Suggestions have been made about the pathways by which spirituality might affect the recovery trajectory for survivors of traumatic events. Spirituality may improve posttrauma outcomes through:

1. Reduction of behavioral risks through healthy religious lifestyles (e.g., less drinking or smoking)

2. Expanded social support through involvement in spiritual communities

3. Enhancement of coping skills and helpful ways of understanding the trauma that results in meaning-making

4. Physiological mechanisms such as activation of the "relaxation response" through prayer or meditation

Feelings of isolation, loneliness, and depression related to grief and loss may be lessened by the social support of a spiritual community. Being part of a spiritual community places survivors among caring individuals who may provide encouragement and emotional support, as well as possible instrumental support in the form of physical or even financial assistance in times of trouble.

## What Issues Most Often Involve Spirituality?

### Making Meaning of the Trauma Experience

Spiritual beliefs may influence the trauma survivor's ability to make meaning out of the trauma experience. In turn, the meaning drawn can have a significant impact on the survivor's symptoms and functioning. Several studies have indicated that negative thoughts or attributions about God, such as "God has abandoned me," and "God is punishing me," or, being angry at God are associated with a number of poor clinical outcomes. Research suggests that these types of thoughts can be associated with poorer physical and mental health, and increased use of substances. One study of Veterans being treated for PTSD found that negative religious coping and lack of forgiveness were both associated with worse PTSD and depression symptoms.

Recovery of meaning in life may be achieved through changed ways of thinking, involvement in meaningful activities, or through rituals experienced as part of religious or spiritual involvement. Some researchers have suggested that traumatic events frequently challenge one's core beliefs about safety, self-worth, and the meaning of life. For individuals whose core values are spiritually grounded, traumatic events may give rise to questions about the fundamental nature of the relationship between the creator and humankind. Survivors may question their belief in a loving, all-powerful God when the innocent are subjected to traumatic victimization. In this way, traumatic experiences may become a starting point for discussion of the many ways in which survivors define what it is to have "faith."

## Guilt and Moral Injury

Additionally, in certain types of traumatic events, such as war, an individual can be both victim and perpetrator of trauma. For example, a soldier during their war-zone service could be exposed to the injury and death of others, be wounded himself or herself, and have a role in killing the enemy. It is also possible for two core elements of a person's worldview—for example, patriotism, and faith—to be in conflict, creating doubt and uncertainty about the right course of action. These experiences can sometimes lead to long-lasting difficult spiritual and moral questions. The result may be the loss of faith, increased guilt and self-blame, and alienation from other people and from God. Individuals may experience a disconnection between the beliefs they were raised with, their expectations about what military service would be like, and their actual war-zone experiences.

## Grief and Bereavement

Grief and loss can be significant issues that survivors must cope with in the aftermath of trauma. In U.S. society, spirituality is frequently utilized to cope with traumatic death and loss. Researchers noted after the 9/11 terrorist attacks that 90 percent of respondents reported turning to "prayer, religion, or spiritual feelings" as a coping mechanism. In general, research suggests there is a positive association between spirituality and grief recovery for survivors of traumatic loss. Researchers suggest that for many spirituality provides a frame through which survivors can "make sense" of the loss. Additionally, survivors may benefit from supportive relationships often provided by spiritual communities.

# Section 53.4

# *Spirituality and Cancer Care*

This section includes text excerpted from "Spirituality in
Cancer Care (PDQ®)—Patient Version," National
Cancer Institute (NCI), May 18, 2015.

## *Importance of Spirituality in Cancer Care*

### *Religious and Spiritual Values Are Important to Patients Coping with Cancer*

Studies have shown that religious and spiritual values are important to Americans. Most American adults say that they believe in God and that their religious beliefs affect how they live their lives. However, people have different ideas about life after death, belief in miracles, and other religious beliefs. Such beliefs may be based on gender, education, and ethnic background.

Many patients with cancer rely on spiritual or religious beliefs and practices to help them cope with their disease. This is called spiritual coping. Many caregivers also rely on spiritual coping. Each person may have different spiritual needs, depending on cultural and religious traditions. For some seriously ill patients, spiritual well-being may affect how much anxiety they feel about death. For others, it may affect what they decide about end-of-life treatments. Some patients and their family caregivers may want doctors to talk about spiritual concerns, but may feel unsure about how to bring up the subject.

Some studies show that doctors' support of spiritual well-being in very ill patients helps improve their quality of life. Healthcare providers who treat patients coping with cancer are looking at ways to help them with religious and spiritual concerns. Doctors may ask patients which spiritual issues are important to them during treatment as well as near the end of life. When patients with advanced cancer receive spiritual support from the medical team, they may be more likely to choose hospice care and less aggressive treatment at the end of life.

## *Spirituality and Religion May Have Different Meanings*

The terms spirituality and religion are often used in place of each other, but for many people, they have different meanings. Religion may be defined as a specific set of beliefs and practices, usually within an organized group. Spirituality may be defined as an individual's sense of peace, purpose, and connection to others, and beliefs about the meaning of life. Spirituality may be found and expressed through an organized religion or in other ways. Patients may think of themselves as spiritual or religious or both.

## *Serious Illness, Such as Cancer, May Cause Spiritual Distress*

Serious illnesses like cancer may cause patients or family caregivers to have doubts about their beliefs or religious values and cause much spiritual distress. Some studies show that patients with cancer may feel that they are being punished by God or may have a loss of faith after being diagnosed. Other patients may have mild feelings of spiritual distress when coping with cancer.

## Spirituality and Quality of Life

### *Spiritual and Religious Well-Being May Help Improve Quality of Life*

It is not known for sure how spirituality and religion are related to health. Some studies show that spiritual or religious beliefs and practices create a positive mental attitude that may help a patient feel better and improve the well-being of family caregivers. Spiritual and religious well-being may help improve health and quality of life in the following ways:

- Decrease anxiety, depression, anger, and discomfort

- Decrease the sense of isolation (feeling alone) and the risk of suicide

- Decrease alcohol and drug abuse

- Lower blood pressure and the risk of heart disease

- Help the patient adjust to the effects of cancer and its treatment

- Increase the ability to enjoy life during cancer treatment

- Give a feeling of personal growth as a result of living with cancer

Increase positive feelings, including:

- Hope and optimism
- Freedom from regret
- Satisfaction with life
- A sense of inner peace
- Spiritual and religious well-being may also help a patient live longer

### *Spiritual Distress May Also Affect Health*

Spiritual distress may make it harder for patients to cope with cancer and cancer treatment. Healthcare providers may encourage patients to meet with experienced spiritual or religious leaders to help deal with their spiritual issues. This may improve their health, quality of life, and ability to cope.

## *Spiritual Assessment*

A spiritual assessment is a method or tool used by doctors to understand the role that religious and spiritual beliefs have in the patient's life. This may help the doctor understand how these beliefs affect the way the patient responds to the cancer diagnosis and decisions about cancer treatment. Some doctors or caregivers may wait for the patient to bring up spiritual concerns. Others may use an interview or a questionnaire.

### *A Spiritual Assessment Explores Religious Beliefs and Spiritual Practices*

A spiritual assessment may include questions about the following:

- Religious denomination, if any
- Beliefs or philosophy of life
- Important spiritual practices or rituals
- Using spirituality or religion as a source of strength
- Being part of a community of support
- Using prayer or meditation
- Loss of faith

- Conflicts between spiritual or religious beliefs and cancer treatments

- Ways that healthcare providers and caregivers may help with the patient's spiritual needs

- Concerns about death and afterlife

The healthcare team may not ask about every issue the patient feels is important. Patients should bring up other spiritual or religious issues that they think may affect their cancer care.

# Chapter 54

# *Relaxation Techniques*

## *What Are Relaxation Techniques?*

Relaxation techniques include a number of practices such as progressive relaxation, guided imagery, biofeedback, self-hypnosis, and deep breathing exercises. The goal is similar in all: to produce the body's natural relaxation response, characterized by slower breathing, lower blood pressure, and a feeling of increased wellbeing.

Meditation and practices that include meditation with movements, such as yoga and tai chi, can also promote relaxation.

Stress management programs commonly include relaxation techniques. Relaxation techniques have also been studied to see whether they might be of value in managing various health problems.

Relaxation techniques are skills, and like other skills, they need practice. People who use relaxation techniques frequently are more likely to benefit from them. Regular, frequent practice is particularly important if you're using relaxation techniques to help manage a chronic health problem. Continuing use of relaxation techniques is more effective than short-term use.

Relaxation techniques include the following:

### *Autogenic Training*

In autogenic training, you learn to concentrate on the physical sensations of warmth, heaviness, and relaxation in different parts of your body.

Text in this chapter is excerpted from "Relaxation Techniques for Health," National Center for Complementary and Integrative Health (NCCIH), April 20, 2017.

### Biofeedback-Assisted Relaxation

Biofeedback techniques measure body functions and give you information about them so that you can learn to control them. Biofeedback-assisted relaxation uses electronic devices to teach you to produce changes in your body that are associated with relaxation, such as reduced muscle tension.

### Deep Breathing or Breathing Exercises

This technique involves focusing on taking slow, deep, even breaths.

### Guided Imagery

For this technique, people are taught to focus on pleasant images to replace negative or stressful feelings. Guided imagery may be self-directed or led by a practitioner or a recording.

### Progressive Relaxation

This technique, also called Jacobson relaxation or progressive muscle relaxation, involves tightening and relaxing various muscle groups. Progressive relaxation is often combined with guided imagery and breathing exercises.

### Self-Hypnosis

In self-hypnosis programs, people are taught to produce the relaxation response when prompted by a phrase or nonverbal cue (called a "suggestion").

## What the Science Says about the Effectiveness of Relaxation Techniques

Researchers have evaluated relaxation techniques to see whether they could play a role in managing a variety of health conditions, including the following:

### Anxiety

Studies have shown relaxation techniques may reduce anxiety in people with ongoing health problems such as heart disease or inflammatory bowel disease (IBD), and in those who are having medical procedures such as breast biopsies or dental treatment. Relaxation techniques have also been shown to be useful for older adults with anxiety.

On the other hand, relaxation techniques may not be the best way to help people with generalized anxiety disorder (GAD). GAD is a mental health condition, lasting for months or longer, in which a person is often worried or anxious about many things and finds it hard to control the anxiety. Studies indicate that long-term results are better in people with GAD who receive a type of psychotherapy called cognitive-behavioral therapy (CBT) than in those who are taught relaxation techniques.

## Asthma

There hasn't been enough research to show whether relaxation techniques can relieve asthma symptoms in either adults or children.

## Childbirth

Relaxation techniques such as guided imagery, progressive muscle relaxation, and breathing techniques may be useful in managing labor pain. Studies have shown that women who were taught self-hypnosis have a decreased need for pain medicine during labor. Biofeedback hasn't been shown to relieve labor pain.

## Depression

An evaluation of 15 studies concluded that relaxation techniques are better than no treatment in reducing symptoms of depression but are not as beneficial as psychological therapies such as CBT.

## Epilepsy

There's no reliable evidence that relaxation techniques are useful in managing epilepsy.

## Fibromyalgia (FM)

Studies of guided imagery for fibromyalgia (FM) have had inconsistent results. A 2013 evaluation of the research concluded that electromyographic (EMG) biofeedback, in which people are taught to control and reduce muscle tension, helped to reduce FM pain, at least for short periods of time. However, EMG biofeedback didn't affect sleep problems, depression, fatigue, or health-related quality of life in people with FM, and its long-term effects haven't been established.

## *Headache*

**Biofeedback.** Biofeedback has been studied for both tension headaches and migraines. An evaluation of high-quality studies concluded that there's conflicting evidence about whether biofeedback can relieve tension headaches. Studies have shown decreases in the frequency of migraines in people who were using biofeedback. However, it's unclear whether biofeedback is better than a placebo.

**Other relaxation techniques.** Relaxation techniques other than biofeedback have been studied for tension headaches. An evaluation of high-quality studies found conflicting evidence on whether relaxation techniques are better than no treatment or a placebo. Some studies suggest that other relaxation techniques are less effective than biofeedback.

## *Heart Disease*

In people with heart disease, studies have shown relaxation techniques can reduce stress and anxiety and may also have beneficial effects on physical measures such as heart rate.

## *High Blood Pressure*

Stress can lead to a short-term increase in blood pressure, and the relaxation response has been shown to reduce blood pressure on a short-term basis, allowing people to reduce their need for blood pressure medication. However, it's uncertain whether relaxation techniques can have long-term effects on high blood pressure.

## *Insomnia*

There's evidence that relaxation techniques can be helpful in managing chronic insomnia. Relaxation techniques can be combined with other strategies for getting a good night's sleep, such as maintaining a consistent sleep schedule; avoiding caffeine, alcohol, heavy meals, and strenuous exercise too close to bedtime; and sleeping in a quiet, cool, dark room.

## *Irritable Bowel Syndrome (IBS)*

An evaluation of research results by the American College of Gastroenterology (ACG) concluded that relaxation techniques have not been shown to help IBS. However, other psychological therapies, including CBT and hypnotherapy, are associated with overall symptom improvement in people with IBS.

### Menopause Symptoms

Relaxation techniques have been studied for hot flashes and other symptoms associated with menopause, but the quality of the research isn't high enough to allow definite conclusions to be reached.

### Menstrual Cramps

Some research suggests that relaxation techniques may be beneficial for menstrual cramps, but definite conclusions can't be reached because of the small number of participants in the studies and the poor quality of some of the research.

### Nausea

An evaluation of the research evidence concluded that some relaxation techniques, including guided imagery and progressive muscle relaxation, are likely to be effective in relieving nausea caused by cancer chemotherapy when used in combination with antinausea drugs.

### Nightmares

Some studies have indicated that relaxation exercises may be an effective approach for nightmares of unknown cause and those associated with posttraumatic stress disorder (PTSD). However, an assessment of many studies concluded that relaxation is less helpful than more extensive forms of treatment (psychotherapy or medication).

### Pain

Evaluations of the research evidence have found promising but not conclusive evidence that guided imagery may help relieve some musculoskeletal pain (pain involving the bones or muscles) and other types of pain. An analysis of data on hospitalized cancer patients showed that those who received integrative medicine therapies, such as guided imagery and relaxation response training, during their hospitalization had reductions in both pain and anxiety.

### Pain in Children and Adolescents

A 2014 evaluation of the scientific evidence found that psychological therapies, which may include relaxation techniques as well as other approaches such as CBT, can reduce pain in children and adolescents with chronic headaches or other types of chronic pain. The evidence is particularly promising for headaches: the effect on pain may last

417

for several months after treatment, and the therapies also help to reduce anxiety.

### Posttraumatic Stress Disorder (PTSD)

Studies of biofeedback and other relaxation techniques for PTSD have had inconsistent results.

### Rheumatoid Arthritis (RA)

There's limited evidence that biofeedback or other relaxation techniques might be valuable additions to treatment programs for rheumatoid arthritis (RA).

### Ringing in the Ears (Tinnitus)

Only a few studies have evaluated relaxation techniques for ringing in the ears. The limited evidence from these studies suggests that relaxation techniques might be useful, especially in reducing the intrusiveness of the problem.

### Smoking Cessation

Limited evidence suggests that guided imagery may be a valuable tool for people who are working to quit smoking. In a study that compared the two techniques, autogenic training was found to be less effective than CBT as a quit-smoking aid. However, this study involved patients in an alcohol detoxification program, so its results may not be applicable to other people. Preliminary research suggests that a guided relaxation routine might help reduce cigarette cravings.

### Temporomandibular Joint Dysfunction (TJD)

Problems with the temporomandibular joint (TJD), the joint that connects the jaw to the side of the head, can cause pain and difficulty moving the jaw. A few studies have shown that programs that include relaxation techniques may help relieve symptoms of TJD.

## What the Science Says about the Safety and Side Effects of Relaxation Techniques

Relaxation techniques are generally considered safe for healthy people. However, occasionally, people report negative experiences such as increased anxiety, intrusive thoughts, or fear of losing control. There have been rare reports that certain relaxation techniques might cause or worsen symptoms in people with epilepsy or certain psychiatric conditions, or with a history of abuse or trauma. People with heart disease should talk to their healthcare provider before doing progressive muscle relaxation.

### Who Teaches Relaxation Techniques?

A variety of professionals, including physicians, psychologists, social workers, nurses, and complementary health practitioners, may teach relaxation techniques. Also, people sometimes learn the simpler relaxation techniques on their own.

### More to Consider

If you have severe or long-lasting symptoms of any kind, see your healthcare provider. You might have a condition that needs to be treated promptly. For example, if depression or anxiety persists, it's important to seek help from a qualified healthcare professional. Tell all your healthcare providers about any complementary or integrative health approaches you use. Give them a full picture of what you do to manage your health. This will help ensure coordinated and safe care.

# Chapter 55

# *Tai Chi and Qi Gong*

## *About Tai Chi and Qi Gong*

Tai chi and qi gong are centuries-old, related mind and body practices. They involve certain postures and gentle movements with mental focus, breathing, and relaxation. The movements can be adapted or practiced while walking, standing, or sitting. In contrast to qi gong, tai chi movements, if practiced quickly, can be a form of combat or self-defense.

## *What the Science Says about the Effectiveness of Tai Chi and Qi Gong*

Research findings suggest that practicing tai chi may improve balance and stability in older people and those with Parkinson disease (PD), reduce pain from knee osteoarthritis (OA), help people cope with fibromyalgia (FM), and back pain, and promote quality of life and mood in people with heart failure and cancer. There's been less research on the effects of qi gong, but some studies suggest it may reduce chronic neck pain (although results are mixed) and pain from FM. Qigong also may help to improve the general quality of life.

Both also may offer psychological benefits, such as reducing anxiety. However, differences in how the research on anxiety was conducted make it difficult to draw firm conclusions about this.

This chapter includes text excerpted from "Tai Chi and Qi Gong: In Depth," National Center for Complementary and Integrative Health (NCCIH), October 2016.

## Falling and Balance

Exercise programs, including tai chi, may reduce falling and the fear of falling in older people. Tai chi also may be more effective than other forms of exercise for improving balance and stability in people with PD.

- A 2012 review determined that tai chi, as well as other groups, and home-based activity programs (which often include balance and strength-training exercises) effectively reduced falling in older people, and tai chi significantly reduced the risk of falling. But the reviewers also found that tai chi was less effective in older people who were at higher risk of falling.

- Fear of falling can have a serious impact on an older person's health and life. In a 2014 review, researchers suggested that various types of exercise, including tai chi, may reduce the fear of falling among older people.

- Findings from a 2012 clinical trial with 195 people showed that practicing tai chi improved balance and stability better than resistance training or stretching in people with mild-to-moderate PD. A 2014 follow-up analysis showed that people who practiced tai chi were more likely to continue exercising during the 3 months following the study compared with those who participated in resistance training or stretching.

## For Pain (Knee Osteoarthritis (OA), Fibromyalgia (FM), Chronic Neck Pain, Back Pain)

There's some evidence that practicing tai chi may help people manage pain associated with knee OA (a breakdown of cartilage in the knee that allows leg bones to rub together), FM (a disorder that causes muscle pain and fatigue), and back pain. Qigong may offer some benefit for chronic neck pain, but results are mixed.

### Knee OA

The results of a small National Center for Complementary and Integrative Health (NCCIH)-funded clinical trial involving 40 participants with knee OA suggested that practicing tai chi reduced pain and improved function better than an education and stretching program. An analysis of seven small and moderately-sized clinical studies concluded that a 12-week course of tai chi reduced pain and improved function in people with this condition.

*FM*

Results from a small NCCIH-supported clinical trial suggested that practicing tai chi was more effective than wellness education and stretching in helping people with fibromyalgia sleep better and cope with pain, fatigue, and depression. After 12 weeks, those who practiced tai chi also had better scores on a survey designed to measure a person's ability to carry out certain daily activities such as walking, housecleaning, shopping, and preparing a meal. The benefits of tai chi also appeared to last longer. A small 2012 NCCIH-supported trial suggested that combining tai chi movements with mindfulness allowed people with fibromyalgia to work through the discomfort they may feel during exercise, allowing them to take advantage of the benefits of physical activity.

The results of a 2012 randomized clinical trial with 100 participants suggested that practicing qigong reduced pain and improved sleep, the ability to do daily activities, and mental function. The researchers also observed that most improvements were still apparent after 6 months.

*Chronic Neck Pain*

The research results on the effectiveness of qi gong for chronic neck pain are mixed, but the people who were studied and the way the studies were done were quite different. A clinical study by German researchers showed no benefit of qigong or exercise compared with no therapy in 117 elderly adults (mostly women) with, on average, a 20-year history of chronic neck pain. Study participants had 24 exercise or qigong sessions over 3 months.

In a 2011 study, some of the same researchers observed that qigong was just as effective as exercise therapy (and both were more effective than no therapy) in relieving neck pain in the 123 middle-aged adults (mostly women) who had chronic neck pain for an average of 3 years. Exercise therapy included throwing and catching a ball, rowing and climbing movements, arm swinging, and stretching, among other activities. People in the study had 18 exercise or qi gong sessions over 6 months.

*Back Pain*

In people who had low-back pain for at least 3 months, a program of tai chi exercises reduced their pain and improved their functioning.

## For Mental Health and Cognitive Function

While a range of research has suggested that exercise helps reduce depression and anxiety, the role of tai chi and qigong for these and other mental health problems is less clear. However, there is evidence that tai chi may boost brain function and reasoning ability in older people. An NCCIH-supported research suggested that practicing tai chi may help reduce stress, anxiety, and depression, and also improve mood and self-esteem. However, in their review, which included 40 studies with more than 3,800 participants, the researchers noted that they couldn't develop firm conclusions because of differences in study designs.

In an NCCIH-supported review, researchers found that the results from 29 studies with more than 2,500 participants didn't offer clear evidence about the effectiveness of tai chi and qigong on such psychological factors as anxiety, depression, stress, mood, and self-esteem. But the researchers noted that most of these studies weren't looking primarily at psychological distress and didn't intentionally recruit participants with mental health issues.

The results from another NCCIH-supported review published in 2014 suggested that practicing tai chi may enhance the ability to reason, plan, remember, and solve problems in older people without evidence of significant cognitive impairment. The data also indicated that tai chi boosted cognitive ability in people who showed signs of mild cognitive impairment (CI) to dementia, but to a lesser degree than in those with no signs of CI.

### For Quality of Life

Much research suggests that physical activity enhances the quality of life. Health providers who treat people with cancer often recommend exercise to reduce illness-related fatigue and improve quality of life. Some studies also suggest that physical activity helps people with heart disease and other chronic illnesses.

### Cancer

Research results indicated that practicing qigong may improve quality of life, mood, fatigue, and inflammation in adults with different types of cancer, compared with those receiving usual care. However, the researchers suggested that the attention received by the qigong participants may have contributed to the positive study findings.

### Heart Disease

Regular practice of tai chi may improve quality of life and mood in people with chronic heart failure, according to a 2011 clinical trial funded by NCCIH. Results from a small study suggested that practicing tai chi improved the ability to exercise and may be an option as cardiac rehabilitation for people who have had a heart attack.

*Other*

An NCCIH-supported research review examined the effects of tai chi and qigong on the quality of life of adults who were healthy, elderly, were breast cancer or stroke survivors or had a chronic disease. The analysis suggested that practicing tai chi or qigong may improve quality of life in healthy and chronically ill people.

## What the Science Says about Safety of Tai Chi and Qi Gong

Tai chi and qigong appear to be safe practices. An NCCIH-supported review noted that tai chi is unlikely to result in serious injury but it may be associated with minor aches and pains. Women who are pregnant should talk with their healthcare providers before beginning tai chi, qi gong, or any other exercise program.

## Training, Licensing, and Certification

Tai chi instructors don't have to be licensed, and the practice isn't regulated by the federal government or individual states. There's no national standard for qigong certification. Various tai chi, and qi gong organizations offer training and certification programs—with differing criteria and levels of certification for instructors.

## More to Consider

If you are considering to try tai chi or qigong consider the following:

- Learning tai chi or qigong from a video or book does not ensure that you're doing the movements correctly or safely.
- If you have a health condition, talk with your healthcare provider before starting tai chi or qigong.
- Ask a trusted source (such as your healthcare provider) to recommend a tai chi or qigong instructor. Find out about the training and experience of any instructor you're considering.
- Tell all your healthcare providers about any complementary or integrative health approaches you use. Give them a full picture of what you do to manage your health. This will help ensure coordinated and safe care.

# Chapter 56

# *Yoga*

## *Chapter Contents*

## Section 56.1

# *Yoga: An Overview*

This section includes text excerpted from "Yoga: In Depth,"
National Center for Complementary and Integrative
Health (NCCIH), June 2013. Reviewed May 2018.

Yoga in its full form combines physical postures, breathing exercises, meditation, and a distinct philosophy. There are numerous styles of yoga. Hatha yoga, commonly practiced in the United States and Europe, emphasizes postures, breathing exercises, and meditation. Hatha yoga styles include Ananda, Anusara, Ashtanga, Bikram, Iyengar, Kripalu, Kundalini, Viniyoga, and others.

## *Use of Yoga for Health in the United States*

According to the National Health Interview Survey (NHIS), which included a comprehensive survey on the use of complementary health approaches by Americans, yoga is the sixth most commonly used complementary health practice among adults. More than 13 million adults practiced yoga. According to a survey by NHIS, use of yoga among adults increased by 1 percent (or approximately 3 million people). The survey also found that more than 1.5 million children practiced yoga in the previous year.

Many people who practice yoga do so to maintain their health and well-being, improve physical fitness, relieve stress, and enhance the quality of life. In addition, they may be addressing specific health conditions, such as back pain, neck pain, arthritis, and anxiety.

## *What the Science Says about Yoga*

Research suggests that a carefully adapted set of yoga poses may reduce low-back pain and improve function. Other studies also suggest that practicing yoga (as well as other forms of regular exercise) might improve quality of life; reduce stress; lower heart rate and blood pressure; help relieve anxiety, depression, and insomnia; and improve overall physical fitness, strength, and flexibility. But some research suggests yoga may not improve asthma, and studies looking at yoga and arthritis have had mixed results.

A National Center for Complementary and Integrative Health (NCCIH)-funded study of 90 people with chronic low-back pain found that participants who practiced Iyengar yoga had significantly less disability, pain, and depression after 6 months. In a 2011 study, also funded by NCCIH, researchers compared yoga with conventional stretching exercises or a self-care book in 228 adults with chronic low-back pain. The results showed that both yoga and stretching were more effective than a self-care book for improving function and reducing symptoms due to chronic low-back pain. Conclusions from another 2011 study of 313 adults with chronic or recurring low-back pain suggested that 12 weekly yoga classes resulted in better function than usual medical care

However, studies show that certain health conditions may not benefit from yoga. A 2011 systematic review of clinical studies suggests that there is no sound evidence that yoga improves asthma. A 2011 review of the literature reports that few published studies have looked at yoga and arthritis, and of those that have, results are inconclusive. The two main types of arthritis—osteoarthritis (OA) and rheumatoid arthritis (RA)—are different conditions, and the effects of yoga may not be the same for each. In addition, the reviewers suggested that even if a study showed that yoga helped osteoarthritic finger joints, it may not help osteoarthritic knee joints.

## Side Effects and Risks

Yoga is generally low-impact and safe for healthy people when practiced appropriately under the guidance of a well-trained instructor. Overall, those who practice yoga have a low rate of side effects, and the risk of serious injury from yoga is quite low. However, certain types of stroke, as well as pain from nerve damage are among the rare possible side effects of practicing yoga.

Women who are pregnant and people with certain medical conditions, such as high blood pressure, glaucoma (a condition in which fluid pressure within the eye slowly increases and may damage the eye's optic nerve), and sciatica (pain, weakness, numbness, or tingling that may extend from the lower back to the calf, foot, or even the toes), should modify or avoid some yoga poses.

### Key Facts

Studies in people with chronic low-back pain suggest that a carefully adapted set of yoga poses may help reduce pain and improve function (the ability to walk and move). Studies also suggest that practicing yoga (as well as other forms of regular exercise) might have other health benefits such as reducing heart rate and blood pressure and may also help relieve anxiety and depression. Other research suggests yoga is not helpful for asthma, and studies looking at yoga and arthritis have had mixed results. People with high blood pressure, glaucoma, or sciatica, and women who are pregnant should modify or avoid some yoga poses.

Ask a trusted source (such as a healthcare provider or local hospital) to recommend a yoga practitioner. Contact professional organizations for the names of practitioners who have completed an acceptable training program. Tell all your healthcare providers about any complementary health approaches you use. Give them a full picture of what you do to manage your health. This will help ensure coordinated and safe care.

## Section 56.2

# *Yoga for Relief from Low-Back Pain*

This section includes text excerpted from "Yoga Similar to Physical Therapy in Helping Low-Back Pain in a Diverse Urban Population," National Center for Complementary and Integrative Health (NCCIH), June 19, 2017.

The results of a National Center for Complementary and Integrative Health (NCCIH)-funded study show yoga and physical therapy offers similar pain-relief and functional benefits to people with low socioeconomic status who had chronic low-back pain. These improvements were greater than self-education; however, they were not considered significant. These findings suggest that a structured yoga program may be an alternative to physical therapy for people with chronic low-back pain, depending on individual preferences, availability, and cost.

The year-long study, which enrolled racially diverse adults with low socioeconomic status, was conducted at Boston University and included researchers from the University of Pittsburgh, Group Health Research Institute in Seattle, the University of Washington, and the RAND Corporation. It was published in the *Annals of Internal Medicine*.

Some studies suggest yoga helps with symptoms of chronic low-back pain. But the evidence has been sparse on whether yoga's benefits extend across diverse populations, including racial, or ethnic minorities, those with lower socioeconomic status, or those with challenges in obtaining medical care because of health disparities.

In the first 12-week phase of the study, researchers randomly assigned 320 predominantly low-income, racially diverse adults aged 18–64 with chronic low-back pain (of no specific cause) to one of three groups:

- One group participated in a 75-minute yoga class, once per week, taught by a yoga instructor, along with home practice.

- Another group received individual physical therapy of up to 15 one-hour sessions delivered by a physical therapist and combined with home practice.

- The final group received an education handbook on self-care for back pain; every 3 weeks, they received brief newsletters that summarized the main points from assigned chapters. Members of this group also received periodic check-in calls.

The researchers measured participants' average pain intensity and disability related to back pain at the study's start and then at 6, 12, 26, 40, and 52 weeks.

In the next phase of the study, members of the yoga and physical therapy groups who had attended at least one of their classes or sessions were randomly assigned to new groups. For example, the yoga participants were assigned to either home practice or drop-in yoga classes, and the physical therapy participants to either home practice only or five "booster" sessions of physical therapy. The education group continued reviewing their materials and receiving check-in calls.

The researchers found that for pain and function, yoga and physical therapy had similar results, and both were better than the education group. Further, at 12 weeks, the yoga and physical therapy groups were less likely than the education group to use any pain medication. Improvements in the yoga and physical therapy groups were maintained at the end of the 52 weeks. The benefits of these two groups appeared to be associated with the number of classes/sessions participants attended.

Additional analyses of these data are planned, including on cost effectiveness, work productivity, and perceived depression and anxiety.

## Section 56.3

# *Parkinson Disease: The Benefits of Yoga*

This section includes text excerpted from "For Veterans with Parkinson's Disease: The Benefits of Yoga," U.S. Department of Veterans Affairs (VA), April 20, 2017.

Yoga is very popular and is cited as a favorite nonmedical therapy by many people living with Parkinson disease (PD). People are often fearful of getting started in a yoga class since there is often an incorrect portrayal of yoga in the media as being only for flexible, skinny ballet dancers. Yoga, on the contrary, is a very adaptable practice, with both functional and psychosocial benefits, that can be suited to a wide variety of abilities.

Yoga has become synonymous with holding and moving between a series of static postures (called asanas); however, this physical practice (called hatha yoga) is only one part of the larger lifestyle of yoga framework that includes branches such as philosophy, chanting, and selfless service. Hatha yoga combines physical postures to address strength, flexibility, balance and mind-body-breath connection. Breathing practices (pranayama) and meditation are included to develop greater self-awareness and can have a tremendous benefit on the mental state.

## *What Yoga Can Do*

Yoga:

- Strengthens your core, especially your transverse abdominal muscles

- Lengthens your psoas muscle a thick muscle that runs from under your armpits to your hips and connects your legs to your torso

- Encourages gentle backbends to open upper spine

- Creates self-awareness, and good habits, around how you hold your body in a standing posture

## *What We Know about Yoga in Parkinson Disease (PD)*

A review of the scientific literature shows a few studies that support hatha yoga for people with PD. This is an area of research that is just starting to build evidence. What studies do exist suggest modest benefits for:

- **Mobility.** The issue of mobility has important implications for fall prevention in PD. Yoga participation can improve functional mobility and influences how a person with PD walks. Standing yoga poses target the hip extensor, knee extensor, and ankle plantar flexor, which support center of gravity during walking and may improve overall stability.

- **Balance.** Balance training is an important component of PD therapy, because 40 percent of nursing home admissions are preceded by a fall. Research shows yoga-related improvements in balance (tandem, one-leg) and an associated decrease in a person's fear of falling; this can also help keep people with PD active in their communities.

- **Strength.** Gains in lower-body strength occur for PD patients following yoga practice and are associated with improved postural stability. Yoga requires isometric contraction (i.e., the joint angle and muscle length do not change) of specific muscle groups to stabilize the body as one performs the postures, and may mimic isokinetic contractions (i.e., variable resistance to a movement performed at constant speed) when performing controlled systemic movements from one pose to the next. These mechanisms may be the reason why yoga improves muscular strength.

- **Flexibility.** Improvements in flexibility and range of motion (ROM) are important since rigidity is a common clinical manifestation in PD. Research shows improvements in flexibility/ROM of the shoulder, hip, and spine. Stooped posture is common in PD and can be related to short spinal flexors and weak spinal extensors; improved shoulder and spinal flexibility from yoga support a more upright posture. Greater hip mobility from yoga may translate into improvements in shuffling gait which can be commonly seen in PD.

433

- **Mood and sleep.** The psychosocial benefits associated with yoga are important for disease management, as they are not often addressed with classic medications used to replace the neurotransmitter dopamine in PD. Many classic medications used to treat anxiety are not safe in PD patients. The calming effect of yoga (by enhancing parasympathetic output) may lessen perceived stress, enhance relaxation, and benefit sleep in PD. Many patients with PD have apathy and fatigue which anecdotally are helped with yoga. Since the mind and the body are very connected in PD, any mental state benefits are tangibly translated into motor benefits. A yoga class can offer a support group, improved confidence, and self-efficacy. Caregivers can also participate and reap the rewards in the psychological realm as well.

Not everyone is lucky enough to live near a yoga instructor who has a deep understanding of PD—this makes it important to educate yourself, both about your specific PD needs and how yoga postures can help, so you can feel comfortable and confident with utilizing the yoga resources that are available in your own community.

### Yoga Can Benefit People with PD Both Physically and Cognitively!

Yoga is both physically and cognitively engaging by focusing on body-awareness during complex body positions. Yoga postures improve physical strength, flexibility, and balance. Yoga postures are also considered skill-acquisition exercises and can benefit our brains thinking patterns and processes to make our movements more efficient and effective.

Yoga helps to increase muscle mass that is usable in everyday life by focusing on functional movements. For example, one-leg balance poses (i.e., tree pose) are helpful for climbing stairs; chair pose builds core and leg strength to help you get up out of bed and/or out of a seated position.

### Yoga Is Actually a Form of Cueing/Attentional Training

The ability to move in PD is not lost; rather the brain mechanisms that initiate movement are defective. Attentional training/cueing may provide a nonautomatic drive for movement, which may compensate for this faulty brain circuitry and improve performance. Yoga breaks up complex sequences and/or postures into component parts, enabling a person to focus their attention on individual aspects of the posture and improve performance. Specific external cues given during a yoga class can also benefit performance in persons with PD.

- Utilize visual cues (i.e., watch the yoga instructor or use a mirror) to help you coordinate your movement.

- Utilize props (i.e., blocks, straps, chairs) to get the experience of the full movement safely, and then take supports away as you progress.

- Talk to your yoga instructor about giving you hands-on adjustments while performing the poses. Subtle adjustments can help you with proper alignment and ensure you are not putting your body in a position that could be painful or result in injury.

- Focus on one aspect of the pose at a time to maintain your attention on your body in the present moment.

### Know That Yoga Can Both Improve and Aggravate Your PD Symptoms!

To avoid aggravating your symptoms, let your yoga instructor know that long holds may increase stiffness or muscle cramping. Instead of holding postures in stillness, try to move into the posture on an inhale breath, and relax out of the posture on an exhale breath. Yoga postures can be beneficial and improve rigidity, stiffness, and slowness, especially in the chest muscles and spine. Focusing on yoga poses that safely extend the spine and/or deep diaphragmatic breathing exercises can create space in the chest and improve posture. Many of the floor poses in yoga allow you to practice getting up safely off the floor. This practice can increase confidence, reduce the fear of falling and increase the likelihood that you can get back up on your own if you do fall. Practice in the company of a caregiver first at least twice per day. You can use two stable supports one on either side at first if needed.

### Use Yoga as an Opportunity to Focus on Posture

Stooped posture in PD is common. It is attributed to shortened contracted spine flexors and weak extensors of the spine. Asymmetry of stiffness can lead to misalignment and can lead to misuse and disuse of muscles that can further worsen posture.

435

# Part Six

# Manipulative and Body-Based Therapies

# Chapter 57

# *The Alexander Technique*

The Alexander technique is an educational method that helps individuals learn to relieve harmful tension in their bodies by correcting faulty movement and posture habits. This method has been used for more than 100 years and is said to be a unique and effective technique of mind-body re-education. The process identifies patterns and movements that are inefficient and result in the accumulation of tension. It is not a set of passive treatments but a method for changing how one thinks and responds.

The technique was created by Frederick Matthias Alexander, an Australian teacher and actor. It began as a method for singers and actors to improve their vocal training. But Alexander discovered that the basis for all vocal education was dependent on developing a highly efficient respiratory system, which led him to focus his process on the breathing mechanism. Some students who had come to Alexander for vocal training recognized that their respiratory difficulties were getting better over time. The improvements were periodically noted by medical doctors and eventually led to the refinement of the Alexander technique.

## *Basic Concepts of the Alexander Technique*

In his writings, Alexander laid out the terminology for his method's basic concepts:

- **Primary control.** Alexander called the relationship between the head, neck, and back primary control. He believed that this relationship was critical in determining overall body function and movement.

- **Recognizing a habit.** Over the years people develop certain habits, some good and others bad. A teacher who is trained in the Alexander technique helps students recognize these habits in order to begin changing them for the better.

- **Direction.** Humans have an innate ability to send messages from the brain to the muscles through the nervous system. The Alexander technique shows how this ability can be used to promote better muscular function.

- **Inhibition.** Individuals react automatically and habitually to stimuli. The Alexander technique aims to train students to use the gap between stimulus and response to choose a productive course of action. Alexander called this inhibition because students are taught to circumvent, or inhibit, their habitual responses.

- **Faulty sensory appreciation.** Certain habits can affect the accuracy of kinesthetic feedback that may prevent an individual from making positive change. The first step in initiating correction is being taught to recognize these faulty habits.

## Learning the Alexander Technique

Proponents of the Alexander technique say that it is a practical and unique way of stopping or changing detrimental habits. Students learn to refrain from habitual patterns that are not useful and develop movements that are natural and spontaneous. The teacher guides the students through movement, coordination patterns, and posture and helps them visualize their body movements. The learning procedure helps students gain a natural perspective about their own sense of coordination. The teacher uses verbal and gentle hands-on guidance to enable the students to experience natural and easy movements without the interference of their current habits. When the process is repeated and expanded, the students' internal coordination becomes more accurate. This helps them respond to stimuli in a coordinated and nonstressful manner.

## Advantages of the Alexander Technique

Teachers, students, and other advocates of the Alexander technique have identified a number of benefits of the method:

- **Improved posture.** By recognizing habits that hinder normal and spontaneous movements and unlearning habits caused by tension, the Alexander technique enables individuals to develop and maintain good posture.

- **Skill enhancement.** Many professionals, like athletes and performing artists, use the Alexander technique to improve their performance in their respective fields.

- **Pain relief.** The technique can help identify and unlearn habitual patterns that lead to musculoskeletal pain caused by excess tension. People tend to tense up during episodes of pain which further aggravates the condition. The technique is said to help relieve neck, back, and joint pain for long periods.

- **Ability to deal with stress.** The technique teaches individuals to deal with any anxiety-producing stimulus by using unique movements designed to reduce tension and empower an individual to handle pressure more effectively.

### *References*

1. "Alexander Technique," Health & Wellness, University of New Hampshire (UNH), n.d.

2. "Alexander Technique: The Insider's Guide," Alexander Technique Center of Washington, February 1, 2002.

3. "Frequently Asked Questions: Alexander Technique Basics," American Society for the Alexander Technique (AmSAT) September 28, 2010.

4. "What Is the Alexander Technique: What Are the Benefits of Lessons or Classes?" The Complete Guide to the Alexander Technique, March 16, 2012.

# Chapter 58

# *Aquatic Therapy (Hydrotherapy)*

Aquatic therapy, also called aquatic physical therapy, has been in use for centuries and is based on the application of skilled physical practice in an aquatic environment. Although predominantly used in clinical settings for the management and rehabilitation of chronic conditions, the practice is gaining acceptance in athletic settings, particularly in areas such as recovery and rehabilitation from orthopedic dysfunction and sports injuries. The zero-gravity environment that water provides is used to intervene in a variety of conditions—including sensory integration and motor control deficits, fine motor deficits, poor social participation skills, and poor strength/endurance—to accomplish the activities of daily living.

The therapy is provided by a trained therapist and features exercise-based treatment in an aquatic environment. The buoyancy of water provides a controlled environment in which increased range of motion by all major muscle groups is possible at all angles. Water also provides a low-impact environment for exercising muscles with less strain than is for similar muscular activity on land. Treatment, which may include total or partial immersion. and helps patients maintain or improve muscular coordination, strength, flexibility, and endurance.

"Aquatic Therapy (Hydrotherapy)," © 2018 Omnigraphics. Reviewed May 2018.

## How Water Works

The physical properties of water make it a conducive therapeutic medium for a variety of chronic conditions. The natural buoyancy and drag resistance of the water makes it possible for patients to remain afloat and while experiencing a decreased effect of gravity on painful joints and muscles. The hydrostatic pressure of water stabilizes the patient and prevents falls while exercising—an important aspect of ensuring patient compliance with exercise regimens. Waves and turbulence can be simulated in pools to provide varying degrees of resistance or manipulation; this allows therapists and patients set specific exercise goals and achieve desired outcomes.

Warm water can also alleviate pain, elevate mood, improve sleep, and lower stress levels in people with depression or chronic illness, and in those seeking quick rehabilitation. Studies have also shown improved pulmonary and cardiovascular functions with aquatic therapy, particularly in patients who cannot participate in traditional land-based rehabilitation as a result of orthopedic constraints.

## Indications for Aquatic Therapy

Rehabilitation through aquatic therapy generally focuses on improving motor functions associated with disability, illness, or injury. Aquatic therapy may also be recommended for treating musculoskeletal pain and pressure ulcers. In pediatric populations, it is widely used as an intervention to improve motor skills in children with developmental disorders such as cerebral palsy or autism spectrum disorders. It may also be indicated in respiratory and circulatory disorders and is regarded as an ideal non-weight-bearing exercise during pregnancy. Prenatal aquatic therapy helps to maintain a moderate or greater intensity of exercise throughout the third trimester. Aquatic interventions are used for a wide variety of conditions, including impaired sensory and motor functions, spasticity, balance deficits, trauma, and to address motor learning and processing disorders. Special populations that require rehabilitation in neurodegenerative disorders also benefit from aquatic intervention; these populations include Parkinson disease, multiple sclerosis, amyotrophic lateral sclerosis, and Huntington disease.

## Modes of Aquatic Therapy

Modes of aquatic therapy differ, but the four main modes are deepwater running, shallow-water running, water calisthenics, and underwater treadmill exercise. Each mode has its own biomechanical requirements and induces its own distinct physiological and functional responses. Physiological responses include factors such as oxygen consumption and degree of exertion, while biomechanical factors include the length or frequency of underwater strides as compared with land-based therapeutic exercise. For instance, deepwater running that does not include ground contact elicits a lower oxygen consumption than other modes of aquatic therapy.

Deepwater jogging or running mimics running on land and is popularly used to maintain fitness levels after an injury. Deepwater running is usually practiced using a flotation device (buoyancy vest or belt), which keeps the body afloat and without ground contact while executing underwater running biomechanics. Shallow-water running, on the other hand, typically includes contact with the ground and is done in shallow water below mid-chest level without the aid of buoyancy aids. Patients walk or run and propel themselves through the water. Water calisthenics includes a variety of aerobic conditioning and resistance-training exercises and is usually executed in the shallow end of a pool. Walking and running are not included in water calisthenics. Underwater treadmill exercise uses a submerged treadmill belt and may include adjustable water depth and treadmill speed in order to control exercise intensity.

## Some Popular Techniques of Aquatic Therapy

While dozens of techniques are used in aquatic therapy, some are more popular than others. These include:

- **Tai Chi:** A therapy based on qi gong (a holistic system of traditional Chinese medicine that combines the elements of coordinated breathing, body posture, movements, and meditation) and tai chi chuan (a Chinese system of internal martial arts based on spiritual and mental aspects).

- **Bad Ragaz Ring Method:** Developed by Swiss physiotherapists, this form of aquatic therapy is based on proprioceptive neuromuscular facilitation that involves targeting specific muscle groups for improving strength and flexibility through a series of contraction and stretching movements. This is a therapist-assisted regime performed with patients lying supine on the water surface supported by rings or floats around their necks, arms, knees, and pelvis. This type of aquatic therapy finds use in the treatment of arthritic conditions, soft tissue injury, and cerebrovascular accident. It is also recommended for postfracture or postsurgery rehabilitation.

- **Halliwick Aquatic Therapy:** Developed in the 1940s by James McMillan, a hydromechanics engineer, this patient-specific aquatic therapy is based on the use of a ten-point structured-learning program that helps people with no experience in swimming progress toward complete independence in the water. Also referred to as water specific therapy, the ten-point program is used to address specific limitations resulting from disability or injury. The water provides a medium for developing specific areas, including a range of movements, strength, stamina, and respiratory function. Water can also serve as a medium for sensory-integration to enhance functional independence and motor learning. Working in groups can also enhance psychological well-being and self-esteem by helping to develop social skills.

- **Watsu:** A form of passive aquatic therapy, this form of aquatic therapy is a one-to-one routine performed in chest-deep water that takes the patient into a state of deep meditation and relaxation. Watsu focuses on the application of manual pressure for manipulation and mobilization of joints and is believed to have physical and emotional benefits for a variety of orthopedic and neurological disorders. During a typical session, the therapist supports the back-floating receiver and performs a routine comprising breath coordination, gentle massage, muscle stretches, and Shiatsu, a type of Japanese bodywork based on traditional Chinese medicine.

## *Aquatic Therapist*

An aquatic therapist works on the principle of specificity and chooses the most advantageous mode of therapy for a particular patient. Ideally, the therapist chooses a mode that is associated with minimal pain and impact, ease of mobility, and maximum relaxation while eliciting the same biomechanical and physiological responses as a parallel land-based exercise therapy. Although aquatic therapy interventions are typically held in a fairly shallow pool, this therapy is not entirely risk-free and safety standards must be maintained in order to provide a safe environment for the patient. Toward this end, aquatic therapy practitioners should be trained in first aid, cardiopulmonary resuscitation (CPR), oxygen administration, automated external defibrillation, and risk awareness related to blood-borne pathogens.

## *The Lowdown on Aquatic Therapy*

Aquatic therapy has been shown to be an effective intervention for improving joint flexibility and functional ability, and also for decreasing pain in certain rheumatic diseases and orthopedic conditions. Its popularity as an alternative therapy notwithstanding, aquatic therapy and some of its aspects, including its role in rehabilitation medicine, still require high-quality research. While most studies to date have focused on the physiological aspects of aquatic therapy, there is a dearth of research on the biomechanical implications of this therapy. Methodologies differ as well. The absence of standardized protocols for evaluating the impact of various modes of aquatic therapy on rehabilitation creates challenges and questions regarding the veracity of published findings in this field.

### *References*

1.  "Aquatherapy for Neurodegenerative Disorders," U.S. National Library of Medicine (NLM), 2014.

2.  "The Effects of Aquatic Exercise on Pulmonary Function in Patients with Spinal Cord Injury," U.S. National Library of Medicine (NLM), 2014.

3.  "What Is Aquatic Therapy?" National Rehabilitation Information Center (NARIC), June 2016.

# Chapter 59

# *Chiropractic Care*

Chiropractic is a healthcare profession that focuses on the relationship between the body's structure—mainly the spine—and it's functioning. Although practitioners may use a variety of treatment approaches, they primarily perform adjustments (manipulations) to the spine or other parts of the body with the goal of correcting alignment problems, alleviating pain, improving function, and supporting the body's natural ability to heal itself.

The term "chiropractic" combines the Greek words "cheir" (hand) and "praxis" (practice) to describe a treatment done by hand. Hands-on therapy—especially adjustment of the spine—is central to chiropractic care. Chiropractic is based on the notion that the relationship between the body's structure (primarily that of the spine) and its function (as coordinated by the nervous system) affects health.

Spinal adjustment/manipulation is a core treatment in chiropractic care, but it is not synonymous with chiropractic. Chiropractors commonly use other treatments in addition to spinal manipulation, and other healthcare providers (e.g., physical therapists or some osteopathic physicians) may use spinal manipulation.

## Use in the United States

In the United States, chiropractic is often considered a complementary health approach. According to the National Health Interview

This chapter includes text excerpted from "Chiropractic: In Depth," National Center for Complementary and Integrative Health (NCCIH), February 2012. Reviewed May 2018.

Survey (NHIS), which included a comprehensive survey of the use of complementary health approaches by Americans, about 8 percent of adults (more than 18 million) and nearly 3 percent of children (more than 2 million) had received chiropractic or osteopathic manipulation in the past 12 months. Additionally, an analysis of NHIS cost data found that adults in the United States spent approximately $11.9 billion out-of-pocket on visits to complementary health practitioners—$3.9 billion of which was spent on visits to practitioners for chiropractic or osteopathic manipulation.

Many people who seek chiropractic care have low-back pain. People also commonly seek chiropractic care for other kinds of musculoskeletal pain (e.g., neck, shoulder), headaches, and extremity (e.g., hand or foot) problems.

An analysis of the use of complementary health approaches for back pain, based on data from the NHIS, found that chiropractic was by far the most commonly used therapy. Among survey respondents who had used any of these therapies for their back pain, 74 percent (approximately 4 million Americans) had used chiropractic. Among those who had used chiropractic for back pain, 66 percent perceived "great benefit" from their treatments.

## Treatment

During the initial visit, chiropractors typically take a health history and perform a physical examination, with a special emphasis on the spine. Other examinations or tests such as X-rays may also be performed. If chiropractic treatment is considered appropriate, a treatment plan will be developed.

During follow-up visits, practitioners may perform one or more of the many different types of adjustments and other manual therapies used in chiropractic care. Given mainly to the spine, a chiropractic adjustment involves using the hands or a device to apply a controlled, rapid force to a joint. The goal is to increase the range and quality of motion in the area being treated and to aid in restoring health. Joint mobilization is another type of manual therapy that may be used.

Chiropractors may combine the use of spinal adjustments and other manual therapies with several other treatments and approaches such as:

- Heat and ice
- Electrical stimulation
- Relaxation techniques

- Rehabilitative and general exercise
- Dietary supplements
- Counseling about diet, weight loss, and other lifestyle factors

## What the Science Says

Researchers have studied spinal manipulation for a number of conditions ranging from back, neck, and shoulder pain to asthma, carpal tunnel syndrome (CTS), fibromyalgia (FM), and headaches. Much of the research has focused on low-back pain and has shown that spinal manipulation appears to benefit some people with this condition.

A review of scientific evidence on manual therapies for a range of conditions concluded that spinal manipulation/mobilization may be helpful for several conditions in addition to back pain, including migraine and cervicogenic (neck-related) headaches, neck pain, upper- and lower-extremity joint conditions, and whiplash-associated disorders. The review also identified a number of conditions for which spinal manipulation/mobilization appears not to be helpful (including asthma, hypertension, and menstrual pain) or the evidence are inconclusive (e.g., FM, mid-back pain, premenstrual syndrome (PMS), sciatica, and temporomandibular joint (TMJ) disorders).

## Safety

- Side effects from spinal manipulation can include temporary headaches, tiredness, or discomfort in the parts of the body that were treated.
- There have been rare reports of serious complications such as stroke, cauda equina syndrome (a condition involving pinched nerves in the lower part of the spinal canal), and worsening of herniated discs, although cause and effect are unclear.
- Safety remains an important focus of ongoing research:
  - A study of treatment outcomes for 19,722 chiropractic patients in the United Kingdom concluded that minor side effects (such as temporary soreness) after cervical spine manipulation were relatively common, but that the risk of a serious adverse event was "low to very low" immediately or up to 7 days after treatment.
  - A study that drew on 9 years of hospitalization records for the population of Ontario, Canada analyzed 818 cases of

451

vertebrobasilar artery (VBA) stroke (involving the arteries that supply blood to the back of the brain). The study found an association between visits to a healthcare practitioner and subsequent VBA stroke, but there was no evidence that visiting a chiropractor put people at greater risk than visiting a primary care physician. The researchers attributed the association between healthcare visits and VBA stroke to the likelihood that people with VBA dissection (torn arteries) seek care for related headache and neck pain before their stroke.

## *Practitioners: Education and Licensure*

Chiropractic colleges accredited by the Council on Chiropractic Education (CCE) offer Doctor of Chiropractic (D.C.) degree programs. (CCE is the agency certified by the U.S. Department of Education (ED) to accredit chiropractic colleges in the United States.) Admission to a chiropractic college requires a minimum of 90 semester hour credits of undergraduate study, mostly in the sciences.

Chiropractic training is a 4-year academic program that includes both classroom work and direct experience caring for patients. Coursework typically includes instruction in the biomedical sciences, as well as in public health and research methods. Some chiropractors pursue a 2- to 3-year residency for training in specialized fields.

Chiropractic is regulated individually by each state and the District of Columbia. All states require completion of a Doctor of Chiropractic degree program from a CCE-accredited college. Examinations administered by the National Board of Chiropractic Examiners (NBCE) are required for licensing and include a mock patient encounter. Most states require chiropractors to earn annual continuing education credits to maintain their licenses. Chiropractors' scope of practice varies by state in areas such as the dispensing or selling of dietary supplements and the use of other complementary health approaches such as acupuncture or homeopathy.

## *If You Are Thinking about Seeking Chiropractic Care*

If you are thinking about seeking chiropractic care then you should:

- Ask about the chiropractor's education and licensure.

- Mention any medical conditions you have, and ask whether the chiropractor has specialized training or experience in the condition for which you are seeking care.

- Ask about typical out-of-pocket costs and insurance coverage. (Chiropractic is covered by many health maintenance organizations and private health plans, Medicare, and state workers' compensation systems.)

- Tell the chiropractor about any medications (prescription or over-the-counter (OTC)) and dietary supplements you take. If the chiropractor suggests a dietary supplement, ask about potential interactions with your medications or other supplements.

- Tell all of your healthcare providers about any complementary health approaches you use. Give them a full picture of what you do to manage your health. This will help ensure coordinated and safe care.

# Chapter 60

# *Craniosacral Therapy*

Osteopathic doctor and professor of biomechanics John E. Upledger was assisting in a surgical procedure in 1970 when he witnessed a rhythmic movement in the dural tube of the cranium. His subsequent analysis of the mechanism of this movement led him to develop craniosacral therapy (CST). William Sutherland, one of Dr. Upledger's students, studied the movements of the bones in the skull and then developed another therapy called cranial osteopathy. There are similarities and differences between these two types of therapies.

## What Is Craniosacral Therapy?

CST is a method of improving the body's ability to heal itself. The therapy uses gentle pressure on the joints in the cranium to increase circulation of cerebrospinal fluid around the brain and spinal cord. The improved flow of cerebrospinal fluid improves central nervous system function, which, in turn, improves the function of the entire body. CST can be used in isolation or in conjunction with other medical therapies.

## What Conditions Does Craniosacral Therapy Address?

CST is used to treat various medical conditions related to pain and dysfunction, including:

- Brain and spinal cord injuries
- Concussion and traumatic brain injury

---

"Craniosacral Therapy," © 2018 Omnigraphics. Reviewed May 2018.

- Attention deficit disorder (ADD) / Attention deficit hyperactivity disorder (ADHD)
- Temporomandibular joint syndrome (TMJ)
- Orthopedic problems
- Immune disorders
- Migraines and headaches
- Central nervous system disorders
- Posttraumatic stress disorder
- Chronic neck and back pain
- Stress- and tension-related disorders
- Motor-coordination impairments
- Infant and childhood disorders
- Learning disabilities
- Chronic fatigue
- Fibromyalgia
- Scoliosis
- Autism

## Procedure of Craniosacral Therapy

The central nervous system is primarily governed by the brain and spinal cord, which, in turn, are protected by the craniosacral system of membranes and fluid that surround them. When the body experiences stress and strain, pressure exerted on its tissues affect the craniosacral system, which works best when all body parts move in craniosacral rhythm.

When body tissues are not moving well, trained therapists who specialize in CST use gentle hand movements to relax the tissues of the craniosacral system and improve cerebrospinal fluid flow. In this way, CST helps the body to correct itself by improving its ability to heal quickly.

## Nature of Craniosacral Therapy

CST is technique oriented. The CST therapists act as witnesses to a healing process that is more about being than doing. Therapists place their hands on their clients' body, exert pressure, and then follow the body's movements as they wait for a release of tension or pain to happen.

The therapists remain neutral during this process and believe that this neutrality allows their clients to activate their own inner wisdom. In this way, therapist and client work together to ease pressure over areas of tension in the body and increase craniosacral system function.

## Craniosacral Therapy and Musculoskeletal Pain

Internal conflicts caused by trauma create patterns of tension in the body, and symptoms occur when the body is overwhelmed. Treating symptoms alone can provide temporary relief, but reducing the internal patterns of tension, as CST does, allows the entire body to function better. This is why CST is used to treat a variety of pain conditions, neurological and circulatory issues, digestive issues, problems with other internal organs, and most especially musculoskeletal pain.

CST requires just a light touch to remove internal tension in the body. However, there are situations when CST must not be used:

- When there is intracranial pressure, or

- If the structure of the membrane around the brain and the spinal cord has been compromised.

Conditions that can cause these situations include:

- Epidural leaks from lumbar puncture,

- Open cavity head wound,

- Acute stroke,

- Severe concussion with consequent swelling of the brain, and

- Unstable cerebral aneurysm.

## Chronic versus Acute Inflammation

The body responds differently to acute and chronic inflammation. It rebuilds itself in response to trauma, which typically causes acute inflammation. However, in cases of chronic inflammation, the body simultaneously rebuilds itself and tears itself apart.

When acute inflammation is present in the body, immune cells in the tissue continue to move in response to the craniosacral rhythm. The tissue is restricted, but the immune cells move well. But the movements of both the immune cells and the tissue are restricted when chronic inflammation is present.

457

The CST therapists "tune into" the movement of immune cells in the body's tissue to see if the cells are moving in tandem with the craniosacral rhythm.

Immune cells release histamine when inflammation is present. This causes capillary beds to open up, which allows the immune cells to move into the surrounding tissue. When this happens, the therapist will feel those cells moving in response to the craniosacral rhythm.

### References

1. "Craniosacral Therapy: Does It Work?" Healthline Media UK Ltd, July 17, 2017.

2. "CST FAQs," Upledger Institute International, 2018.

3. "Craniosacral Therapy: An Ideal Modality for Treating Inflammation," Massage Magazine, Inc. December 21, 2017.

# Chapter 61

# *Feldenkrais Method*

The Feldenkrais method is a therapy system that uses movement to help people learn new and effective ways of living a holistic life. The method was developed by Moshe Feldenkrais, a physicist and engineer, who synthesized insights from biomechanics, psychology, motor development, and martial arts to develop an effective and practical application that can help people reconnect with their health through movement.

Feldenkrais was born into a Hasidic family and community. A serious injury that impaired his walking prompted him to explore the connection between body movement and healing. This not only restored his ability to walk, but also led him to many breakthrough discoveries in human movement. Before his death in 1984, Feldenkrais trained about 300 practitioners to continue his work, and now around 6,000 Feldenkrais practitioners are at work around the world. The method continues to influence other disciplines, such as education, psychology, child development, sports, gerontology, and occupational therapy, and has also helped develop the new field of somatic education.

Feldenkrais method was influenced by Moshe Feldenkrais involvement in jiu jitsu, a martial art. Feldenkrais incorporated the views of neurosurgeon Karl H. Pribram and cyberneticist Heinz Von Foerster. Esther Thelen, human development researcher also influenced Feldenkrais Method. Moshe Feldenkrais said that humans move according to their perceived self-image, so his method employs different strategies to improve posture, coordination, flexibility, and athletic ability. It

"Feldenkrais Method," © 2018 Omnigraphics. Reviewed May 2018.

also intended to help relieve chronic pain, restricted movement, back pain, and other common ailments. Neurological and psychological problems are also resolved using this type of therapy. The Feldenkrais method employs new ways of moving by expanding one's perception and awareness to enable a person to be more aware of his or her habits and body tension and move accordingly.

The Feldenkrais method teaches that personal history, cultural background, upbringing, injuries, and illness make people adopt a set of behaviors, both physical and psychological. Sometimes these behaviors become so dysfunctional or outmoded that they get embedded deep into the nervous system and create unnecessary physical and psychological limitations. It analyses the person's cultural and biological aspects of movement, posture, learning, and habits to see how they limit his or her potential. The method also engages organic learning and movement to enable freedom from habitual patterns and allows new methods of movement, thinking, and feeling to emerge.

## *Formats of the Feldenkrais Method*

The Feldenkrais method is taught in two formats:

- Functional integration (FI)
- Awareness through movement (ATM)

### *Functional Integration (FI)*

Functional integration (FI), also known as Feldenkrais private sessions, is a one-to-one approach between the teacher and individual student. The teacher helps the student in movement lessons through gentle and noninvasive touch as the primary means of communication. The FI lessons are quite flexible, allowing the student to take it at his or her own pace and as their needs demand. The lessons are done by the student sitting, standing, or lying on a specially designed table. The teacher uses touch to reflect how the student organizes current body movements and patterns. The instructor then analyses and teaches more effective movement patterns for the student. The teacher creates a comfortable environment for the student so that learning becomes easier, then focuses on the student's abilities and needs, with more forceful procedures being employed as necessary.

FI lessons relate to how much a student desires to learn, their intent, and their need for the lesson. The lessons are customized according to the student's unique requirements, and they learn how to integrate the learned movements into their daily lives. FI is a gentle and subtle method widely recognized to heal minor aches and pains, musculoskeletal problems, neurological problems, tension, and child developmental issues.

### *Awareness through Movement (ATM)*

Similar to tai chi or gentle yoga, ATM reengages the nervous system. People usually pick up certain habits and behaviors when they are infants and later abandon them. Through ATM, the old habits are replaced by new skills and awareness through engaging a person's entire body. ATM is generally taught in group classes in which students walk, stand, sit, or lie on the floor as the instructor takes them through a series of carefully planned movements intended to retrain neuromuscular patterns.

### *References*

1. "About Feldenkrais Method," The Feldenkrais Institute, April 30, 2009.

2. "About the Feldenkrais Method," Feldenkrais.com, June 17, 2017.

3. "Feldenkrais Method," Goodtherapy.org, July 19, 2016.

4. Fry, Rich. "The Feldenkrais Method," Flowingbody.com, n.d.

# Chapter 62

# *Kinesiotherapy*

## *History of Kinesiotherapy*

Kinesiotherapy (KT) is the application of scientifically based exercise principles adapted to enhance the strength, endurance, coordination, range of motion, and mobility of individuals with functional limitations or those requiring extended physical conditioning. Kinesiotherapy (formerly corrective therapy) is an allied health profession whose origins can be traced back to 1943.

The roots of this profession began during World War II when corrective physical reconditioning units were established to accelerate the return of urgently needed troops to active duty following injury. Corrective therapists, as a result, became a part of the U.S. Armed Forces' rehabilitation effort employing exercise and mobility programming. As the demand for these physical reconditioning specialists grew, early leaders in rehabilitation recognized the need to organize and accredit these new specialists accordingly through a structured educational curriculum.

---

This chapter contains text excerpted from the following sources: Text under the heading "History of Kinesiotherapy" is excerpted from "Kinesiotherapist at Richmond VA Medical Center," U.S. Department of Veterans Affairs (VA), May 12, 2015; Text under the heading "What Kinesiotherapist Do" is excerpted from "Kinesiotherapist," U.S. Bureau of Labor Statistics (BLS), U.S. Department of Labor (DOL), December 2014. Reviewed May 2018; Text beginning with the heading "Treatment Settings" is excerpted from "Kinesiotherapy Fact Sheet," U.S. Department of Veterans Affairs (VA), March 2018.

Since that time, the discipline has expanded into both the public and private sectors. Kinesiotherapists apply advanced skills, certifications, and specialty training in their practice across the continuum of care for members with a wide spectrum of neurologic, orthopedic, mental health, surgical, and medical conditions, including special populations such as stroke, spinal cord injury (SCI), traumatic brain injury (TBI), amputation, homeless, and geriatric patients. Advanced skills include, but not limited to, driver rehabilitation, cardiopulmonary rehabilitation, geriatric rehabilitation, psychiatric rehabilitation, polytrauma rehabilitation, prosthetic, orthotic and amputation rehabilitation as well as functional capacity evaluations, therapeutic aquatics, wheelchair seating, and SCI rehabilitation.

## What Kinesiotherapists Do

Job duties for kinesiotherapists vary, depending on where they work—and sometimes within the facility itself. Responsibilities usually include assessing and treating patients, among other tasks. Kinesiotherapists work under a physician's direction, often with other specialists, such as a nurse, a dietitian, and a social worker.

### Assessment

To determine what exercises and training may be beneficial, a kinesiotherapist first evaluates patients to assess their physical abilities and activity levels. This assessment allows the kinesiotherapist to decide how much help, if any, patients need each day for routine tasks, such as walking, eating, and getting into and out of bed.

Home-care providers also do an environmental assessment of the patient's residence to ensure safety. This includes evaluating a home's potential safety risks—such as stairs, unsafe furniture, and nonworking smoke detectors—and recommending corrective action.

### Treatment

Kinesiotherapists base a patient's treatment plan on what they learned during the assessment. Emphasizing the physical and psychological benefits of exercise, they focus on reconditioning and physical education. Treatment is tailored to each patient's needs and situation. For example, Laura Hines a kinesiotherapist had a patient with mobility problems who was limited to crawling in his own home. The patient could stand for only brief periods, so Laura created a plan that would help him rebuild strength gradually. "I started him on a treadmill for a few minutes at a time, because he needed to rest in between," she says. Eventually, through reconditioning exercises with Laura's guidance, the patient became fully mobile not just inside his house but out and about as well.

### Other Duties

In addition to tasks related to assessment and treatment, kinesiotherapists have some administrative duties. These include documenting patient visits; ordering equipment, such as adaptive-eating utensils or wheelchairs; and participating in outreach activities. Some kinesiotherapists' other responsibilities are related to the work but specific to their patient population.

## Treatment Settings

Kinesiotherapy provides a full scope of services. Treatment settings include inpatient settings (including medical centers and community living centers), outpatient clinics, and telerehabilitation.

## Kinesiotherapy Training

Kinesiotherapists are highly trained healthcare professionals. Entry-level education requirements include a bachelor's degree in kinesiotherapy or exercise science with an emphasis in kinesiotherapy. This education must include or be supplemented by clinical practice in a VA approved training program or its equivalent.

Kinesiotherapy promotes an environment for clinical education. There are on average, about 60 KT students participating in clinical internship across the VHA each year.

## Clinical Training Partnerships

The Council on Professional Standards for Kinesiotherapy (COPS-KT) signed a Memorandum of Understanding (MoU) on January 31, 2012 to begin clinical training for masters prepared exercise science majors who have completed the core educational requirements in kinesiotherapy.

## Advanced Training

Many Kinesiotherapists have advanced skills, certification and training in specialty areas. Advanced skills include driver rehabilitation, cardiopulmonary rehabilitation, geriatrics, orthopedics, polytrauma, and amputation. Kinesiotherapy advanced training also includes functional capacity evaluations, therapeutic aquatics, wheelchair seating, and spinal cord injury (SCI).

# Chapter 63

# *Massage Therapy*

## *Chapter Contents*

# Section 63.1

# *Massage Therapy: An Overview*

This section includes text excerpted from "Massage Therapy
for Health Purposes," National Center for Complementary and
Integrative Health (NCCIH), June 2016.

The term "massage therapy" includes many techniques and the type
of massage given usually depends on your needs and physical condition. It dates back thousands of years. References to massage appear
in ancient writings from China, Japan, India, and Egypt.

In general, massage therapists work on muscle and other soft tissue
to help you feel better. In Swedish massage, the therapist uses long
strokes, kneading, deep circular movements, vibration, and tapping.
Sports massage combines techniques of Swedish massage and deep
tissue massage to release chronic muscle tension. It's adapted to the
needs of athletes. Myofascial trigger point therapy focuses on trigger
points—areas that are painful when pressed and are associated with
pain elsewhere in the body.

Massage therapy is sometimes done using essential oils as a form
of aromatherapy.

## What the Science Says about the Effectiveness of Massage

A lot of the scientific research on massage therapy is preliminary or
conflicting, but much of the evidence points toward beneficial effects on
pain and other symptoms associated with a number of different conditions. Much of the evidence suggests that these effects are short term and
that people need to keep getting massages for the benefits to continue.

Researchers have studied the effects of massage for many conditions. Some that they have studied more extensively are the following:

### *Pain*

A research review and 2011 National Center for Complementary
and Integrative Health (NCCIH)-funded clinical trial concluded that

massage may be useful for chronic low-back pain. It may also help with chronic neck pain, an NCCIH-funded clinical trial reported. According to a 2012 NCCIH-funded study massage may help with pain due to osteoarthritis (OA) of the knee. Studies suggest that for women in labor, massage provided some pain relief and increased their satisfaction with other forms of pain relief, but the evidence isn't strong, a 2012 review concluded.

### *Cancer*

Numerous research reviews and clinical studies have suggested that at least for the short term, massage therapy for cancer patients may reduce pain, promote relaxation, and boost mood. However, the National Cancer Institute (NCI) urges massage therapists to take specific precautions with cancer patients and avoid massaging:

- Open wounds, bruises, or areas with skin breakdown

- Directly over the tumor site

- Areas with a blood clot in a vein

- Sensitive areas following radiation therapy

### *Mental Health*

A meta-analysis of 17 clinical trials concluded that massage therapy may help to reduce depression. A brief, twice-weekly yoga and massage sessions for 12 weeks were associated with a decrease in depression, anxiety, and back and leg pain in pregnant women with depression, a 2012 NCCIH-funded clinical trial showed. Also, the women's babies weighed more than babies born to women who didn't receive the therapy. However, a 2013 research review concluded that there's not enough evidence to determine if massage helps pregnant mothers with depression.

A review concluded that massage may help older people relax. For generalized anxiety disorder (GAD), massage therapy was no better at reducing symptoms than providing a relaxing environment and deep breathing lessons, according to a small NCCIH-supported clinical trial.

### *Fibromyalgia (FM)*

A review concluded that massage therapy may help temporarily reduce pain, fatigue, and other symptoms associated with fibromyalgia

(FM), but the evidence is not definitive. The authors noted that it's important that the massage therapist not cause pain.

## Headaches

Clinical trials on the effects of massage for headaches are preliminary and only somewhat promising.

## Human Immunodeficiency Virus (HIV) / Acquired Immunodeficiency Syndrome (AIDS)

Massage therapy may help improve the quality of life for people with human immunodeficiency virus (HIV) or acquired immunodeficiency syndrome (AIDS), a review of four small clinical trials concluded.

## Infant Care

Massaging preterm infants using moderate pressure may improve weight gain, a review suggested. We don't have enough evidence to know if massage benefits healthy infants who are developing normally, a 2013 review determined.

## Other Conditions

Researchers have studied massage for the following but it's still unclear if it helps:

- Behavior of children with autism or autism spectrum disorders (ASD)
- Immune function in women with breast cancer
- Anxiety and pain in patients following heart surgery
- Quality of life and glucose levels in people with diabetes
- Lung function in children with asthma

## What the Science Says about the Safety and Side Effects of Massage Therapy

Massage therapy appears to have few risks when performed by a trained practitioner. However, massage therapists should take some precautions in people with certain health conditions. In some cases, pregnant women should avoid massage therapy. Talk with your healthcare provider before getting a massage if you're pregnant.

470

People with some conditions such as bleeding disorders or low blood platelet counts should avoid having forceful and deep tissue massage. People who take anticoagulants (also known as blood thinners) also should avoid them. Massage should not be done in any potentially weak area of the skin, such as wounds.

Deep or intense pressure should not be used over an area where the patient has a tumor or cancer unless approved by the patient's healthcare provider.

## *More to Consider*

If you are thinking of trying massage therapy then:

- Do not use massage therapy to replace conventional care or to postpone seeing a healthcare provider about a medical problem.

- If you have a medical condition and are unsure whether massage therapy would be appropriate for you, discuss your concerns with your healthcare provider, who may also be able to help you select a massage therapist.

- Ask about the training, experience, and credentials of the massage therapist you are considering. Also ask about the number of treatments that might be needed, the cost, and insurance coverage.

- Tell all your healthcare providers about any complementary and integrative health approaches you use. Give them a full picture of what you do to manage your health. This will ensure coordinated and safe care.

Section 63.2

# *Lymphatic Drainage Massage*

"Lymphatic Drainage Therapy,"
© 2015 Omnigraphics. Reviewed May 2018.

Lymphatic drainage therapy is a manual massage technique intended to reduce fluid buildup and swelling that may occur due to problems with the lymph nodes. Lymph is a clear, watery fluid that flows through a network of tissues, organs, and vessels known as the lymphatic system. The main components of the lymphatic system include the bone marrow, spleen, and thymus, as well as lymph nodes located in the neck, armpits, chest, and groin.

The lymph nodes play a vital role in the functioning of the immune system. They filter out harmful substances that are carried in the lymph fluid, such as bacteria and viruses, and attack and destroy them with white blood cells called lymphocytes. If a person has an infection, injury, or a disease like cancer, the lymph nodes may become tender and swollen as they aid in the immune response.

When the lymph nodes are compromised by disease or surgically removed, the lymphatic system may lose its ability to drain fluid from a nearby region of the body, resulting in a condition called lymphedema. Problems involving the lymph nodes in the armpit, for instance, may result in painful fluid buildup and swelling in the arm. Lymphatic drainage therapy was developed to treat lymphedema and related conditions.

## *Causes and Symptoms of Lymphedema*

Lymphedema can be related to several different factors. Primary lymphedema, which is rare, can arise at birth as a result of a malformed or dysfunctional lymphatic system. The more common condition, secondary lymphedema, can result from anything that obstructs or causes damage to the lymphatic system, including infection, injury, cancer, surgery, or radiation therapy.

Among the most common causes of secondary lymphedema are cancer and cancer treatments. When surgeons operate to remove a malignancy, they often remove lymph nodes in the area of the tumor to determine whether cancer cells are present in the lymphatic system. If the cancer has spread to the lymph nodes, the patient faces a higher risk that the disease will come back following surgery. The degree to which the cancer has affected the lymph nodes determines its stage of advancement and the type of treatment that the patient requires. Cancer in the lymph nodes, surgical removal of the lymph nodes, and radiation therapy designed to kill cancer cells can all cause lymphedema.

Regardless of the cause, the symptoms of lymphedema include swelling of the hands, arms, feet, legs, or any other part of the body; loss of mobility in the affected joints and limbs; redness, itching, and tightening of the skin; and general feelings of heaviness and discomfort.

## Massage Therapy for Lymph Drainage

Chronic lymphedema has no cure, but there are a number of methods that can be used to help manage its severity and symptoms. One option is lymphatic drainage or manual massage therapy. Developed in Europe in the 1930s, it is intended to improve the natural flow of lymph and the drainage of fluids from body parts affected by lymphedema.

The manual massage technique involves gentle rubbing, tapping, and stroking of the skin using a specific speed, pressure, and pattern. The goal is to stimulate the movement of lymph out of congested areas, bypassing the damaged lymph vessels, and channel it into healthy vessels so that it can return to systemic circulation.

Manual massage treatments should begin with a certified therapist, although patients can learn to perform the technique on themselves. Generally, it does not involve risks when done correctly. However, the technique should not be used on open wounds, broken skin, or tissues that have been exposed to radiation therapy. It is also not suitable if the patient has a deep vein thrombosis (blood clot).

Proponents claim that manual massage therapy can lead to improvements in many different medical conditions, including poor circulation, injuries, burns, nervous system disorders, arthritis, pregnancy-related swelling, varicose veins, stress, and insomnia. A few studies have indicated that women with lymphedema related to breast cancer treatment may experience a reduction in swelling following manual massage therapy. But the efficacy of the treatment must be demonstrated in larger, controlled studies for it to gain acceptance in the mainstream medical community.

### References

1. American Cancer Society (ACS). "Lymph Nodes and Cancer," 2015.

2. Dr. Vodder School International. "Manual Lymphatic Drainage," 2015.

3. National Cancer Institute (NCI). "Lymphedema for Health Professionals: Manual Lymphedema Therapy," 2015.

## Section 63.3

# *Reflexology*

"Reflexology (Zone Therapy)"
© 2015 Omnigraphics. Reviewed May 2018.

Reflexology is based on the idea that applying pressure to specific points on the feet, hands, or ears will produce beneficial effects on the corresponding body organs and a person's general health. It is utilized worldwide as a complementary and alternative treatment method for a variety of conditions, such as anxiety, asthma, cancer, diabetes, headaches, premenstrual syndrome, and stress.

Reflexology is also known as zone therapy. According to proponents of the method, the body is divided into ten longitudinal zones, with five located on each side of the body. Each zone within the body is represented by a certain point on the hands or feet. Practitioners claim to be able to detect abnormalities in the organs of each zone by feeling the corresponding areas on the hands or feet. Once the problem has been identified, the reflexologist puts pressure on the reflex points in order to stimulate a flow of energy, blood, nutrients, and nerve impulses to the zone.

Reflexology has experienced a rapid increase in popularity in Europe and Asia. In several countries, in fact, local governing bodies and private companies have begun employing reflexologists to treat their staff members. The practice has been credited with helping to increase job satisfaction and reduce absenteeism in some of these organizations

## Origin and Development of Reflexology

Reflexology has been practiced since ancient times. It is depicted in a pictograph on the Egyptian tomb of Ankhmahor that dates to 2330 BCE, for instance, as well as in symbols engraved on the feet of Buddha statues in India and China. The earliest discussion of reflexology in print appears in the Yellow Emperor's Classic of Internal Medicine, a Chinese text written around 1,000 BCE. Marco Polo is credited with introducing reflexology methods in Europe in the 1300s by translating Chinese massage instructions into Italian.

The so-called Father of Zone Therapy in the United States was Dr. William H. Fitzgerald. In 1913, he introduced the idea that putting pressure on certain points on the feet and hands could exert an anesthetic effect on other parts of the body. He used the zone therapy technique to relieve pain from injuries or minor medical procedures. Fitzgerald's work was expanded by Dr. Shelby Riley, who also suggested pressure points on the outer ear. Another important contribution was made by Eunice D. Ingham, a physiotherapist who mapped the body's reflex zones in the 1940s.

## Reflexology Points and Areas

Although the practice of reflexology varies in different parts of the world, most practitioners agree on the major reflex points. Reflexologists use maps to represent the correspondence between these points on the feet, hands, and ears and different bodily systems. Each foot represents a vertical half of the body, for instance, with points on the left foot corresponding to organs on the left side of the body and points on the right foot corresponding to organs on the right side of the body. For instance, the liver, which is located on the right side of the abdomen, is represented by an area on the right foot.

## Research on Reflexology

Medical research into the effectiveness of reflexology has yielded mixed results. Most patients find reflexology therapy relaxing, and many report that it provides such health benefits as relieving pain, reducing anxiety, improving mood, and enhancing sleep. Studies funded by the National Institutes of Health (NIH) have supported the anecdotal evidence that reflexology may help alleviate pain and reduce the psychological stress associated with injury and illness. As a result, reflexology treatments are increasingly being used as part of the palliative care of people with cancer.

On the other hand, the mainstream medical community generally rejects the idea that reflexology can effectively diagnose and treat potentially serious medical conditions, such as asthma, diabetes, or cancer. A systematic review of controlled studies concluded that reflexology had failed to demonstrate effectiveness in treating any medical condition. Critics argue that there is no scientific evidence to support claims that reflexology practitioners can identify problems or improve the function of bodily systems by putting pressure on reflex points. They point out that medical research has never established any nerve connection or flow of energy between reflex points and other parts of the body.

Although reflexology is not considered harmful and may aid some patients with the psychological aspects of healing, doctors warn that it should only be used in addition to, rather than in place of, appropriate medical treatment.

### References

1. Barrett, Stephen. "Reflexology: A Close Look." Quackwatch, 2015.

2. Bauer, Brent A. "What Is Reflexology? Can It Relieve Stress?" Mayo Clinic, 2015.

3. Teagarden, Karen. "Reflexology." Taking Charge of Your Health and Wellbeing, University of Minnesota Center for Spirituality and Healing, 2013.

# Chapter 64

# *Pilates*

## *What Is Pilates?*

Pilates is a fitness regimen for building flexibility, strength, endurance, and coordination. The emphasis is on improving core strength and fitness without adding muscle bulk. Pilates involves controlled movements done on a mat or with equipment. It improves physical and mental well-being, strengthens muscles, and tones the body, while also strengthening the torso and providing better posture and good health. Pilates strongly emphasizes technique, and despite outward appearances it is not as easy as doing crunches or other core-strengthening exercises. The moves look simple, but execution requires precision and control. The exercises have names such as "The 100," "The Elephant," and "The Swan" and are usually done in a specific order, one after the other.

The method was developed by Joseph H. Pilates, a German bodybuilder, gymnast, and physical trainer, who overcame childhood disease and fragility to become an accomplished athlete in various sports. Working as a nurse in Great Britain during World War I, he designed equipment and a system of exercises for rehabilitating immobilized soldiers and other patients. After immigrating to the United States in the 1920s, Pilates taught these exercises in a studio in New York.

"Pilates," © 2018 Omnigraphics. Reviewed May 2018.

## What Are the Types of Pilates Exercises?

Pilates exercises can be generally categorized into two types:

1. The first requires primarily just a floor mat and a training routine and is designed to use body weight for resistance. Of the 500 exercises that were originally developed for Pilates, 34 are mat-based movements. In addition to the mat, these exercises utilize other traditional Pilates equipment, such as magic circles and hand weights, or nonstandard gear like gym balls, stretch bands, and foam rollers.

2. The second type employs specialized equipment, such as "Reformer," "Cadillac," "Wunda Chair," "Spine Corrector," and "Ladder Barrel," which were designed by Pilates himself. This equipment uses a system of pulleys, springs, handles, and straps to provide resistance or support based on the requirements of the exercise.

Both kinds of exercises can be adapted for varying degrees of fitness and ability. If exercising on the mat turns out to be difficult for some people, the equipment offers alternative ways to exercise.

## How Does Pilates Work?

Pilates can be practiced with a mat at home—possibly with the guidance of a home video—at a gymnasium or studio with special equipment, or at a class with a trainer. Typically, classes last for 45 minutes to an hour. Pilates, which can be practiced for a few days per week along with aerobics, is considered a medium-intensity regimen, and though you will not necessarily work up a sweat, your muscles will get a thorough workout. Pilates focuses on concentration and breathing, as well as strengthening the core of the body, arms, and legs. It can also improve flexibility and joint mobility while strengthening the muscles and helping maintain a healthy body weight.

## Who Can Do Pilates?

Pilates is suitable for people of all ages and fitness levels, from beginners to athletes. The equipment can be calibrated for support, to help beginners and people with health conditions, or for resistance in the case of athletes who want to challenge themselves. As with any exercise routine, it's a good idea to consult a healthcare professional if you have an injury or a medical condition before you begin working out.

## What Are the Health Benefits of Pilates?

The benefits of Pilates can include improved posture, balance, muscle tone, joint mobility, and relief from stress and tension. Pilates has been shown to be particularly beneficial for athletes and dancers, because it helps develop overall body strength and flexibility and reduces the risk of injury. While there is scientific evidence to support many of these benefits, there has not been enough rigorous scrutiny for definitive conclusions. More standardized research in this area is needed in order to verify the benefits scientifically.

## What Are the Benefits of Pilates for People with Health Conditions?

Pilates has the advantage of being adaptable to a variety of individual needs. In many cases, it has been a useful addition to aerobics for people with heart disease, hypertension, and high cholesterol. For people with arthritis, it can be a beneficial strength-training program. Pilates may also be a good choice for lower back pain, helping to strengthen the muscles that support the back. Pregnant women who are already working out with Pilates should be able to continue, with their doctor's approval, as long as modifications are made to accommodate the pregnancy. It is important to understand that people with any medical condition should participate in a Pilates program only after consultation with a healthcare professional.

## How Is Pilates Different from Yoga?

Pilates and yoga are different methods of exercises, but both offer similar benefits, such as improved posture, strength, balance, flexibility, and good breathing techniques. Although both systems promote physical and mental health, yoga tends to focus more on meditation and relaxation. Pilates makes use of equipment but yoga does not, and Pilates uses flow of movement, while yoga features static poses.

## How Should You Choose a Pilates Class?

Pilates classes are often taught in a studio with equipment or in open areas with mats, and they usually last for about an hour. Ideally, equipment-based Pilates should be taught on a one-to-one basis and mat exercises in small groups to ensure personal attention. If you are joining a group class for equipment training, make sure you gain sufficient familiarity with the equipment before attempting to use it on your own. There are no legal requirements or qualifications needed to become a Pilates instructor. As a result, it's important to choose a teacher or class leader based on experience, recommendations, and personal rapport. Good instructors should have up to 450 hours of experience over a span of several years.

### References

1. "A Guide to Pilates," NHS Choices, May 18, 2015.

2. "Pilates," The Nemours Foundation, February 2014.

3. Robinson, Kara Mayer. "Pilates," WebMD, 2017.

# Chapter 65

# *Rolfing Structural Integration*

## *What Is Rolfing Structural Integration (SI)?*

Rolfing® is a system of movement education and body manipulation that reorganizes connective tissues, known as fascia. The connective tissues support, stabilize, and surround all the muscles, nerves, bones, and organs in the body. The system aims to align the entire body with the Earth's gravity by manipulating the particular fascia that affect posture and structure in a positive manner. The Rolfing method does not see the body as a collection of separate parts, but rather a network of connected tissues and works on them to realign, release, and balance the whole body. The main goal of Rolfing structural integration (SI) is to restore flexibility, revitalize energy, and help one regain balance and vitality.

## *Origin of Rolfing SI*

Rolfing SI was named after its founder, Dr. Ida P. Rolf. In 1920, she received her doctorate in biochemistry from Columbia University and furthered her study of the human body through her work in organic chemistry at the Rockefeller Institute. Her interest and research were mainly oriented towards methods that emphasized the effect of structure on function, such as osteopathy, yoga, and chiropractic. Rolf combined her research with other scientific knowledge about the

---

"Rolfing Structural Integration," © 2018 Omnigraphics. Reviewed May 2018.

body's structural order to develop Rolfing SI and began practicing the technique on clients.

During her lifetime, Rolf taught her methods to many students at the Esalen Institute in Big Sur, California, and since her death in 1979, these students and other practitioners have continued to use the methods and expand on them. At present, this method is practiced in about 27 countries, and there are more than 1,200 certified Rolfers worldwide. Although there have been few objective scientific studies validating the effectiveness of Rolfing, through the years many thousands of individuals claim to have benefited from structural integration.

## How Does Rolfing SI Work?

The system aims to align and balance body structures until the entire body functions and coordinates smoothly. Its primary focus is on the fascial system, which is like an internal wire-network for the entire body. If something goes wrong, such as one set of wires being out of place or becoming rigid, the result can be sore muscles, joint pain, or a shift in posture. The Rolfing method tries to ease tension and bring back balance and alignment to the entire body. Rolf's insights led her to believe that when body structures are balanced in gravity, they function more effectively and remain at ease.

If there are internal misalignments, the Rolfing system uses mild, direct pressure to release tension in the fascia and allow for rejuvenation of health through the re-establishment of balance. The deep, slow strokes of Rolfing stimulate intra-fascial mechanoreceptors that enable the nervous system to be triggered and reduce strain on the muscles.

Rolfing SI seeks to restore alignment to body systems that are out of place. For example, when positioned correctly the legs are aligned to the hips, shoulders to the rib cage, and joints and related tissue are integrated into one another with the body positioned over the feet. The Rolfing method allows the healthy level of muscle contraction to be established and alleviates pain.

## How Does Rolfing Differ from Massage?

Although Rolfing involves hands-on manipulation by a practitioner, it differs from deep tissue massage. While massage is purely aimed at relaxing the muscles, Rolfing seeks to improve body alignment and functionality. It concentrates on and affects body posture and structure for longer periods. The method may also speed up recovery from injury, rigid muscle tension, movement around joints, and any secondary pain.

Rolfing is typically administered via "The Ten," a series of ten sessions divided into three groups or units. The first group strives to loosen surface layers of connective tissue in the shoulders, arms, ribcage, spine, hips, and feet. The next unit concentrates on the core area between the pelvis and the head. And the final group of sessions focuses on progress made in previous steps and integrating a sense of permanent order and balance in the body.

## Benefits of Rolfing SI

Some of the major benefits attributing to Rolfing are listed below.

- People have experienced a reduction in pain, improved flexibility, and posture, as well as a deep sense of body awareness with the Rolfing method.

- Rolfing can permanently alter a person's posture, stability, and structure.

- The Rolfing method restores balance to the body by releasing unnecessary tension.

- An estimated one million people have undergone Rolfing treatment, including dancers, athletes, and businesspeople.

- Proponents say that Rolfing results in the more efficient use of muscles, helps the body conserve energy, and creates refined patterns of movement.

- Rolfing is said to help neurological function and reduce the spinal misalignment of individuals with lordosis, or curvature of the spine.

## Who Should Use Rolfing SI?

Dr. Rolf had a global vision that imagined a more structurally efficient human species through the application of Rolfing. Therefore, she believed all children and adults should receive Rolfing SI since all bodies have some degree of disorder and imbalance. People with a history of injury or trauma from accidents and people with minor injuries that interfere with their daily activities are also said to benefit from the method. People without injuries also can use Rolfing because it is intended to help enhance overall body functionality and condition. It is also said to have helped some people attain enhanced spiritual and emotional well-being.

### References

1. "How Does Rolfing Structural Integration Work?" Rolf Institute of Structural Integration, August 10, 2012.

2. Lynn, Judy. "Rolfing and MS: Bliss or Pain?" Multiple Sclerosis News Today, January 17, 2018.

3. "What Is Rolfing?" Action Potential, October 14, 2010.

4 "What Is Rolfing Structural Integration?" Rolf Institute of Structural Integration, September 20, 2017.

# Chapter 66

# *Tui Na*

Tui na is a form of massage therapy that originated in China around 2,500 years ago. Its name comes from the Chinese words for two of the motions commonly used by practitioners, *tui* (meaning "push") and *na* ("squeeze"). Tui na incorporates elements from several different forms of traditional Chinese medicine (TCM) and martial arts, including qi gong, shiatsu, acupuncture, fire cupping, and tai chi.

Although it employs manual manipulation techniques similar to those used in other types of body massage—such as pressing, kneading, tapping, rolling, gliding, and shaking—tui na tends to focus on identifying and addressing specific problems rather than on promoting simple relaxation. The goal for the tui na therapist is to find and correct imbalances in the flow of energy through the patient's body, known as *qi*. According to TCM, obstructions or deficiencies in the qi can contribute to many chronic health issues. Tui na therapists use manual techniques to access the qi, harmonize the flow of energy through the body, and thus restore the patient to good health.

## The Tui Na Treatment Process

Proponents of tui na believe that the qi must be in balance for a person to have positive energy and enjoy good health. The tui na treatment process thus focuses on enhancing the flow of qi through the body in channels called *meridians*. Therapists are trained to access the qi by massaging vital points along the meridians. They may employ a variety of manual techniques designed to remove obstructions in the

---

"Tui Na," © 2015 Omnigraphics. Reviewed May 2018.

flow of energy, such as kneading, rolling, rubbing, gliding, pulling, rocking, rotating, vibrating, and shaking. Some tui na practitioners also incorporate acupressure or spinal manipulation techniques into the treatment process.

A typical tui na therapy session lasts between 30 and 60 minutes. The client usually wears loose clothing and lies on a massage table or floor mat. The practitioner begins by examining the client to identify problem areas, whether specific pain sites or obstructions in the flow of qi. Then the therapist applies manual massage techniques to acupressure points, energy meridians, and muscles and joints to treat the problems. The client usually feels relaxed but energized at the end of the treatment. Depending on the severity of the problems, the client may need to return for additional sessions.

## Benefits of Tui Na

Proponents claim that tui na massage therapy can lead to improvements in many different health conditions, including arthritis, sciatica, muscle spasms, chronic pain, insomnia, digestive problems, constipation, headaches, and stress. They believe that restoring the free flow of energy through the body relaxes muscles, relieves pain, improves circulation, and creates a feeling of vitality and emotional well-being.

While tui na may aid in the healing process for some patients, doctors warn that it should only complement, rather than replace, conventional medical treatment for potentially serious health conditions. Critics argue that there is no scientific evidence to support the existence of qi or the claim that tui na can improve the function of bodily systems. In addition, since tui na is more vigorous and intense than many other forms of massage, it may not be appropriate for everyone.

### References

1. Hafner, Christopher. "Tui Na," Center for Spirituality and Healing, University of Minnesota, 2013.

2. Henderson, Jan. "What Is Tui Na?" *Balance Flow Health and Bodyworks*, 2014.

3. Pacific College of Oriental Medicine. "Benefits of Tui Na Massage," 2014.

# Part Seven

# Energy-Based Therapies

# Chapter 67

# *Feng Shui*

Feng shui is an ancient philosophical system of Chinese origin that dates back to 1700 BC. It is based on the concept that people who live in harmony with their environment can lead healthier, happier, more productive lives. Feng shui is the art of designing the physical environment so that it balances various elements of nature. Achieving this balance is believed to enhance the flow of qi (pronounced "chee"), the central energy or life force that is present in all things. When qi flows gently and smoothly through a person's surroundings, it may exert a positive influence on their health, relationships, and worldly success.

## *History of Feng Shui*

In ancient China, the principles of feng shui were widely used to select, orient, design, and decorate living spaces. Citizens relied upon the system to choose locations to build homes, grow crops, and bury departed family members. The dynasties that ruled over China applied this "art of placement" to the construction of palaces, government buildings, and even entire cities.

Over time, the principles associated with feng shui expanded to include nuances from astronomy, astrology, philosophy, cosmology, and metaphysics. During the Cultural Revolution of 1966–76, however, Chinese Communist leaders purged the country of many traditional elements of Chinese culture. Although the practice of feng shui was

---

"Feng Shui," © 2015 Omnigraphics. Reviewed May 2018.

suppressed in mainland China, the discipline gained prominence in the United States and elsewhere in the world.

## *Principles of Feng Shui*

Wherever it is practiced, feng shui incorporates the same basic principles:

**Qi.** In traditional Chinese culture, qi is the life force or energy flow that permeates all living things and connects them to the natural environment. Qi is the core principle of feng shui as well as traditional Chinese medicine and martial arts. In the practice of feng shui, people strive to arrange their surroundings to remove obstructions, create harmony, and keep qi flowing smoothly.

**Yin and Yang.** Feng shui also incorporates the principle of polarity or duality. Under this principle, everything in nature is comprised of two opposing, yet interconnected forces. These two forces cannot exist without each other, and they can be regarded as parts of a whole circle. Yin is considered to be a female force, and it is often characterized as soft, gentle, and nurturing. Yang, on the other hand, is considered to be a male force, characterized as hard, active, and aggressive. In feng shui, people strive to balance opposing forces—light and dark, straight and curvy, etc.—in an effort to promote harmony in their environment.

**Connectedness.** This principle is based on the idea that the environment can influence people, just as people can influence their environment. Due to this connectedness, organizing one's surroundings through the practice of feng shui is believed to have an impact on other aspects of one's life, such as health and success.

**The Five Elements.** Feng shui divides the environment into five elements: fire, earth, metal, water, and wood. The five elements are believed to relate to each other as they do in nature, in what are known as productive cycles and destructive cycles. Arranging surroundings with feng shui means striving to attain a balance between the various elements. When one element is emphasized too heavily, it can obstruct the flow of qi and make the surroundings feel uncomfortable. Each element is associated with a certain shape, color, and set of characteristics or attributes:

1.  **Fire** is represented by a triangle and the color red. Among the qualities associated with the fire element are passion, enthusiasm, expressiveness, inspiration, boldness, and

leadership. In the environment, objects that incorporate the fire element include candles, fireplaces, and lamps.

2.   **Earth** is represented by a square, and its main colors are brown and yellow. It is associated with such attributes as balance, stability, grounding, and practicality. Objects that bring the earth element into the environment might include hardwood floors, granite countertops, or clay pots.

3.   **Metal** is represented by a circle, and its main colors are silver, gold, and white. Metal energy is associated with activities of the mind, such as strength, focus, and clarity of thought. This element can be featured in the environment through the use of wrought iron furniture or light fixtures, metal picture frames, or electronic devices like clocks or televisions.

4.   **Water** is represented by wavy lines and the colors blue and black. It is regarded as a mystical element that symbolizes spirituality, reflection, movement, and flow. It can be incorporated into the environment in the form of water-filled glass vases, aquariums, fountains, or objects that have a swirling pattern.

5.   **Wood** is represented by a rectangle and the color green. Among the attributes of wood-energy are growth, vitality, and creativity. Objects that bring wood energy into the environment include anything made of wood, such as furniture or flooring, as well as live plants and flowers—especially bamboo.

6.   The **bagua** is an important tool used in the practice of feng shui. It is an octagonal or rectangular chart containing nine equal spaces that correspond to the following critical aspects of life:

- Power and wealth

- Fame and reputation

- Love and relationships

- Children and legacy

- Compassion and travel

- Work and career

- Knowledge and wisdom

- Health and community
- Well-being and balance

The bagua is used to determine which physical part of a home, office, shop, or restaurant relates to each attribute. This information can help people decide how to decorate or place favorite personal possessions within a space in order to enhance the flow of qi.

The first step in using the bagua involves orienting it to space, with the main entrance in the middle of the bottom row. Next, feng shui experts suggest conceptualizing the floor plan of the space as nine squares that match the ones on the bagua. Finally, they recommend decorating and accessorizing each area with objects that activate the specific energy or attributes of the corresponding square on the bagua. For example, diplomas and trophies should be placed in the area that represents fame and reputation, while family photos and children's drawings should be placed in the area that represents children and legacy. Proponents of feng shui believe that people who use these principles to organize their surroundings will achieve greater balance and experience positive changes in their lives.

### References

1. Jones, Katina Z. *The Everything Feng Shui Book*, New York: F+W Media, 2011.

2. Olmstead, Carol. "Basics," *Feng Shui for Real Life*, 2015.

Chapter 68

# *Magnet Therapy*

Magnets are often marketed for different types of pain, such as foot or back pain resulting from arthritis and fibromyalgia (FM). Made from metal or alloys, magnets vary considerably in their strength. Magnets marketed for pain are usually encased in a wrap or sold in a product that is placed against the skin near where the pain is felt. Different types of magnets have been studied for pain.

- **Static or permanent magnets.** Static magnets have magnetic fields that do not change. The activity of electrons in the metal causes it to be magnetic. These magnets usually aren't very strong and are often put in products such as shoe insoles, headbands, bracelets, and more.

- **Electromagnets.** This type of magnet is created when an electrical current charges the metal, making it magnetic. Devices with electromagnets in them are also marketed for health purposes.

### *Bottom Line*

Research studies don't support the use of static magnets for any form of pain. Electromagnets may help with osteoarthritis (OA) but

This chapter contains text excerpted from the following sources: Text in this chapter begins with excerpts from "Magnets for Pain," National Center for Complementary and Integrative Health (NCCIH), December 27, 2017; Text under the heading "Before Considering Using Magnet Therapy" is excerpted from "Magnets," National Center for Complementary and Integrative Health (NCCIH), February 2013. Reviewed May 2018.

it's unclear if they can relieve the pain enough to improve quality of life and day-to-day functioning, a 2013 research review concluded. For OA, small machines or mats are used to deliver electromagnetic fields to the whole body or to certain joints.

In 2013 the U.S. Food and Drug Administration (FDA) approved a device that uses strong electromagnets to treat migraines by stimulating nerve cells in the brain, a process called transcranial magnetic stimulation (TMS). TMS may help other pain conditions as well.

## Safety

Some magnets may interfere with medical devices, such as pacemakers and insulin pumps. Beyond interference with medical devices, there isn't much good information on the possible side effects of magnets, but few problems have been reported.

Children may swallow or accidentally inhale small magnets, which can be deadly. Do not use static magnets or electromagnets that you can buy without a prescription to postpone seeing a healthcare provider about pain or any other medical problem.

## Before Considering Using Magnet Therapy

If you are considering using magnets:

- Scientific evidence does not support the use of magnets for pain relief.

- Do not use magnets as a replacement for conventional medical treatment or as a reason to postpone seeing your healthcare provider about any health problem.

- Magnets may not be safe for some people, such as those who use pacemakers or insulin pumps, as magnets may interfere with the devices. Otherwise, magnets are generally considered safe when applied to the skin.

- Tell all your healthcare providers about any complementary health approaches you use. Give them a full picture of what you do to manage your health. This will help ensure coordinated and safe care.

# Chapter 69

# *Polarity Therapy*

Polarity therapy is based on ancient therapeutic techniques and focuses on restoring energy balance in the body. The therapy was discovered by Dr. Randolph Stone in the nineteenth century, and draws from the energy principles of qi and prana, a combination of both Eastern and Western practices. Dr. Stone integrated his knowledge on the nervous system, human anatomy, the muscular network, and the cerebrospinal fluid system to create polarity therapy. This therapy does not produce physical fitness, but rather the expression of the soul that wants to find peace, happiness, and well-being.

## *What Is Polarity Therapy?*

Polarity therapy is based on the belief that the body has the ability to heal itself when stimulated properly. Good health and well-being are achieved when there is a free flow of energy. Treating this implies rooting out any issues that impede the free flow of energy in order to restore stability at a physical, emotional, and psychological level. This involves various steps, but chief among them are traditional touch massage, adjustments in nutrition and diet, and physical exercise.

Polarity therapy is based on three levels of touch:

- Satva, or soft touching
- Rajas, or rocking motion
- Tamas, or dispersing movement

"Polarity Therapy," © 2018 Omnigraphics. Reviewed May 2018.

The therapist uses a gentle touch in *satva* touching, which allows the body to achieve a state of complete relaxation and inaction. *Rajas* touching aims to stimulate and change the frequencies of life energy within the client and achieve balance, while the *tamas* touch focuses on magnetic reactions within the body.

## What Are the Principles behind Polarity Therapy?

Polarity therapy is based on the principle that energy flows from the head to the feet. The body is surrounded by an energy field that is based on the Ayurvedic chakras and the traditional Chinese principle of yin and yang. The human energy field is influenced by touch, exercise, diet, relationships, and life experiences. Balancing the effects of these influences is achieved through yoga, counseling, diet, and bodywork.

According to the beliefs of polarity therapy, the body is affected by stress and trauma whenever an interruption in the energy flow of the body occurs.

Polarity therapy posits that there are three types of energy fields in the body:

- Long-line currents that run north to south in the body.

- Transverse currents that run east-west in the body.

- Spiral currents that start at the navel and expand outward.

## Procedure of Polarity Therapy

Each session of polarity therapy begins with an open discussion that allows a polarity therapist to assess a patient's medical condition while helping them to explore their feelings and attitudes toward life. The primary questions are

- How is your illness connected to your life situations?

- How can you resolve issues and free your thoughts?

- Are you ready to experience positive energy in your life?

- Are you willing to let go of the negative energy in your life?

As patient and therapist begin to explore the answers to these questions, the polarity therapist is able to locate energy blockages and the process of healing begins. It is important to remember that polarity therapy does not treat illnesses, though. Instead, patients are developing self-awareness and deep inner peace. The therapy also helps clients recover balance and stability in their lives.

Polarity therapy includes four main techniques:

1.  The therapist begins by asking a few questions that will help clients assess themselves and find the answers to their problems.

2.  After this discussion, the therapist will place his or her hands on a patient's head, feet, hands, or body to restore energy flow to the body. This is done through a gentle rocking movement to induce sleep.

3.  The sessions vary based on the individual needs of the patient but the therapist is required to continue communicating in. specific ways with the patient.

4.  Toward the end of the session, the therapist will advise the patient to follow a particular dietary plan and perform some specific physical exercises.

The polarity therapist locates energy blockages by following this process. After identifying the areas of pain and discomfort, she or he uses various techniques to realign the energy fields by incorporating physical movements and exercises.

## *Benefits of Polarity Therapy*

Polarity therapy is believed to heal the following health conditions:

*   Migraines and stress headaches

*   Depression and anxiety

*   Irritable bowel syndrome (IBS)

*   Chronic fatigue syndrome (CFS)

*   Allergies

*   Anxiety

*   Back pain

*   Arthritis

Polarity therapy is said to improve the function of the immune system and ward off diseases. It is also believed to improve range of motion, increase energy levels, alleviate pain, and reduce stress and inflammation.

## Contraindications of Polarity Therapy

The Satva touch in the polarity therapy can be used to treat a number of health-related conditions. However, the Rajas and Tamas are considered inappropriate for the treatment of some health problems. Moreover, only a professional with proper credentials can decide what level of treatment is appropriate for the patient. The American Polarity Therapy Association (APTA) requires 155 hours of training for a beginner massage therapist. It is advised that the patient research a potential polarity therapist before considering treatment of the same.

## Research Conducted into the Efficacy of Polarity Therapy

Studies on polarity therapy have shown the following results:

- 45 women with breast cancer were found to show lower levels of fatigue after undergoing chemotherapy and radiation treatments.
- 38 patients suffering from anxiety, sleep disorders, poor quality of life, and depression showed a drastic reduction in stress levels.

Polarity therapy has been proven to be effective in helping people regain their health and well-being. Administered along with a healthy diet, physical exercise, and lifestyle counseling, polarity therapists can help patients solve the emotional issues that are connected to their physical ailments.

## How to Find a Polarity Therapy Practitioner

The APTA offers information on how to find a qualified practitioner of polarity therapy.

### References

1. "Polarity Therapy," Massagetique.com, 2018.
2. "Polarity Therapy," University of New Hampshire Health and Wellness, 2018.
3. "The Benefits of Polarity Therapy and Energy Balancing," Verywell, 2018.
4. "Polarity Therapy," Cupping Resource, 2018.

# Chapter 70

# *Reiki*

## What Is Reiki?

Reiki is a complementary health approach in which practitioners place their hands lightly on or just above a person, with the goal of facilitating the person's own healing response.

- Reiki is based on an Eastern belief in an energy that supports the body's innate or natural healing abilities. However, there isn't any scientific evidence that such an energy exists.

- Reiki has been studied for a variety of conditions, including pain, anxiety, fatigue, and depression.

## What the Science Says about the Effectiveness of Reiki

Several groups of experts have evaluated the evidence on Reiki, and all of them have concluded that it's uncertain whether Reiki is helpful.

Only a small number of studies of Reiki have been completed, and most of them included only a few people. Different studies looked at different health conditions making it hard to compare their results. Many of the studies didn't compare Reiki with both sham (simulated) Reiki and with no treatment. Studies that include both of these comparisons are usually the most informative.

This chapter includes text excerpted from "Reiki: In Depth," National Center for Complementary and Integrative Health (NCCIH), October 2015.

## What the Science Says about the Safety of Reiki

Reiki appears to be generally safe. In studies of Reiki, side effects were no more common among participants who received Reiki than among those who didn't receive it.

### More to Consider

If you are considering trying it:

- Reiki should not be used to replace conventional care or to postpone seeing a healthcare provider about a health problem. If you have severe or long-lasting symptoms, see your healthcare provider. You may have a health problem that needs prompt treatment.

- Tell all your healthcare providers about any complementary health approaches you use. Give them a full picture of what you do to manage your health. This will help ensure coordinated and safe care.

# Chapter 71

# *Shiatsu*

Shiatsu, which is a Japanese word meaning "finger pressure," is a form of therapeutic bodywork. Practitioners use their fingers, thumbs, and palms to knead, press, tap, and stretch various parts of the body in a rhythmic sequence. In most forms of shiatsu, the goal is to correct imbalances in the flow of energy through the body, known as qi (pronounced "chee") in Japanese and Chinese medical traditions. According to these traditions, obstructions or deficiencies in the qi can contribute to many chronic health issues, such as headaches, muscular pain, digestive problems, or frequent colds. Shiatsu therapists use manual techniques to access the qi, harmonize the flow of energy through the body, and thus restore the client to good health.

## *History of Shiatsu*

The person often credited as the founder of modern shiatsu therapy is Tokujiro Namikoshi, who was born in Japan in 1905. He began using hands-on therapy techniques at the age of seven to treat his mother's rheumatoid arthritis. He eventually developed a theory of bodywork that he called shiatsu and established a school to train shiatsu therapists. Namikoshi introduced shiatsu to the United States in the 1950s, and from there it spread around the world. Although shiatsu evolved from anma, a massage system popularized in the 1600s by acupuncturist Sugiyama Waichi, it integrated this traditional Japanese form of manual therapy with modern medical knowledge. The Japanese

---

"Shiatsu," © 2015 Omnigraphics. Reviewed May 2018.

Ministry of Health recognized shiatsu as a distinct form of therapeutic treatment in 1964.

Over the years, many shiatsu practitioners developed their own therapeutic styles. Some approaches emphasize stimulation of acupressure points, while others concentrate on influencing the flow of qi. Although the techniques may differ slightly, they all share the same basic goals. Some of the common variations include:

- Five-Element Shiatsu

- Hara Shiatsu

- Macrobiotic Shiatsu

- Meridian Shiatsu

- Oha Shiatsu

- Quantum Shiatsu

- Tao Shiatsu

- Tsubo Shiatsu

- Water Shiatsu

- Zen Shiatsu

## *The Shiatsu Treatment Process*

Regardless of the style used, a shiatsu treatment typically begins with an assessment of the state of the client's qi. The practitioner performs this evaluation in order to determine what obstructions or sources of imbalance might be present. This process allows the therapist to design a treatment plan that will address the problems, restore the balance, and improve the client's health.

Following the initial assessment, the practitioner uses manual techniques—including pressing, kneading, rubbing, tapping, and stretching—to access the client's qi. The qi is believed to flow through pathways in the body called meridians. Practitioners attempt to influence the flow of energy by manipulating locations known as vital points. If the client is experiencing a great deal of stress or anxiety, the therapist may employ techniques designed to disperse energy. On the other hand, if the client is experiencing fatigue or depression, the practitioner may use techniques designed to restore energy.

Unlike some other types of massage therapy, shiatsu is performed through clothing and without the use of oils. The person undergoing treatment usually lies on a low massage table or on a pad on the floor. A typical session lasts between 60 and 90 minutes. Although shiatsu is considered a low-risk treatment, it may not be appropriate for people who have recently undergone surgery, have skin rashes, open wounds, or injuries, or who are in the advanced stages of pregnancy.

## Research on Shiatsu

Most people find shiatsu therapy to be very soothing and relaxing. Anecdotal evidence suggests that it can offer some health benefits, such as alleviating pain from injuries or arthritis and reducing the psychological stress associated with illness. Proponents claim that it is also effective in relieving headaches, reducing anxiety, enhancing sleep, improving digestion, and treating the symptoms of premenstrual syndrome.

While shiatsu may aid in the healing process for some patients, doctors emphasize that it should complement, rather than replace, appropriate medical treatment. The mainstream medical community generally rejects the idea that shiatsu can effectively prevent, diagnose, or treat potentially serious medical conditions. Critics argue that there is no scientific evidence to support the existence of qi or the claim that shiatsu can improve the function of bodily systems.

### References

1.  Canadian Shiatsu Society of British Columbia. "About Shiatsu," n.d.

2.  Pelava, Cari Johnson. "What Is Shiatsu?" *Taking Charge of Your Health and Well-Being, Center for Spirituality and Healing*, University of Minnesota, 2013.

# Chapter 72

# *Therapeutic Touch*

## *What Is Therapeutic Touch?*

Therapeutic touch, sometimes called "laying on of hands," is a type of therapy that practitioners say promotes relaxation, pain relief, healing, and the restoration of balanced energy fields. Although it is based on ancient principles, modern therapeutic touch was developed in the 1970s by Dolores Krieger, a professor of nursing, and Dora Kunz, a natural healer and a theosophy. And although the effectiveness of therapeutic touch remains controversial, their methods have since been taught to many thousands of people, including health professionals and lay practitioners.

Despite the name, practitioners of therapeutic touch generally place their hands two to four inches over an individual's body, passing them from head to toe in order to identify energy that is out of balance. By doing so, the practitioner interacts with the individual's energy field and can consciously direct or modulate the person's energies. According to proponents, mind, body, and emotions are components of a complex energy field. The therapy works on the principle that when these three (mind, body, and emotions) are balanced they are an indication of good health, whereas when there is an imbalance the result is bad health.

---

## Energy Field

In the ancient health systems of such civilizations as India and China, an energy field is known as life energy. It is present throughout the body and is responsible for the maintenance of psychological, physiological, and spiritual functions. In the Indian Ayurvedic system, it is called "prana," and in traditional Chinese medicine (TCM) it is "qi." In these and many other cultures, correcting disruptions or imbalances in the life energy is a key part of healthcare.

## How Is Therapeutic Touch Performed?

A typical session of therapeutic touch will last for approximately 15–30 minutes, during which the individual will sit in a chair or lie down, fully clothed. The session starts with the practitioner asking the client about his or her healing goals and the problems being faced. Then the practitioner uses sweeping hand motions above the individual to identify and attempt to balance the energy field in and around the body. The following are some of the steps that may be followed by the practitioner during a therapeutic touch session:

- **Centering.** The practitioner focuses to a level of calm.

- **Assessment.** The client's energy field is appraised.

- **Intervention.** If an imbalance is identified, the practitioner clears and mobilizes the individual's energy field and redirects energy to achieve wholeness and balance in the field.

- **Evaluation and closure.** The practitioner evaluates the effectiveness of the treatment. If the individual has any questions, the practitioner answers them and asks for feedback.

## Benefits of Therapeutic Touch

Therapeutic touch aims to help an individual discover his or her own healing process and restore wholeness at physical, mental, and emotional levels. The two most reliable and immediate effects of therapeutic touch are said to be pain relief and relaxation. The therapy helps in stimulating the body's natural healing but does not necessarily claim to cure any illness.

Some of the benefits of therapeutic touch, as described by practitioners and clients, are discussed below.

- Therapeutic touch is said to be effective on people of all ages.

- Therapeutic touch stimulates cell growth.

- The process can relieve tension headaches and reduce pain, including that stemming from burns, osteoarthritis (OA), or surgery.

- It helps improve joint function in people affected by arthritis.

- It can reduce stress in patients with cancer and heart disease.

- Some research suggests that the therapy helps reduce cholesterol levels, improve breathing, and lower blood pressure.

- Therapeutic touch can ease difficult pregnancies.

- Along with conventional medical treatment, the therapy can help patients with such other conditions as lupus, chronic pain, Alzheimer disease (AD), addictions, allergies, sleep apnea, fibromyalgia (FM), bronchitis, and restless legs syndrome (RLS).

- Some people experience significant emotional and spiritual change after the therapy. They may gain more self-confidence and self-control.

## Risks of Therapeutic Touch

Since therapeutic touch is noninvasive and is not generally used as a major form of treatment for any serious health conditions, it comes with very few risks. After a therapeutic touch session, the individual can feel lightheaded, thirsty, and may need to urinate. In most cases, the light-headedness may last for around 15 minutes, and the individual can feel thirsty for a few days. However, some therapeutic practitioners say the therapy can cause mild fever and some inflammation, and some have found that too much energy can cause increased pain and leave the individual frustrated, anxious, and restless. Practitioners also suggest that therapeutic touch should not be done in areas of the body affected with cancer.

If an individual has been abused physically or sexually in the past, it is best discussed with the practitioner before the session begins, even though the therapy does not involve touching. Children, the elderly, and extremely sick people should be treated only for a short period of time, according to some therapeutic practitioners.

### References

1. "Therapeutic Touch," University of Maryland Medical Center (UMMC), February 4, 2016.

2. "Therapeutic Touch," University of Minnesota, October 29, 2008.

3. "Therapeutic Touch: Topic Overview," WebMD, December 22, 2007.

4. "Understanding Therapeutic Touch," Therapeutic Touch Network of Ontario (TTNO), September 1, 2007.

# Part Eight

# Alternative Treatments for Specific Diseases and Conditions

# Chapter 73

# *Asthma and CAM*

Asthma is a chronic disease that affects your airways. Your airways are tubes that carry air in and out of your lungs. If you have asthma, the inside walls of your airways become sore and swollen. That makes them very sensitive, and they may react strongly to things that you are allergic to or find irritating. When your airways react, they get narrower and your lungs get less air.

Symptoms of asthma include:

- Wheezing

- Coughing, especially early in the morning or at night

- Chest tightness

- Shortness of breath

Not all people who have asthma have these symptoms. Having these symptoms doesn't always mean that you have asthma. Your doctor will diagnose asthma based on lung function tests, your medical history, and a physical exam. You may also have allergy tests. When your asthma symptoms become worse than usual, it's called an

This chapter contains text excerpted from the following sources: Text in this chapter begins with excerpts from "Asthma," MedlinePlus, National Institutes of Health (NIH), January 2, 2017; Text beginning with the heading "Complementary Health Approaches for Asthma" is excerpted from "Asthma: In Depth," National Center for Complementary and Integrative Health (NCCIH), April 2013. Reviewed May 2018.

asthma attack. Severe asthma attacks may require emergency care, and they can be fatal.

Asthma is treated with two kinds of medicines:

1. Quick-relief medicines to stop asthma symptoms

2. Long-term control medicines to prevent symptoms

## Complementary Health Approaches for Asthma

Most people are able to control their asthma with conventional therapies and by avoiding the substances that can set off asthma attacks. Even so, some people turn to complementary health approaches in their efforts to relieve symptoms. According to the National Health Interview Survey (NHIS), which included a comprehensive survey on the use of complementary health approaches by Americans, asthma ranked 13th as a condition prompting use of complementary health approaches by adults; 1.1 percent of respondents (an estimated 788,000 adults) said they had used a complementary approach for asthma in the past year. In the NHIS survey, which included adults and children, asthma ranked eighth among conditions prompting the use of complementary health approaches by children but did not appear in a similar ranking for adults.

## What the Science Says about Complementary Health Approaches and Asthma

According to reviewers who have assessed the research, there is not enough evidence to support the use of any complementary health approaches for the relief of asthma.

- Several studies have looked at actual or true acupuncture—stimulation of specific points on the body with thin metal needles—for asthma. Although a few studies showed some reduction in medication use and improvements in symptoms and quality of life, the majority showed no difference between actual acupuncture and simulated or sham acupuncture on asthma symptoms. At this point, there is little evidence that acupuncture is an effective treatment for asthma.

- There has been renewed patient interest in breathing exercises or retraining to reduce hyperventilation, regulate breathing, and achieve a better balance of carbon dioxide and oxygen in the blood. A review of seven randomized controlled trials found a trend toward improvement in symptoms with breathing techniques but not enough evidence for firm conclusions.

- A 2011 study examined the placebo response in patients with chronic asthma and found that patients receiving a placebo (placebo inhaler and simulated acupuncture) reported significant improvement in symptoms such as chest tightness and perception of difficulty breathing. However, lung function did not improve in these patients. This is an important distinction because although the patients felt better, their risk for becoming very sick from untreated asthma was not lessened.

## Considering Complementary Health Approaches for Asthma!

If you are considering complementary health approaches for asthma:

- Conventional medical treatments are very effective for managing asthma symptoms. See your healthcare provider to discuss a comprehensive medical treatment plan for your asthma.

- Do not use any complementary approaches to postpone seeing your healthcare provider about asthma-like symptoms or any health problem.

- Do not replace conventional treatments for asthma with unproven products or practices.

- Keep in mind that dietary supplements can act in the same way as drugs. They can cause health problems if not used correctly or if used in large amounts, and some may interact with medications you take. Your healthcare provider can advise you. If you are pregnant or nursing a child, or if you are considering giving a child a dietary supplement, it is especially important to consult your (or your child's) healthcare provider.

- Tell all your healthcare providers about any complementary health approaches you use. Give them a full picture of what you do to manage your health. This will help ensure coordinated and safe care.

# Chapter 74

# *Cancer and CAM*

Cancer is a term for diseases in which abnormal cells divide without control. Cancer cells can invade nearby tissues and spread to other parts of the body through the bloodstream and the lymph system. Although cancer is the second leading cause of death in the United States, improvements in screening, detection, treatment, and care have increased the number of cancer survivors, and experts expect the number of survivors to continue to increase in the coming years.

People with cancer want to do everything they can to combat the disease, manage its symptoms, and cope with the side effects of treatment. Many turn to complementary health approaches, including natural products, such as herbs (botanicals) and other dietary supplements, and mind and body practices, such as acupuncture, massage, and yoga.

## *Key Facts*

- **Symptom management.** A substantial amount of scientific evidence suggests that some complementary health approaches may help to manage some symptoms of cancer and side effects of treatment. For other complementary approaches, the evidence is more limited.

This chapter includes text excerpted from "Cancer: In Depth," National Center for Complementary and Integrative Health (NCCIH), July 2014. Reviewed May 2018.

- **Disease treatment.** At present, there is no convincing evidence that any complementary health approach is effective in curing cancer or causing it to go into remission

- **Cancer prevention.** A 2012 study indicated that taking a multivitamin/mineral supplement may slightly reduce the risk of cancer in older men. No other complementary health approach has been shown to be helpful in preventing cancer.

## About Complementary Health Approaches

Complementary health approaches are a group of diverse medical and healthcare systems, practices, and products whose origins come from outside of mainstream medicine. They include such products and practices as herbal supplements, other dietary supplements, meditation, spinal manipulation, and acupuncture.

The same careful scientific evaluation that is used to assess conventional therapies should be used to evaluate complementary approaches. Some complementary approaches are beginning to find a place in cancer treatment—not as cures, but as additions to treatment plans that may help patients cope with disease symptoms and side effects of treatment and improve their quality of life.

## Use of Complementary Health Approaches for Cancer

Many people who've been diagnosed with cancer use complementary health approaches.

- According to the National Health Interview Survey (NHIS), which included a comprehensive survey on the use of complementary health approaches by Americans, 65 percent of respondents who had ever been diagnosed with cancer had used complementary approaches, as compared to 53 percent of other respondents. Those who had been diagnosed with cancer were more likely than others to have used complementary approaches for general wellness, immune enhancement, and pain management.

- Other surveys have also found that use of complementary health approaches is common among people who've been diagnosed with cancer, although estimates of use vary widely. Some data indicate that the likelihood of using complementary approaches varies with the type of cancer and with factors such as sex, age, and ethnicity. The results of surveys from 18 countries show that use of complementary approaches by people who had been diagnosed with cancer was more common in North America than in Australia/New Zealand or Europe and that use had increased since the 1970s and especially since 2000.

- Surveys have also shown that many people with cancer don't tell their healthcare providers about their use of complementary health approaches. In the NHIS, survey respondents who had been diagnosed with cancer told their healthcare providers about 15 percent of their herb use and 23 percent of their total use of complementary approaches. In other studies, between 32–69 percent of cancer patients and survivors who used dietary supplements or other complementary approaches reported that they discussed these approaches with their physicians. The differences in the reported percentages may reflect differences in the definitions of complementary approaches used in the studies, as well as differences in the communication practices of different groups of patients.

## What the Science Says about the Safety and Side Effects of Complementary Health Approaches for Cancer

- Delaying conventional cancer treatment can decrease the chances of remission or cure. Don't use unproven products or practices to postpone or replace conventional medical treatment for cancer.

- Some complementary health approaches may interfere with cancer treatments or be unsafe for cancer patients. For example, the herb St. John's wort, which is sometimes used for depression, can make some cancer drugs less effective.

- Other complementary approaches may be harmful if used inappropriately. For example, to make massage therapy safe for people with cancer, it may be necessary to avoid massaging places on the body that are directly affected by the disease or its treatment (for example, areas where the skin is sensitive following radiation therapy).

- People who've been diagnosed with cancer should consult the healthcare providers who are treating them for cancer before using any complementary health approach for any purpose— whether or not it's cancer-related.

# What the Science Says about the Effectiveness of Complementary Health Approaches for Cancer

No complementary health product or practice has been proven to cure cancer. Some complementary approaches may help people manage cancer symptoms or treatment side effects and improve their quality of life.

## *Incorporating Complementary Health Approaches into Cancer Care*

The Society for Integrative Oncology (SIO) issued evidence-based clinical practice guidelines for healthcare providers to consider when incorporating complementary health approaches in the care of cancer patients. The guidelines point out that, when used in addition to conventional therapies, some of these approaches help to control symptoms and enhance patients' well-being. The guidelines warn, however, that unproven methods shouldn't be used in place of conventional treatment because delayed treatment of cancer reduces the likelihood of a remission or cure.

No complementary health product or practice has been proven to cure cancer. Some complementary approaches may help people manage cancer symptoms or treatment side effects and improve their quality of life.

## *Complementary Health Approaches for Cancer Symptoms and Treatment Side Effects*

Some complementary health approaches, such as acupuncture, massage therapy, mindfulness-based stress reduction, and yoga, may help people manage cancer symptoms or the side effects of treatment. However, some approaches may interfere with conventional cancer treatment or have other risks. People who have been diagnosed with cancer should consult their healthcare providers before using any complementary health approach.

- **Acupuncture.** There is substantial evidence that acupuncture can help to manage treatment-related nausea and vomiting in cancer patients. There isn't enough evidence to judge whether acupuncture relieves cancer pain or other symptoms such as treatment-related hot flashes. Complications from acupuncture are rare, as long as the acupuncturist uses sterile needles and proper procedures. Chemotherapy and radiation therapy weaken the body's immune system, so it's especially important for acupuncturists to follow strict clean-needle procedures when treating cancer patients.

- **Ginger.** Studies suggest that the herb ginger may help to control nausea related to cancer chemotherapy when used in addition to conventional antinausea medication

- **Massage therapy.** Studies suggest that massage therapy may help to relieve symptoms experienced by people with cancer, such as pain, nausea, anxiety, and depression. However, investigators haven't reached any conclusions about the effects of massage therapy because of the limited amount of rigorous research in this field. People with cancer should consult their healthcare providers before having massage therapy to find out if any special precautions are needed. The massage therapist shouldn't use deep or intense pressure without the healthcare providers' approval and may need to avoid certain sites, such as areas directly over a tumor or those where the skin is sensitive following radiation therapy.

- **Mindfulness-based stress reduction.** There is evidence that mindfulness-based stress reduction, a type of meditation training, can help cancer patients relieve anxiety, stress, fatigue, and general mood and sleep disturbances, thus improving their quality of life. Most participants in mindfulness studies have been patients with early-stage cancer, primarily breast cancer, so the evidence favoring mindfulness training is strongest for this group of patients.

- **Yoga.** Preliminary evidence indicates that yoga may help to improve anxiety, depression, distress, and stress in people with cancer. It also may help to lessen fatigue in breast cancer patients and survivors. However, only a small number of yoga studies in cancer patients have been completed, and some of the research hasn't been of the highest quality. Because yoga involves physical activities, it's important for people with cancer to talk with their healthcare providers in advance to find out whether any aspects of yoga might be unsafe for them.

- **Hypnosis, relaxation therapies, and biofeedback.** Various studies suggest possible benefits of hypnosis, relaxation therapies, and biofeedback to help patients manage cancer symptoms and treatment side effects.

- **Herbal supplements.** A review of the research literature on herbal supplements and cancer concluded that although several herbs have shown promise for managing side effects and symptoms such as nausea and vomiting, pain, fatigue, and insomnia, the scientific evidence is limited, and many clinical trials haven't been well designed. Use of herbs for managing symptoms also raises concerns about potential negative interactions with conventional cancer treatments.

## Complementary Health Approaches for Cancer Prevention

A large 2012 clinical trial has shown that taking a multivitamin/ mineral supplement may slightly reduce the risk of cancer in older men. No other complementary health approach has been shown to be helpful in preventing cancer, and some have been linked with increased health risks.

**Vitamin and mineral supplements.** The results of a study of older men completed in 2012 indicate that taking a multivitamin/mineral supplement slightly reduces the risk of cancer. In this study, which was part of the Physicians' Health Study II (a complex trial that tested several types of supplements), more than 14,000 male U.S. physicians were randomly assigned to take a multivitamin/mineral supplement or a placebo (an identical-appearing product that did not contain vitamins and minerals) for 11 years. Those who took the supplement had 8 percent fewer total cancers than those who took the placebo.

Other studies of vitamins and minerals—most of which evaluated supplements containing only one or a few nutrients—haven't found protective effects against cancer. Some of these studies identified possible risks of supplementing with high doses of certain vitamins or related substances. Examples of research results include the following:

- In another part of the Physicians' Health Study II, supplementing with relatively high doses of either vitamin E or vitamin C did not reduce the risks of prostate cancer or total cancer in men aged 50 or older. Men taking vitamin E had an increased risk of hemorrhagic stroke (a type of stroke caused by bleeding in the brain).

- A 2010 meta-analysis of 22 clinical trials found no evidence that antioxidant supplements (vitamins A, C, and E; beta carotene; and selenium) help to prevent cancer.

- Two large-scale studies found evidence that supplements containing beta carotene increased the risk of lung cancer among smokers.

- The Selenium and Vitamin E Cancer Prevention Trial (SELECT), funded by the National Cancer Institute (NCI), the National Center for Complementary and Integrative Health (NCCIH), and other agencies at the National Institutes of Health (NIH), showed that selenium and vitamin E supplements, taken either alone or together, did not prevent prostate cancer. It also showed that vitamin E supplements, taken alone, increased the risk of prostate cancer in healthy men. There was no increase in prostate cancer risk when vitamin E and selenium were taken together. The doses of selenium and vitamin E used in this study were much higher than those typically included in multivitamin/ mineral supplements.

- Although substantial evidence suggests that calcium may help protect against colorectal cancer, the evidence of potential benefit from calcium in supplement form is limited and inconsistent. Therefore, NCI doesn't recommend the use of calcium supplements to reduce the risk of colorectal cancer.

**Other Natural Products.** A systematic review of 51 studies with more than 1.6 million participants found "insufficient and conflicting" evidence regarding an association between consuming green tea and cancer prevention. Several other natural products, including ginkgo biloba, isoflavones, noni, pomegranate, and grape seed extract, have been investigated for possible cancer-preventive effects, but the evidence on these substances is too limited for any conclusions to be reached.

## Beware of Cancer Treatment Frauds

The U.S. Food and Drug Administration (FDA) and the Federal Trade Commission (FTC) have warned the public to be aware of fraudulent cancer treatments. Cancer treatment frauds aren't new, but over the years it has become easier for the people who market them to reach the public using the Internet.

Some fraudulent cancer treatments are harmful by themselves, and others can be indirectly harmful because people may delay seeking medical care while they try them, or because the fraudulent product interferes with the effectiveness of proven cancer treatments.

The people who sell fraudulent cancer treatments often market them with claims such as "scientific breakthrough," "miraculous cure," "secret ingredient," "ancient remedy," "treats all forms of cancer," or "shrinks malignant tumors." The advertisements may include personal stories from people who've taken the product, but such stories—whether or not they're real—aren't reliable evidence that a product is effective. Also, a money-back guarantee isn't proof that a product works.

## Considering a Complementary Health Approach!

If you have been diagnosed with cancer and are considering a complementary health approach:

- Cancer patients need to make informed decisions about complementary health approaches.

- Gather information about the complementary health product or practice that interests you, and then discuss it with your healthcare providers. If you've been diagnosed with cancer, it's especially important to talk with your healthcare providers before you start using any new complementary health approach. If you're already using a complementary approach, tell your healthcare providers about it, even if your reason for using it has nothing to do with cancer. Some approaches may interfere with standard cancer treatment or may be harmful when used along with standard treatment. Examples of questions to ask include:

  - What is known about the benefits and risks of this product or practice? Do the benefits outweigh the risks?

  - What are the potential side effects?

  - Will this approach interfere with conventional treatment?

  - Can you refer me to a practitioner?

- Do not use any health product or practice that has not been proven safe and effective to replace conventional cancer care or as a reason to postpone seeing your healthcare provider about any health problem.

- Tell all your healthcare providers about any complementary health approaches you use. Give them a full picture of what you do to manage your health. This will help ensure coordinated and safe care.

## *Keep in Mind*

- Unproven products or practices should not be used to replace or delay conventional medical treatment for cancer.

- Some complementary approaches can interfere with standard cancer treatments or have special risks for people who've been diagnosed with cancer. Before using any complementary health approach, people who've been diagnosed with cancer should talk with their healthcare providers to make sure that all aspects of their care work together.

- Tell all your healthcare providers about any complementary health approaches you use. Give them a full picture of what you do to manage your health. This will help ensure coordinated and safe care.

# Chapter 75

# *Chronic Pain and CAM*

Chronic pain is pain that lasts more than several months (variously defined as 3–6 months, but certainly longer than "normal healing"). It's a very common problem. Results from the 2012 National Health Interview Survey (NHIS) show that:

- About 25.3 million U.S. adults (11.2%) had pain every day for the previous 3 months.

- Nearly 40 million adults (17.6%) had severe pain.

- Individuals with severe pain had worse health, used more healthcare, and had more disability than those with less severe pain.

Chronic pain becomes more common as people grow older, at least in part because health problems that can cause pain, such as osteoarthritis (OA), become more common with advancing age. Not all people with chronic pain have a physician-diagnosed health problem, but among those who do, the most frequent conditions by far are low-back pain or OA, according to a national survey. Other common diagnoses include rheumatoid arthritis (RA), migraine, carpal tunnel syndrome (CTS), and fibromyalgia (FM). The annual economic cost of chronic pain in the United States, including both treatment and lost productivity, has been estimated at nearly $635 billion.

This chapter includes text excerpted from "Chronic Pain: In Depth," National Center for Complementary and Integrative Health (NCCIH), September 2016.

Chronic pain may result from an underlying disease or health condition, an injury, medical treatment (such as surgery), inflammation, or a problem in the nervous system (in which case it is called "neuropathic pain"), or the cause may be unknown. Pain can affect the quality of life and productivity, and it may be accompanied by difficulty in moving around, disturbed sleep, anxiety, depression, and other problems.

## What the Science Says about Complementary Health Approaches for Chronic Pain

The scientific evidence suggests that some complementary health approaches may help people manage chronic pain. This chapter highlights the research status of some approaches used for common kinds of pain.

### Chronic Pain: In General

Some research has looked at the effects of complementary approaches on chronic pain in general rather than on specific painful conditions.

- **Yoga, tai chi, and music.** A 2014 evaluation of studies on active self-care complementary approaches (approaches that individuals can do themselves after being taught the technique) found that there is some evidence in favor of using yoga, tai chi, and music for self-management of chronic pain symptoms, but not enough to justify a strong recommendation for their use. The evidence is insufficient, according to this evaluation, to allow conclusions to be reached about other self-care approaches such as mindfulness/meditation, relaxation techniques, and qigong.

- **Mindfulness-based interventions.** A 2016 evaluation of the research on mindfulness-based interventions found they may be helpful for patients with chronic pain, with effectiveness similar to that of cognitive-behavioral approaches.

- **Hypnosis.** Research shows that hypnosis is moderately effective in managing chronic pain, when compared to usual medical care. However, the effectiveness of hypnosis can vary substantially from one person to another.

- **Cannabinoids.** There's some evidence that cannabinoids (substances from marijuana) might be helpful for chronic neuropathic or cancer pain.

## Low-Back Pain

- **Acupuncture.** A 2012 combined analysis of data from several studies conclude that acupuncture is a reasonable option to consider for chronic low-back pain. How acupuncture works to relieve pain is unclear. Current evidence suggests other factors—like expectation and belief—that are unrelated to acupuncture needling may play important roles in the beneficial effects of acupuncture on pain. A 2016 review of studies conducted in the United States found evidence that acupuncture can help some patients manage low-back pain.

- **Massage.** Massage might provide short-term relief from low-back pain, but the evidence is not of high quality. Massage has not been shown to have long-term benefits on low-back pain.

- **Progressive relaxation.** There is some evidence that progressive relaxation may help relieve low-back pain, but studies on this topic have not been of the highest quality

- **Spinal manipulation.** Spinal manipulation appears to be as effective as other therapies commonly used for chronic low-back pain, such as physical therapy, exercise, and standard medical care.

- **Yoga.** Studies have shown that yoga can be helpful for low-back pain in the short term and may also be helpful over longer periods of time.

- **Herbal products.** A 2014 evaluation of research on herbal products for low-back pain found preliminary evidence that devil's claw and white willow bark, taken orally (by mouth), may be helpful for back pain. Cayenne, comfrey, Brazilian arnica, and lavender essential oil may be helpful when used topically (applied to the skin).

- **Prolotherapy.** Studies of prolotherapy (a treatment involving repeated injections of irritant solutions) for low-back pain have had inconsistent results.

## Osteoarthritis (OA)

- **Acupuncture.** A 2012 combined analysis of data from several studies indicated that acupuncture can be helpful and a reasonable option to consider for OA pain. After that analysis was completed, a 2014 Australian study showed that both needle and laser acupuncture were modestly better than no treatment at relieving knee pain from OA but not better than simulated (sham) laser acupuncture. These results generally agree with previous studies, which showed that acupuncture is consistently better than no treatment but not necessarily better than simulated acupuncture at relieving OA pain.

- **Massage.** A small amount of research suggests that massage may help reduce OA symptoms

- **Traditional Chinese medicines (TCM).** Tai chi may improve pain in people with knee OA. Qigong may have similar benefits, but little research has been done on it.

- **Yoga.** It's uncertain whether yoga is helpful for OA.

- **Glucosamine, chondroitin, and S-adenosyl-L-methionine (SAMe).** Studies of glucosamine, chondroitin, and S-adenosyl-L-methionine (SAMe) for knee OA pain have had conflicting results.

- **Dimethyl sulfoxide (DMSO) or methylsulfonylmethane (MSM).** There isn't enough research on dimethyl sulfoxide (DMSO) or methylsulfonylmethane (MSM) for OA pain to allow conclusions to be reached.

## Rheumatoid Arthritis (RA)

- **Mind and body practices.** The amount of research on mind and body practices for RA pain is too small for conclusions to be reached about their effectiveness.

- **Dietary supplements.** Dietary supplements containing omega-3 fatty acids, gamma-linolenic acid (GLA), or the herb thunder god vine may help relieve RA symptoms.

## Headache

- **Acupuncture.** A 2012 combined analysis of data from several studies indicate that acupuncture can be helpful and a reasonable option to consider for headache pain. How acupuncture works to relieve pain is unclear. Current evidence suggests that many factors—like expectation and belief—that are unrelated to acupuncture needling may play important roles in the beneficial effects of acupuncture on pain.

- **Biofeedback, massage, relaxation techniques, spinal manipulation, and tai chi.** Because the evidence is limited or inconsistent, it's uncertain whether biofeedback, massage, relaxation techniques, spinal manipulation, and tai chi are helpful for headaches

- **Butterbur, feverfew, magnesium, riboflavin, and coenzyme $Q_{10}$.** Guidelines from the American Academy of Neurology (AAN) and the American Headache Society (AHS) classify butterbur as effective; feverfew, magnesium, and riboflavin as probably effective; and coenzyme $Q_{10}$ as possibly effective for preventing migraines.

### Neck Pain

- **Acupuncture.** Acupuncture hasn't been studied as extensively for neck pain as for some other conditions. A large study in Germany found that people who received acupuncture for neck pain had better pain relief than those who didn't receive acupuncture. Several studies have compared actual acupuncture with simulated acupuncture, but the amount of research is limited. No current guidelines recommend acupuncture for neck pain.

- **Massage therapy.** A 2016 review of studies performed in the United States found that massage therapy may provide short-term relief from neck pain, especially if massage sessions are relatively lengthy and frequent.

- **Spinal manipulation.** Spinal manipulation may be helpful for neck pain.

### Fibromyalgia (FM)

- It's uncertain whether **acupuncture** is helpful for FM pain.

- **Tai chi, yoga, mindfulness, and biofeedback.** Although some studies of tai chi, yoga, mindfulness, and biofeedback for FM symptoms have had promising results, the evidence is too limited to allow definite conclusions to be reached about whether these approaches are helpful.

- **Natural products.** There is insufficient evidence that any natural products can relieve FM pain, with the possible exception of vitamin D supplements, which may reduce pain in people with FM who have low vitamin D levels.

- Studies of **homeopathy** have not demonstrated that it is beneficial for FM.

### *Irritable Bowel Syndrome (IBS)*

- **Hypnotherapy and probiotics.** Although no complementary health approach has definitively been shown to be helpful for irritable bowel syndrome (IBS), some research results for hypnotherapy and probiotics have been promising.

- **Peppermint oil.** There's only weak evidence supporting the idea that peppermint oil might be helpful for IBS.

- **Acupuncture.** Studies of acupuncture for irritable bowel syndrome have not found actual acupuncture to be more helpful than simulated acupuncture.

### *Other Types of Pain*

- Various complementary approaches have been studied for other types of chronic pain, such as facial pain, nerve pain, chronic pelvic pain, elbow pain, pain associated with endometriosis, CPS, pain associated with gout, and cancer pain. There's promising evidence that some complementary approaches may be helpful for some of these types of pain, but the evidence is insufficient to clearly establish their effectiveness.

### *Other Complementary Approaches*

- **Reiki.** There is a lack of high-quality research to definitively evaluate whether Reiki is of value for pain relief.

- **Static magnets.** Although static magnets are widely marketed for pain control, the evidence does not support their use.

## What the Science Says about Safety and Side Effects

As with any treatment, it's important to consider safety before using complementary health approaches. Safety depends on the specific approach and on the health of the person using it. If you're considering or using a complementary approach for pain, check with your healthcare providers to make sure it's safe for you.

### Safety of Mind and Body Approaches

- Mind and body approaches, such as acupuncture, hypnosis, massage therapy, mindfulness/meditation, relaxation techniques, spinal manipulation, tai chi / qi gong, and yoga, are generally safe for healthy people if they're performed appropriately.

- People with medical conditions and pregnant women may need to modify or avoid some mind and body practices.

- Like other forms of exercise, mind and body practices that involve movements, such as tai chi and yoga, can cause sore muscles and may involve some risk of injury.

- It's important for practitioners and teachers of mind and body practices to be properly qualified and to follow appropriate safety precautions.

### Safety of Natural Products

- "Natural" doesn't always mean "safe." Some natural products (dietary supplements) may have side effects and may interact with medications.

- The U.S. Food and Drug Administration (FDA) has warned the public about several dietary supplements promoted for arthritis or pain that were tainted with prescription drugs.

## Guidelines for the Treatment of Chronic Pain Conditions

National health professional organizations have issued guidelines for treating several chronic pain conditions. Some mention ways in which certain complementary health approaches can be incorporated into treatment plans. Others discourage the use of certain complementary approaches.

The American College of Rheumatology (ACR) mentions several complementary approaches in its guidelines for the management of OA of the hip or knee. For OA of the knee, the guidelines mention tai chi as one of several nondrug approaches that might be helpful. The same guidelines, however, discourage using the dietary supplements glucosamine and chondroitin for OA of the hip or knee.

The American College of Gastroenterology (ACG) included probiotics/prebiotics, peppermint oil, and hypnotherapy in its evaluation of approaches for managing IBS. The ACG found only weak evidence that any of these approaches may be helpful.

## Considering Complementary Health Approaches for Chronic Pain!

If you are considering complementary health approaches for chronic pain:

- Do not use an unproven product or practice to replace conventional care or to postpone seeing a healthcare provider about chronic pain or any other health problem.

- Learn about the product or practice you are considering, especially the scientific evidence on its safety and whether it works.

- Talk with the healthcare providers you see for chronic pain. Tell them about the product or practice you are considering and ask any questions you may have. They may be able to advise you on its safety, use, and likely effectiveness.

- If you are considering a practitioner-provided complementary health practice such as spinal manipulation, massage, or acupuncture, ask a trusted source (such as your healthcare provider or a nearby hospital) to recommend a practitioner. Find out about the training and experience of any practitioner you are considering. Ask whether the practitioner has experience working with your pain condition.

- If you are considering dietary supplements, keep in mind that they can cause health problems if not used correctly, and some may interact with prescription or nonprescription medications or other dietary supplements you take. Your healthcare provider can advise you. If you are pregnant or nursing a child, or if you are considering giving a child a dietary supplement, it is especially important to consult your (or your child's) healthcare provider.

- Tell all your healthcare providers about any complementary or integrative health approaches you use. Give them a full picture of what you do to manage your health. This will help ensure coordinated and safe care.

# Chapter 76

# *Cognitive Decline and CAM*

Thinking, reasoning, and remembering are cognitive functions. Dementia is when those functions decrease much more significantly than what occurs with normal aging. In older people, the most common cause of dementia is Alzheimer disease (AD). An incurable disease, it slowly impairs your memory and thinking skills and, eventually, the ability to care for yourself. Researchers are investigating a variety of complementary health approaches, as well as diets, for preventing or slowing the progression of dementia, including AD.

## *What the Science Says about Complementary Health Approaches for Cognitive Decline*

Researchers have explored many complementary health approaches for preventing or slowing dementia, including AD. There is no strong evidence that any complementary health approach or diet can prevent cognitive impairment.

Following are some of the complementary health approaches that have been studied in over the years.

- **Fish oil/omega-3s.** Among the nutritional and dietary factors studied to prevent cognitive decline in older adults, the most consistent positive research findings are for omega-3 fatty acids,

---

This chapter includes text excerpted from "Cognitive Function, Dementia, and Alzheimer's Disease," National Center for Complementary and Integrative Health (NCCIH), September 24, 2017.

often measured as how much fish people ate. However, taking omega-3 supplements did not have any beneficial effects on the cognitive functioning of older people without dementia.

- **Ginkgo.** A National Center for Complementary and Integrative Health (NCCIH)-funded study of the well-characterized ginkgo supplement EGb-761 found that it didn't lower the incidence of dementia, including AD, in older adults. Further analysis of the same data showed that ginkgo did not slow cognitive decline, lower blood pressure, or reduce the incidence of hypertension. In this clinical trial, known as the Ginkgo Evaluation of Memory study, researchers recruited more than 3,000 volunteers age 75 and older who took 240 mg of ginkgo daily. Participants were followed for an average of approximately 6 years.

- **B-vitamins.** Results of short-term studies suggest that B-vitamin supplements do not help cognitive functioning in adults age 50 or older with or without dementia. The vitamins studied were $B_{12}$, $B_6$, and folic acid, taken alone or in combination.

- **Curcumin**, which comes from turmeric, has anti-inflammatory and antioxidant properties that might affect chemical processes in the brain associated with AD, laboratory studies have suggested. However, the few clinical trials (studies done in people) that have looked at the effects of curcumin on AD have not found a benefit.

- **Melatonin.** People with dementia can become agitated and have trouble sleeping. Supplements of melatonin, which is a naturally occurring hormone that helps regulate sleep, are being studied to see if they improve sleep in some people with dementia. However, in one study researchers noted that melatonin supplements may worsen mood in people with dementia.

For caregivers, taking a mindfulness meditation class or a caregiver education class reduced stress more than just getting time off from providing care, a small, 2010 NCCIH-funded study showed.

## Side Effects and Risks

Don't use complementary approaches as a reason to postpone seeing a healthcare provider about memory loss. Treatable conditions, such as depression, bad reactions to medications, or thyroid, liver, or kidney problems, can cause memory impairment.

Keep in mind that although many dietary supplements (and some prescription drugs) come from natural sources, "natural" does not always mean "safe."

Some dietary supplements have been found to interact with medications, whether prescription or over-the-counter (OTC). For example, the herbal supplement St. John's wort interacts with many medications, making them less effective. Your healthcare provider can advise you.

Many people, particularly older individuals, worry about forgetfulness and whether it is the first sign of dementia or AD. In fact, forgetfulness has many causes. It can also be a normal part of aging or related to various treatable health issues or to emotional problems, such as stress, anxiety, or depression. The National Institute on Aging (NIA) has a lot of information on the aging brain as well as cognitive function, dementia, and AD. Although no treatment is proven to stop dementia or AD, some conventional drugs may limit worsening of symptoms for a period of time in the early stages of the disease.

# Chapter 77

# *Coronary Heart Disease and Chelation Therapy*

## *What Is Coronary Heart Disease (CHD)?*

Coronary heart disease (CHD) is the most common form of heart disease, which is the leading cause of death among American men and women. Each year nearly 380,000 Americans die from CHD. In CHD the coronary arteries, the vessels that provide oxygen-rich blood to the tissues of the heart, become blocked by deposits of a waxy substance called plaque. As plaque builds, the arteries become narrower and less oxygen and nutrients are transported to the heart. CHD can lead to serious problems, such as angina (pain caused by not enough oxygen-carrying blood reaching the heart) and heart attack. A heart attack occurs if the flow of oxygen-rich blood to a section of heart muscle is cut off. If blood flow is not restored quickly, the affected section of heart muscle begins to die. Without quick treatment, a heart attack can lead to serious health problems or death.

Factors that can increase the risk of developing CHD include:

- High blood pressure

- High blood cholesterol levels

This chapter includes text excerpted from "Questions and Answers: The NIH Trials of EDTA Chelation Therapy for Coronary Heart Disease," National Center for Complementary and Integrative Health (NCCIH), September 2016.

- Smoking

- Overweight or obesity

- Physical inactivity

- Diabetes

- Insulin resistance

- Metabolic syndrome (MS)

- Unhealthy diet

- Family history of CHD

- Older age

Symptoms of CHD can include chest pain, shortness of breath, lightheadedness, cold sweats, or nausea, but not everyone with CHD have symptoms.

## What Is Ethylene Diamine Tetra-Acetic Acid (EDTA) Chelation Therapy?

Chelation is a chemical process in which a substance is used to bind molecules, such as metals or minerals, and hold them tightly so that they can be removed from a system, such as the body. In medicine, chelation has been scientifically proven to rid the body of excess or toxic metals. For example, a person who has lead poisoning may be given chelation therapy in order to bind and remove lead from the body before it can cause damage.

In the case of ethylene diamine tetra-acetic acid (EDTA) chelation therapy, the substance that binds and removes metals and minerals is the salts of EDTA, a synthetic, or artificial, amino acid that is delivered intravenously. EDTA was first used in the 1950s for the treatment of heavy metal poisoning. Calcium disodium EDTA chelation removes heavy metals and minerals from the blood, such as lead, iron, copper, and calcium, and is approved by the U.S. Food and Drug Administration (FDA) for use in treating lead poisoning and toxicity from other heavy metals. Rather than testing calcium disodium EDTA, the Trial to Assess Chelation Therapy (TACT) used another salt, disodium EDTA, under the FDA license as an Investigational New Drug (IND). Although disodium EDTA it is not approved by the FDA to treat CHD, some physicians and alternative medicine practitioners have recommended its use in chelation as a way to treat CHD.

## What Are the Possible Side Effects of EDTA Chelation Therapy?

The most common side effect is a burning sensation at the site where EDTA is delivered into a vein. Rare side effects can include fever, headache, nausea, and vomiting. Even rarer are serious and potentially fatal side effects that can include heart failure, a sudden drop in blood pressure, abnormally low calcium levels in the blood (hypocalcemia), permanent kidney damage, and bone marrow depression (meaning that blood cell counts fall). Hypocalcemia and death may occur, particularly if disodium EDTA is infused too rapidly. Reversible injury to the kidneys, although infrequent, has been reported with EDTA chelation therapy. Other serious side effects can occur if EDTA is not administered by a trained health professional.

## How Commonly Is EDTA Chelation Therapy Used?

The National Health Interview Survey (NHIS), conducted by the Centers for Disease Control and Prevention (CDC), found that 111,000 adults 18 years of age and older used chelation therapy as a form of complementary medicine in the previous 12 months.

# Chapter 78

# *Diabetes and CAM*

Diabetes is a disease that occurs when your blood glucose, also called blood sugar, is too high. It can lead to serious health problems if it's not managed well. Between 12–14 percent of U.S. adults have diabetes, but more than 25 percent of people with it are undiagnosed. Taking insulin or other diabetes medicine is often key to treating diabetes, along with making healthy food choices and being physically active.

There are three types of diabetes—type 1, type 2, and gestational. All three involve problems with how your body responds to the hormone insulin. Food supplies your body with glucose, sugar and the main fuel for our bodies. To use glucose, your body needs insulin. If you have type 1 diabetes your body is producing little or no insulin. If you have type 2 your body makes insulin but doesn't respond to it normally. Gestational diabetes affects only pregnant women. It usually goes away after birth, but it increases the mother's risk of developing diabetes later in life.

About 95 percent of people diagnosed with diabetes have type 2. People with type 1, which is usually diagnosed in childhood or early adulthood, must take insulin to survive.

---

This chapter includes text excerpted from "Diabetes and Dietary Supplements: In Depth," National Center for Complementary and Integrative Health (NCCIH), July 2017.

# What the Science Says about the Effectiveness and Safety of Dietary Supplements for Diabetes

## Alpha Lipoic Acid

Alpha lipoic acid is an antioxidant (a substance that may protect against cell damage) being studied for its effect on complications of diabetes, including macular edema, an eye condition that causes blurred vision; unhealthy cholesterol levels; and poor insulin sensitivity. Two 2011 studies of about 570 patients didn't find that the supplement helped with conditions related to diabetes.

### Safety Concerns

High doses of alpha lipoic acid supplements can cause stomach problems.

## Chromium

Found in many foods, chromium is an essential trace mineral. If you have too little chromium in your diet, your body can't use glucose efficiently. Studies have found few or no benefits of chromium supplements for controlling diabetes or reducing the risk of developing it. Taking chromium supplements, along with conventional care, improved blood sugar control in people with diabetes (primarily type 2) who had poor blood sugar control, a 2014 review concluded; however, the improvement was very small. The review included 25 studies with about 1,600 participants.

### Safety Concerns

Chromium supplements may cause stomach pain and bloating, and there have been a few reports of kidney damage, muscular problems, and skin reactions following large doses. The effects of taking chromium long-term haven't been well investigated.

## Herbal Supplements

There is no reliable evidence that any herbal supplements can help to control diabetes or its complications. There are no clear benefits of cinnamon for people with diabetes. Other herbal supplements studied for diabetes include bitter melon, Chinese herbal medicines, fenugreek, ginseng, milk thistle, selenium, and sweet potato. Studies haven't proven that any of these are effective, and some may have side effects.

*Safety Concerns*

There is little conclusive information on the safety of herbal supplements for people with diabetes. Cassia cinnamon, the most common type of cinnamon sold in the United States and Canada, contains varying amounts of a chemical called coumarin, which might cause or worsen liver disease. In most cases, cassia cinnamon doesn't have enough coumarin to make you sick. However, for some people, such as those with liver disease, taking a large amount of cassia cinnamon might worsen their condition. Using herbs such as St. John's wort, prickly pear cactus, aloe, or ginseng with conventional diabetes drugs can cause unwanted side effects.

## Magnesium

Found in many foods, including in high amounts in bran cereal, certain seeds and nuts, and spinach, magnesium is essential to the body's ability to process glucose.

Magnesium deficiency may increase the risk of developing diabetes. A number of studies have looked at whether taking magnesium supplements helps people who have diabetes or who are at risk of developing it. However, the studies are generally small and their results aren't conclusive.

*Safety Concerns*

Large doses of magnesium in supplements can cause diarrhea and abdominal cramping. Very large doses—more than 5,000 mg per day—can be deadly.

## Omega-3s

Taking omega-3 supplements, such as fish oil, hasn't been shown to help people who have diabetes control their blood sugar levels. Research on whether eating fish lowers your risk of getting diabetes is generally negative. However, the effect of eating fish may depend on what type of fish you eat, among other factors. Studies on the effects of eating fish have had conflicting results, two 2012 research reviews with hundreds of thousands of participants showed. Some research from the United States and Europe found that people who ate more fish had a higher incidence of diabetes. Research from Asia and Australia found the opposite—eating more fish was associated with a lower risk of diabetes. There's no strong evidence explaining these differences. Taking omega-3 supplements does not help protect against heart disease in people who have or are at risk of having diabetes, an American Heart Association (AHA) science advisory, based on 5 studies with more than 10,000 participants, stated in 2017. However, it's unclear whether people who have both diabetes and a high risk of developing heart disease would benefit from taking omega-3 supplements.

*Safety Concerns*

Omega-3 supplements don't usually have side effects. When side effects do occur, they typically consist of minor symptoms, such as bad breath, indigestion, or diarrhea. It may interact with drugs that affect blood clotting.

## Vitamins

Studies generally show that taking vitamin C doesn't improve blood sugar control or other conditions in people with diabetes. However, a 2017 research review of 22 studies with 937 participants found weak evidence that vitamin C helped with blood sugar in people with type 2 diabetes when they took it for longer than 30 days. Having low levels of vitamin D is associated with an increased risk of developing a metabolic disorder, such as type 2 diabetes, metabolic syndrome, or insulin resistance, studies and research reviews from the past 5 years have found. But taking vitamin D doesn't appear to help prevent diabetes or improve blood sugar levels for adults with normal levels, prediabetes, or type 2 diabetes, a 2014 research review of 35 studies with 43,407 participants showed.

*Safety Concerns*

Taking too much vitamin D is dangerous and can cause nausea, constipation, weakness, kidney damage, disorientation, and problems with your heart rhythm. You're unlikely to get too much vitamin D from food or the sun.

## Other Supplements

The evidence is still very preliminary on how supplements or foods rich in polyphenols—antioxidants found in tea, coffee, wine, fruits, grains, and vegetables—might affect diabetes.

## Healthy Behaviors: Key to Managing Your Diabetes

### Diet

Develop a meal plan with help from your healthcare providers.

### Physical Activity

Different types and even small amounts of physical activity can help you control diabetes. Physical activity lowers blood sugar, blood pressure, improves blood flow, decreases the risk of falling in older adults, and more. Talk with your healthcare provider before you start a new physical activity program.

## More to Consider

- If you are considering dietary supplements then:

- Talk to your healthcare provider before considering any dietary supplement for yourself, particularly if you're pregnant or nursing, or for a child. Many supplements have not been tested in pregnant women, nursing mothers, or children.

- The U.S. Food and Drug Administration (FDA) is warning consumers not to buy illegally marketed, potentially dangerous products claiming to prevent, treat, or cure diabetes. These products make claims like "lowers your blood sugar naturally" or "inexpensive therapy to fight and eliminate type II diabetes." They may contain harmful ingredients and the label may not tell you what you're actually taking.

- Fraudulent diabetes products can be especially dangerous if you use them instead of proven treatments for diabetes. You can develop serious health complications if you don't follow your doctor's directions for managing diabetes.

- Keep in mind that dietary supplements may interact with medications or other dietary supplements.

- Tell all your healthcare providers about any complementary or integrative health approaches you use. Give them a full picture of what you do to manage your health. This will help ensure coordinated and safe care.

# Chapter 79

# *Fibromyalgia and CAM*

Fibromyalgia (FM) is a common disorder that involves widespread pain, tenderness, fatigue, and other symptoms. It's not a form of arthritis, but like arthritis, it can interfere with a person's ability to perform everyday activities. An estimated 5 million American adults have FM. Between 80–90 percent of people with FM are women, but men and children can also have this condition.

In addition to pain and fatigue, people with FM may have other symptoms, such as cognitive and memory problems, sleep disturbances, morning stiffness, headaches, painful menstrual periods, numbness or tingling of the extremities, restless legs syndrome (RLS), temperature sensitivity, and sensitivity to loud noises or bright lights.

A person may have two or more coexisting chronic pain conditions. Such conditions can include chronic fatigue syndrome (CFS), endometriosis, FM, irritable bowel syndrome (IBS), interstitial cystitis (IC), temporomandibular joint dysfunction (TMJ), and vulvodynia. It's not known whether these disorders share a common cause.

The exact cause of FM is unclear, but it may be related to injury, emotional distress, or viruses that change the way the brain perceives pain. There's no diagnostic test for FM, so healthcare providers diagnose it by examining the patient, evaluating symptoms, and ruling out other conditions.

---

This chapter includes text excerpted from "Fibromyalgia: In Depth," National Center for Complementary and Integrative Health (NCCIH), May 2016.

The U.S. Food and Drug Administration (FDA) has approved several drugs to treat FM, but medication is just one part of conventional medical treatment. Nondrug approaches such as exercise and good sleep habits can also help manage symptoms. Research has repeatedly shown that regular exercise is one of the most effective treatments for FM. People with FM who have too much pain or fatigue to do vigorous exercise should begin with walking or other gentle exercise and build their endurance and intensity slowly.

## What the Science Says about Complementary Health Approaches for Fibromyalgia (FM)

### Mind and Body Practices

#### Acupuncture

Acupuncture is a technique in which practitioners stimulate specific points on the body, known as acupuncture points. This is most often done using needles that penetrate the skin (manual acupuncture), but other techniques, such as using electrical current (electroacupuncture), may also be used. Limited evidence indicates that people with FM who receive acupuncture have improvements in symptoms such as pain and stiffness when compared to those who don't receive it (for example, people on a waiting list). However, acupuncture hasn't been shown to be more effective than simulated acupuncture in relieving FM symptoms. Electroacupuncture may produce better results than manual acupuncture. Acupuncture is generally considered safe when performed by an experienced practitioner using sterile needles. Improperly performed acupuncture can cause potentially serious side effects.

#### Biofeedback

Biofeedback techniques measure body functions and give you information about them so that you can learn to control them. A small number of short-term studies of biofeedback, particularly electromyographic (EMG) biofeedback, in which people learn to control and decrease muscle tension, indicate that it may reduce FM pain. However, the overall evidence on biofeedback is so limited that no definite conclusions can be reached about whether it's helpful for FM symptoms. In studies of EMG biofeedback for FM, some participants reported that the procedure was stressful. No other side effects were reported.

548

*Guided Imagery*

Guided imagery is a technique in which people are taught to focus on pleasant images to replace negative or stressful feelings. Guided imagery may be self-directed or led by a practitioner or a recording. Studies of guided imagery for FM symptoms have had inconsistent results. In some studies, patients who were taught guided imagery had decreases in symptoms such as pain and fatigue, but in other studies, it had no effect. Guided imagery is one of a group of approaches called relaxation techniques. Relaxation techniques are generally considered safe for healthy people. Occasionally, however, people report unpleasant experiences such as increased anxiety.

*Massage Therapy*

Massage therapy includes a variety of techniques in which practitioners manipulate the soft tissues of the body. Several studies have evaluated various types of massage therapy for FM. Most indicated that massage could provide short-term relief of some FM symptoms. However, the current evidence is too limited to be considered conclusive. Experts recommend that massage therapy for FM should not cause pain. It may be necessary to start with a very gentle massage and increase the intensity gradually over time. Massage therapy appears to have few risks when performed by a trained practitioner.

*Meditative Movement Practices (Tai Chi, Qi Gong, and Yoga)*

Tai chi and qi gong, which originated in China, and yoga, which is of Indian origin, all involve a combination of physical postures or movements, a focus on breathing, and meditation or relaxation. Because these three practices have so many features in common, they are sometimes grouped together as meditative movement practices. Exercise is beneficial for people with FM, so meditative movement practices may be helpful because of the physical activity they involve. It's also possible that the meditative component of these practices might help too. Some individual studies of tai chi, qi gong, or yoga for FM symptoms have had promising results. However, there isn't enough high-quality evidence on these approaches to allow definite conclusions to be reached about their effects. Meditative movement practices generally have good safety records when practiced under the guidance of a qualified instructor. Few side effects have been reported in studies of yoga, tai chi, or qigong. However, these practices may need to be modified to make them suitable for people with FM.

### Mindfulness Meditation

Mindfulness meditation is a type of meditation that involves completely focusing on experiences on a moment-to-moment basis. In several studies, mindfulness meditation training has led to short-term improvements in pain and quality of life in people with FM. However, the number of studies is small, and the quality of the evidence is relatively low, so no definite conclusions can be reached. Frequent practice of mindfulness techniques may be important for good results. In a 2014 study of mindfulness for FM, those participants who practiced mindfulness more frequently had a greater reduction in symptoms. Mindfulness and other forms of meditation are generally considered to be safe for healthy people. However, they may need to be modified to make them safe and comfortable for people with some health conditions.

### Other Mind and Body Practices

So little research has been done on chiropractic care and hypnosis for FM that no conclusions can be reached about these practices. An approach called amygdala retraining, which includes various mind and body practices has been proposed as a treatment for FM. Because almost no research has been done on this approach, its effectiveness and safety cannot be evaluated.

## Natural Products

It has been suggested that deficiencies in vitamin D might worsen FM symptoms. In one study of women with FM who had low vitamin D levels, 20 weeks of vitamin D supplementation led to a reduction in pain. Researchers are investigating whether low magnesium levels contribute to FM and if magnesium supplements might help to reduce symptoms. Other natural products that have been studied for FM include dietary supplements such as soy, S-adenosyl-L-methionine (SAMe), and creatine, and topical products containing capsaicin (the substance that gives chili peppers their heat). There's not enough evidence to determine whether these products are helpful. "Natural" doesn't necessarily mean "safe." Natural products can have side effects, and some may interact with medications. Even vitamins and minerals (including vitamin D and magnesium) can be harmful if taken in excessive amounts.

## Other Complementary Approaches

### Balneotherapy

Balneotherapy is the technique of bathing in tap or mineral water for health purposes; it also includes related practices such as mud packs. Although some research has been done on balneotherapy for FM, there's not enough evidence to reach definite conclusions on whether it relieves symptoms. Balneotherapy has a good safety record.

### Homeopathy

Homeopathy is a medical system based on the unconventional idea that a disease can be cured by highly diluted solutions of a substance that causes similar symptoms in healthy people. Studies of homeopathy have not demonstrated that it is beneficial for FM. Highly diluted homeopathic remedies are generally safe. However, not all products labeled as homeopathic are highly dilute; some may contain substantial amounts of ingredients and, therefore, could cause side effects.

### Magnetic Therapies

Static (permanent) magnets are found in magnetic mattress pads, shoe inserts, bracelets, and other products. There's not enough evidence on static magnets to allow any conclusions to be reached. Electromagnets are used in a type of treatment called transcranial magnetic stimulation (TMS), which influences brain activity. The FDA has approved certain TMS devices for treating migraine and treatment-resistant depression. A small number of preliminary studies have evaluated TMS for FM symptoms, and some have had promising results. Magnets and magnetic devices may not be safe for people who have metal implants or medical devices such as pacemakers in their bodies. Headaches have been reported as a side effect in several studies of TMS for FM.

### Reiki

Reiki is a complementary health approach in which practitioners place their hands lightly on or just above a person, with the goal of facilitating the person's own healing response. The National Center for Complementary and Integrative Health (NCCIH)-funded study examined the use of Reiki for FM-related pain. The study showed no effect of Reiki on pain or any of the other outcomes measured in the study (physical and mental functioning, medication use, and visits to healthcare providers). Reiki appears to be generally safe.

## *More to Consider*

If you are considering complementary health approaches for FM then:

- Be aware that some complementary health approaches— particularly dietary supplements—may interact with conventional medical treatments.

- If you're considering a practitioner-provided complementary health approach such as acupuncture, check with your insurer to see if the services will be covered, and ask a trusted source (like your FM healthcare provider or a nearby hospital or medical school) to recommend a practitioner.

- Tell all your healthcare providers about any complementary or integrative health approaches you use. Give them a full picture of what you do to manage your health. This will help ensure coordinated and safe care.

# Chapter 80

# *Flu and Cold and CAM*

Each year, Americans get more than 1 billion colds, and between 5–20 percent of Americans get the flu. The two diseases have some symptoms in common, and both are caused by viruses. However, they are different conditions, and the flu is more severe. Unlike the flu, colds generally don't cause serious complications, such as pneumonia, or lead to hospitalization.

No vaccine can protect you against the common cold, but vaccines can protect you against the flu. Everyone over the age of 6 months should be vaccinated against the flu each year. Vaccination is the best protection against getting the flu.

Prescription antiviral drugs may be used to treat the flu in people who are very ill or who are at high risk of flu complications. They're not a substitute for getting vaccinated. Vaccination is the first line of defense against the flu; antivirals are the second. If you think you've caught the flu, you may want to check with your healthcare provider to see whether antiviral medicine is appropriate for you. Call promptly. The drugs work best if they're used early in the illness.

---

This chapter includes text excerpted from "Flu and Colds: In Depth," National Center for Complementary and Integrative Health (NCCIH), November 2016.

# What the Science Says about Complementary Health Approaches for the Flu

Complementary approaches that have been studied for the flu include the following. In all instances, there's not enough evidence to show whether the approach is helpful.

- American ginseng
- Chinese herbal medicines
- Echinacea
- Elderberry
- Green tea
- Oscillococcinum
- Vitamin C
- Vitamin D

No complementary approach has been shown to prevent the flu or relieve flu symptoms.

# What the Science Says about Complementary Health Approaches for Colds

## American Ginseng

Several studies have evaluated the use of American ginseng (*Panax quinquefolius*) to prevent colds. A 2011 evaluation of these studies concluded that the herb has not been shown to reduce the number of colds that people catch, although it may shorten the length of colds. The researchers who conducted the evaluation concluded that there was insufficient evidence to support the use of American ginseng for preventing colds. Taking American ginseng in an effort to prevent colds means taking it for prolonged periods of time. However, little is known about the herb's long-term safety. American ginseng may interact with the anticoagulant (blood thinning) drug warfarin.

## Echinacea

At least 24 studies have tested echinacea to see whether it can prevent colds or relieve cold symptoms. A comprehensive 2014 assessment of this research concluded that echinacea hasn't been convincingly shown to be beneficial. However, at least some echinacea products might have a weak effect. One reason why it's hard to reach definite conclusions about this herb is that echinacea products vary greatly. They may contain different species (types) of the plant and be made from different plant parts (the above-ground parts, the root, or both). They also may be manufactured in different ways, and some products contain other ingredients in addition to echinacea. Research findings on one echinacea product may not apply to other products. Few side effects have been reported in studies of echinacea. However, some people are allergic to this herb, and in one study in children, taking echinacea was linked to an increase in rashes.

### Garlic

A 2014 evaluation of the research on garlic concluded that there isn't enough evidence to show whether this herb can help prevent colds or relieve their symptoms. Garlic can cause bad breath, body odor, and other side effects. Because garlic may interact with anticoagulant drugs (blood thinners), people who take these drugs should consult their healthcare providers before taking garlic.

### Honey

Honey's traditional reputation as a cough remedy has some science to back it up. A small amount of research suggests that honey may help to decrease nighttime coughing in children. Honey should never be given to infants under the age of 1 year because it may contain spores of the bacterium that causes infant botulism. Honey is considered safe for older children.

### Meditation

Reducing stress and improving general health may protect against colds and other respiratory infections. In a 2012 study funded by the National Center for Complementary and Integrative Health (NCCIH), adults aged 50 and older were randomly assigned to training in mindfulness meditation, which can reduce stress; an exercise training program, which may improve physical health; or a control group that didn't receive any intervention. The study participants kept track of their illnesses during the cold and flu season. People in the meditation group had shorter and less severe acute respiratory infections (most of which were colds) and lost fewer days of work because of these illnesses than those in the control group. Exercise also had some benefit, but not as much as meditation. This study is the first to suggest that meditation may reduce the impact of colds. Because it's the only study of its kind, its results shouldn't be regarded as conclusive.

Meditation is generally considered to be safe for healthy people. However, there have been reports that it might worsen symptoms in people with certain chronic physical or mental health problems. If you have an ongoing health issue, talk with your healthcare provider before starting meditation.

## Probiotics

A 2015 evaluation of 13 studies found some evidence suggesting that probiotics might reduce the number of colds or other upper respiratory tract infections that people catch and the length of the illnesses, but the quality of the evidence was low or very low. In people who are generally healthy, probiotics have a good safety record. Side effects, if they occur at all, usually consist only of mild digestive symptoms such as gas. However, information on the long-term safety of probiotics is limited, and safety may differ from one type of probiotic to another. Probiotics have been linked to severe side effects, such as dangerous infections, in people with serious underlying medical problems.

## Saline Nasal Irrigation

Saline nasal irrigation means rinsing your nose and sinuses with salt water. People may do this with a neti pot (a device that comes from the Ayurvedic tradition) or with other devices, such as bottles, sprays, pumps, or nebulizers. Saline nasal irrigation may be used for sinus congestion, allergies, or colds. There's limited evidence that saline nasal irrigation can help relieve cold symptoms. Studies of this technique have been too small to allow researchers to reach definite conclusions.

Saline nasal irrigation used to be considered safe, with only minor side effects such as nasal discomfort or irritation. However, in 2011, a severe disease caused by an amoeba (a type of microorganism) was linked to nasal irrigation with tap water. The U.S. Food and Drug Administration (FDA) has warned that tap water that is not filtered, treated, or processed in specific ways is not safe for use in nasal rinsing devices and has explained how to use and clean these devices safely.

## Vitamin C

An evaluation of researches done on vitamin C and colds (29 studies involving more than 11,000 people) concluded that taking vitamin C doesn't prevent colds in the general population and shortens colds only slightly. Taking vitamin C only after you start to feel cold symptoms doesn't affect the length or severity of the cold. Unlike the situation in the general population, vitamin C does seem to reduce the number of colds in people exposed to short periods of extreme physical stress (such as marathon runners, and skiers). In studies of these groups, taking vitamin C cut the number of colds in half.

Taking too much vitamin C can cause diarrhea, nausea, and stomach cramps. People with the iron storage disease hemochromatosis should avoid high doses of vitamin C. People who are being treated for cancer or taking cholesterol-lowering medications should talk with their healthcare providers before taking vitamin C supplements.

## Zinc

Zinc has been used for colds in forms that are taken orally (by mouth), such as lozenges, tablets, or syrup, or used intranasally (in the nose), such as swabs, or gels.

### Oral Zinc

A 2012 evaluation of 17 studies of various types of zinc lozenges, tablets, or syrup found that zinc can reduce the duration of colds in adults. Two evaluations of three studies of high-dose zinc acetate lozenges in adults, conducted in 2015 and 2016, found that they shortened colds. Some participants in studies that tested zinc for colds reported that the zinc caused a bad taste or nausea. Long-term use of high doses of zinc can cause low copper levels, reduced immunity, and low levels of high-density lipoproteins (HDL) cholesterol (the "good" cholesterol). Zinc may interact with drugs, including antibiotics and penicillamine (a drug used to treat rheumatoid arthritis (RA)).

### Intranasal Zinc

The use of zinc products inside the nose, such as gels or swabs, may cause loss of the sense of smell, which may be long-lasting or permanent. The FDA warned consumers to stop using several intranasal zinc products marketed as cold remedies because of this risk. Prior to the warnings about effects on the sense of smell, a few studies of intranasal zinc had suggested a possible benefit against cold symptoms. However, the risk of a serious and lasting side effect outweighs any possible benefit in the treatment of a minor illness.

## Other Complementary Approaches

In addition to the complementary approaches described above, several other approaches have been studied for colds. In all instances, there is insufficient evidence to show whether these approaches help to prevent colds or relieve cold symptoms.

- Andrographis (Andrographis paniculata)
- Chinese herbal medicines
- Green tea
- Guided imagery
- Hydrotherapy
- Vitamin D
- Vitamin E

## *More to Consider*

If you are thinking of considering complementary approaches for treating flu or cold, then:

- Complementary health approaches should never be used as a substitute for flu vaccination.
- Tell all your healthcare providers about any complementary health approaches you use. Give them a full picture of what you do to manage your health. This will help ensure coordinated and safe care.

# Chapter 81

# *Headache and CAM*

Headaches are the most common form of pain. They're a major reason why people miss work or school or visit a healthcare provider. This chapter focuses on two types of headache: tension headaches and migraines.

- **Tension headaches**—the most common type of headache—are caused by tight muscles in the shoulders, neck, scalp, and jaw. They may be related to stress, depression, or anxiety and may occur more often in people who work too much, sleep too little, miss meals, or drink alcoholic beverages.

- **Migraine headaches**—which affect about 12 percent of Americans—involve moderate to severe throbbing pain, often on one side of the head. During a migraine, people are sensitive to light and sound and may feel nauseated. Some people have visual disturbances before a migraine—like seeing zigzag lines or flashing lights, or temporarily losing their vision. Anxiety, stress, lack of food or sleep, exposure to light, or hormonal changes (in women) can trigger migraines. Genes that control the activity of some brain cells may play a role in causing migraines.

Researchers have studied complementary health approaches for both.

This chapter includes text excerpted from "Headaches: In Depth," National Center for Complementary and Integrative Health (NCCIH), September 2016.

## What the Science Says about Complementary Health Approaches for Headache

Research has produced promising results for some complementary health approaches for tension headache or migraine. For other approaches, evidence of effectiveness is limited or conflicting.

### *Mind and Body Approaches*

Mind and body approaches that have been studied for headache include acupuncture, biofeedback, massage, relaxation techniques, spinal manipulation, and tai chi.

#### *Acupuncture*

Acupuncture is a technique in which practitioners stimulate specific points on the body, most often by inserting thin needles through the skin.

There have been many studies of acupuncture for headache. The combined results from these studies indicate that acupuncture may help relieve headache pain, but that much of its benefit may be due to nonspecific effects including expectation, beliefs, and placebo responses rather than specific effects of needling.

Acupuncture is generally considered safe when performed by an experienced practitioner using sterile needles. Improperly performed acupuncture can cause potentially serious side effects.

#### *Biofeedback*

Biofeedback measures body functions and gives you information about them so that you can become more aware of those functions and learn to control them. For example, a biofeedback device may show you measurements of muscle tension. By watching how these measurements change, you can become more aware of when your muscles are tense and learn to relax them.

Several types of biofeedback have been studied for headaches, including techniques that help people learn to relax and more specific techniques that focus on changes that occur during headaches.

- **Tension headaches.** Many studies have tested biofeedback for tension headaches, and several evaluations of this research have concluded that biofeedback may be helpful. However, an evaluation that included only the highest quality studies concluded that there is conflicting evidence about whether biofeedback is helpful for tension headaches.

- **Migraines.** Studies have shown decreases in the frequency of migraines in people who were using biofeedback. However, it's unclear whether biofeedback is better than a placebo for migraines.

Biofeedback generally does not have harmful side effects.

## Massage

Massage therapy includes a variety of techniques in which practitioners manipulate the soft tissues of the body. Limited evidence from two small studies suggests massage therapy is possibly helpful for migraines, but clear conclusions cannot be drawn.

Massage therapy appears to have few risks when performed by a trained practitioner. However, people with health conditions and pregnant women may need to avoid some types of massage and should consult their healthcare providers before having massage therapy.

## Relaxation Techniques

Relaxation techniques—such as progressive muscle relaxation, guided imagery, and breathing exercises—are practices that can produce the body's natural relaxation response. Although some experts consider relaxation techniques to be promising for tension headaches, there isn't much evidence to support their effectiveness. An evaluation of high-quality studies on relaxation techniques found conflicting evidence on whether they're better than no treatment or a placebo. Some studies suggest that relaxation techniques are less helpful than biofeedback.

Relaxation techniques generally don't have side effects. However, rare harmful effects have been reported in people with serious physical or mental health conditions.

## Spinal Manipulation

Spinal manipulation is a technique in which practitioners use their hands or a device to apply a controlled force to a joint of the spine. Chiropractors or other health professionals may use this technique.

Spinal manipulation is frequently used for headaches. However, it's uncertain whether manipulation is helpful because studies have had contradictory results.

561

Side effects from spinal manipulation can include temporary headaches, tiredness, or discomfort in the area that was manipulated. There have been rare reports of strokes occurring after manipulation of the upper (cervical) spine, but whether manipulation actually caused the strokes is unclear.

### Tai Chi

Tai chi, which originated in China, combines meditation with slow, graceful movements, deep breathing, and relaxation. One small randomized study has evaluated tai chi for tension headaches. Some evidence of improvements in headache status and health-related quality of life was found among patients on the tai chi program compared to others on a waitlist. These data are too limited to draw meaningful conclusions about whether this practice is helpful for tension headaches.

Tai chi is generally considered to be a safe practice.

## Dietary Supplements

Several dietary supplements have been studied for headaches, particularly for migraine prevention. In 2012, the American Academy of Neurology (AAN) and the American Headache Society (AHS) issued evidence-based guidelines that classified certain dietary supplements as "effective," "probably effective," or "possibly effective" in preventing migraines.

### Butterbur

In their guidelines for migraine prevention, the AAN and the AHS concluded that butterbur is effective and should be offered to patients with migraine to reduce the frequency and severity of migraine attacks.

The most common side effects of butterbur are belching and other mild digestive tract symptoms. Raw butterbur extracts contain pyrrolizidine alkaloids, which can cause liver damage and cancer. Extracts of butterbur that are almost completely free from these alkaloids are available. It is uncertain whether butterbur products, including reduced-alkaloid products, are safe for prolonged use.

### Coenzyme $Q_{10}$

Coenzyme $Q_{10}$ is an antioxidant that cells need to function properly. It's available as a dietary supplement and has been studied for a variety of purposes. The guidelines from the AAN and the AHS say that coenzyme $Q_{10}$ is possibly effective and may be considered for migraine prevention.

No serious side effects of coenzyme $Q_{10}$ have been reported. It may interact with some medications, including the anticoagulant (blood-thinning) medication warfarin (Coumadin).

### *Feverfew*

The guidelines from the AAN and the AHS say that a specific feverfew extract called MIG-99 is probably effective and should be considered for migraine prevention.

Side effects of feverfew may include joint aches, digestive disturbances, and mouth ulcers. It may interact with anticoagulants (blood thinners) and some other medications. Feverfew is not safe for use during pregnancy. Its long-term safety has not been established.

### *Magnesium*

Magnesium deficiency is related to factors that promote headaches, and people who get migraines may have lower levels of magnesium in their bodies than those who do not. The guidelines from the AAN and the AHS say that magnesium is probably effective and should be considered for migraine prevention.

Magnesium supplements can cause diarrhea and may interact with some medications. Because the amounts of magnesium people take for migraines are greater than the Tolerable Upper Intake Level (TUL) for this mineral (the largest amount that's likely to be safe for almost everyone), magnesium supplements for migraine should be used only under the supervision of a healthcare provider.

### *Riboflavin*

The AAN and AHS's guidelines say that riboflavin is probably effective and should be considered for migraine prevention. Riboflavin has minimal side effects, but it can cause an intense yellow discoloration of the urine.

## More to Consider

If you are considering complementary health approaches for treating headache then you should consider the following:

- Most dietary supplements have not been tested in pregnant women, nursing mothers, or children. If you're pregnant or nursing a child, or if you're considering giving a child a dietary supplement, consult your (or your child's) healthcare provider.

- Be aware that some dietary supplements may interact with conventional medical treatments.

- If you're considering a practitioner-provided complementary health practice such as biofeedback or acupuncture, ask a trusted source (such as your healthcare provider or nearby hospital) to recommend a practitioner. Find out about the training and experience of any complementary health practitioner you're considering.

- Tell all your healthcare providers about any complementary or integrative health approaches you use. Give them a full picture of what you do to manage your health. This will help ensure coordinated and safe care.

# Chapter 82

# *Hepatitis C and CAM*

## *About Hepatitis C*

Hepatitis C is a liver disease caused by a virus. It's usually chronic (long-lasting), but most people don't have any symptoms until the virus causes liver damage, which can take 10 or more years to happen. Without medical treatment, chronic hepatitis C can eventually cause liver cancer or liver failure. Hepatitis C is usually treated with a combination of medicines.

Hepatitis C virus is contagious. People usually get the virus through contact with blood from a person who's already infected or, less commonly, through having sex with an infected person. The infection usually becomes chronic. An estimated 2.7–3.9 million people in the United States have chronic hepatitis C.

## *What the Science Says about Dietary Supplements for Hepatitis C*

Several dietary supplements have been studied for hepatitis C, and many people with hepatitis C have tried dietary supplements. The most commonly used supplement for hepatitis C is silymarin (an extract from milk thistle).

This chapter includes text excerpted from "Hepatitis C and Dietary Supplements," National Center for Complementary and Integrative Health (NCCIH), May 2018.

### Silymarin (Milk Thistle)

Milk thistle (scientific name *Silybum marianum*) is a plant from the aster family. Silymarin is an extract from milk thistle. A 2014 evaluation of five studies of silymarin in people with hepatitis C, involving a total of 389 participants, did not show silymarin to be beneficial. The supplement did not improve liver function or decrease levels of the hepatitis C virus. One of these studies, cofunded by the National Center for Complementary and Integrative Health (NCCIH) and the National Institute of Diabetes and Digestive and Kidney Diseases (NIDDK), showed that higher-than-usual doses of silymarin, given for 24 weeks, were no better than a placebo (an inactive substance) in improving a measure of liver function in people who had not responded to drug treatment for chronic hepatitis C. The study, completed in 2012, had 154 participants. Those receiving silymarin also showed no significant differences from participants receiving the placebo in hepatitis C virus levels or quality of life.

Side effects have been uncommon in studies of silymarin in people with hepatitis C. When side effects occurred, they were usually mild digestive problems, like bloating, indigestion, nausea, or diarrhea.

### Probiotics

Probiotics are live microorganisms that are intended to have a health benefit. Research hasn't produced any clear evidence that probiotics are helpful in people with hepatitis C. In healthy people, probiotics usually have only minor side effects if any. However, in people with underlying health problems (for example, weakened immune systems), serious side effects such as infections have occasionally been reported.

### Zinc

Preliminary studies, most of which were conducted outside the United States, have examined the use of zinc for hepatitis C. Zinc supplements might help to correct zinc deficiencies associated with hepatitis C, reduce some symptoms, or improve patients' response to treatment, but the evidence for these possible benefits is limited. Zinc is generally considered to be safe when used appropriately, but it can be toxic if taken in excessive amounts.

### Licorice Root and Glycyrrhizin

Dietary supplements containing glycyrrhizin—a compound found in licorice root—have been tested in a few studies in people with hepatitis

C, but there's currently not enough evidence to determine if they're helpful. Glycyrrhizin or licorice can be dangerous in people with a history of hypertension (high blood pressure), kidney failure, diabetes, or cardiovascular diseases.

### Colloidal Silver

Colloidal silver has been suggested as a treatment for hepatitis C, but there's currently no research to support its use for this or any other purpose. Colloidal silver is known to cause serious side effects, including a permanent bluish discoloration of the skin, called argyria.

### Other Dietary Supplements

Preliminary studies have examined the potential of the following products for treating chronic hepatitis C: TJ-108 (a mixture of herbs used in Japanese Kampo medicine), oxymatrine (an extract from the sophora root), chlorella (a type of algae), black cumin (Nigella sativa), S-adenosyl-L-methionine (SAMe), and thymus extract (from cattle). The limited research on these products hasn't produced convincing evidence that they're helpful for hepatitis C.

A few preliminary studies have looked at the effects of combining supplements such as lactoferrin, SAMe, or zinc with conventional drug therapy for hepatitis C. The evidence isn't sufficient to draw clear conclusions about benefit or safety. Preliminary research has looked at substances that might reduce the risk of liver cancer in people with hepatitis C, including dietary supplements such as carotenoids and vitamin K, but the evidence is too limited for conclusions to be reached.

## More to Consider

If you are considering complementary health approach for treating hepatitis C then consider the following:

- Don't use any complementary health approach to replace conventional treatment for hepatitis C or as a reason to postpone seeing your healthcare provider about any medical problem.

- Be aware that dietary supplements may have side effects or interact with conventional medical treatments.

- If you're pregnant or nursing a child, or if you're considering giving a child a dietary supplement, it's especially important to consult your (or the child's) healthcare provider. Many supplements have not been tested in pregnant women, nursing mothers, or children.

- Tell all your healthcare providers about any complementary or integrative health approaches you use. Give them a full picture of what you do to manage your health. This will help ensure coordinated and safe care.

# Chapter 83

# *HIV and CAM*

## Basics of HIV / AIDS

### *Human Immunodeficiency Virus (HIV)*

HIV is a virus spread through certain body fluids that attacks the body's immune system, specifically the CD4 cells, often called T cells. Over time, HIV can destroy so many of these cells that the body can't fight off infections and disease. These special cells help the immune system fight off infections. Untreated, HIV reduces the number of CD4 cells (T cells) in the body. This damage to the immune system makes it harder and harder for the body to fight off infections and some other diseases. Opportunistic infections or cancers take advantage of a very weak immune system and signal that the person has AIDS. Learn more about the stages of HIV and how to know whether you're infected.

HIV stands for human immunodeficiency virus. It is the virus that can lead to acquired immunodeficiency syndrome, or AIDS, if not treated. Unlike some other viruses, the human body can't get rid of HIV completely, even with treatment. So once you get HIV, you have it for life.

---

This chapter contains text excerpted from the following sources: Text under the heading "Basics of HIV/AIDS" is excerpted from "About HIV & AIDS: What Are HIV and AIDS?" U.S. Department of Health and Human Services (HHS), May 15, 2017; Text beginning with the heading "Alternative Therapy" is excerpted from "HIV/AIDS—Alternative (Complementary) Therapies for HIV/AIDS: Entire Lesson," U.S. Department of Veterans Affairs (VA), February 8, 2018.

HIV attacks the body's immune system, specifically the CD4 cells (T cells), which help the immune system fight off infections. Untreated, HIV reduces the number of CD4 cells (T cells) in the body, making the person more likely to get other infections or infection-related cancers. Over time, HIV can destroy so many of these cells that the body can't fight off infections and disease. These opportunistic infections or cancers take advantage of a very weak immune system and signal that the person has AIDS, the last stage of HIV infection.

No effective cure currently exists, but with proper medical care, HIV can be controlled. The medicine used to treat HIV is called antiretroviral therapy or ART. If taken the right way, every day, this medicine can dramatically prolong the lives of many people infected with HIV, keep them healthy, and greatly lower their chance of infecting others. Before the introduction of ART in the mid-1990s, people with HIV could progress to AIDS in just a few years. Today, someone diagnosed with HIV and treated before the disease is far advanced can live nearly as long as someone who does not have HIV.

### Acquired Immuno Deficiency Syndrome (AIDS)

AIDS is the most severe phase of HIV infection. People with AIDS have such badly damaged immune systems that they get an increasing number of severe illnesses, called opportunistic infections.

This is the stage of HIV infection that occurs when your immune system is badly damaged and you become vulnerable to opportunistic infections. When the number of your CD4 cells falls below 200 cells per cubic millimeter of blood (200 cells/mm3), you are considered to have progressed to AIDS. (In someone with a healthy immune system, CD4 counts are between 500 and 1,600 cells/mm3.) You are also considered to have progressed to AIDS if you develop one or more opportunistic illnesses, regardless of your CD4 count.

Without treatment, people who progress to AIDS typically survive about 3 years. Once you have a dangerous opportunistic illness, life-expectancy without treatment falls to about 1 year. ART can be helpful for people who have AIDS when diagnosed and can be lifesaving. Treatment is likely to benefit people with HIV no matter when it is started, but people who start ART soon after they get HIV experience more benefits from treatment than do people who start treatment after they have developed AIDS.

In the United States, most people with HIV do not develop AIDS because effective ART stops disease progression. People with HIV who are diagnosed early can have a life span that is about the same as someone like them who does not have HIV.

People living with HIV may progress through these stages at different rates, depending on a variety of factors, including their genetic makeup, how healthy they were before they were infected, how much virus they were exposed to and its genetic characteristics, how soon after infection they are diagnosed and linked to care and treatment, whether they see their healthcare provider regularly and take their HIV medications as directed, and different health-related choices they make, such as decisions to eat a healthful diet, exercise, and not smoke.

## Alternative Therapy

Many people use complementary (sometimes known as alternative) health treatments to go along with the medical care they get from their doctor. These therapies are called "complementary" therapies because usually they are used alongside the more standard medical care you receive (such as your doctor visits and the anti-human immunodeficiency virus (HIV) drugs you might be taking).

They are sometimes called "alternative" because they don't fit into the more mainstream, Western ways of looking at medicine and healthcare. These therapies may not fit in with what you usually think of as "healthcare."

Some common complementary therapies include:

- **Physical (body) therapies**, such as yoga, massage, and acupuncture

- **Relaxation techniques**, such as meditation and visualization

- **Herbal medicine** (from plants)

With most complementary therapies, your health is looked at from a holistic (or "whole picture") point of view. Think of your body as working as one big system. From a holistic viewpoint, everything you do—from what you eat to what you drink to how stressed you are—affects your health and well-being.

## Do Alternative Therapies Work?

Healthy people use these kinds of therapies to try to make their immune systems stronger and to make themselves feel better in general. People who have diseases or illnesses, such as HIV, use these therapies for the same reasons. They also can use these therapies to help deal with symptoms of the disease or side effects from the medicines that treat the disease. Many people report positive results from using complementary therapies. In most cases, however, there is not enough research to tell if these treatments really help people with HIV. In this chapter, you can read about some of the more common complementary therapies that people with HIV use. Sometimes these are used alone, but often they are used in combination with one another. For example, some people combine yoga with meditation.

## Physical (Body) Therapies

Physical, or body, therapies include such activities as yoga, massage, and aromatherapy. These types of therapies focus on using a person's body and senses to promote healing and well-being. Here you can learn about examples of these types of therapies.

### Yoga

Yoga is a set of exercises that people use to improve their fitness, reduce stress, and increase flexibility. Yoga can involve breathing exercises, stretching and strengthening poses, and meditation. Many people, including people with HIV, use yoga to reduce stress and to become more relaxed and calm. Some people think that yoga helps make them healthier in general, because it can make a person's body stronger.

If you would like to try yoga, talk to your healthcare provider. There are many different types of yoga and various classes you can take. You can also try out yoga by following a video program. Before you begin any kind of exercise program, always talk with your doctor.

### Massage

Many people believe that massage therapy is an excellent way to deal with the stress and side effects that go along with having an illness, including HIV. During massage therapy, a trained therapist moves and rubs your body tissues (such as your muscles). There are many kinds of massage therapy.

You can try massage therapy for reducing muscle and back pain, headaches, and soreness. Massages also can improve your blood flow (your circulation) and reduce tension. Some people think that massages might even make your immune system stronger.

### Acupuncture

Acupuncture is part of a whole healing system known as traditional Chinese medicine (TCM). During acupuncture treatment, tiny needles (about as wide as a hair) are inserted into certain areas of a person's body. Most people say that they don't feel any pain at all from the needles.

Many people with HIV use acupuncture. Some people think that acupuncture can help treat symptoms of HIV and side effects from the medicine, like fatigue and nausea. Some people say that acupuncture can be used to help with neuropathy (body pain caused by nerve damage from HIV or the medicines used to treat HIV). Others report that acupuncture gives them more energy.

### Aromatherapy

Aromatherapy is based on the idea that certain smells can change the way you feel. The smells used in aromatherapy come from plant oils, and they can be inhaled (breathed in) or used in baths or massages.

People use aromatherapy to help them deal with stress or to help with fatigue. For example, some people report that lavender oil calms them down and helps them sleep better. You can also ask friends or family if they've tried aromatherapy or know someone who has. Please remember! The oils used in aromatherapy can be very strong and even harmful. Always talk with an expert before using these oils yourself.

## Relaxation Techniques

Relaxation therapies, such as meditation and visualization, focus on how a person's mind and imagination can promote overall health and well-being. In this chapter, you can read about some examples of how you can use relaxation therapies to reduce stress and relax.

### Meditation

Meditation is a certain way of concentrating that may allow your mind and body to become very relaxed. Meditation helps people to focus and be quiet. There are many different forms of meditation. Most involve deep breathing and paying attention to your body and mind.

Sometimes people sit still and close their eyes to meditate. Meditation also can be casual. For instance, you can meditate when you are taking a walk or watching a sunrise.

People with HIV can use meditation to relax. It can help them deal with the stress that comes with any illness. Meditation can help you to calm down and focus if you are feeling overwhelmed.

### *Visualization*

Visualization is another method people use to feel more relaxed and less anxious. People who use visualization imagine that they are in a safe, relaxing place (such as the beach). Most of us use visualization without realizing it—for example, when we daydream or remember a fun, happy time in our lives.

Focusing on a safe, comfortable place can help you to feel less stress, and sometimes it can lessen the pain or side effects from HIV or the medicines you are taking. You can ask your doctor where you can learn more about visualization. There are classes you can take, and there are self-help tapes that you can listen to that lead you through the process.

### *Herbal Medicine*

Herbal medicines are substances that come from plants, and they work like standard medicine. They can be taken from all parts of a plant, including the roots, leaves, berries, and flowers.

People with HIV sometimes take these medicines to help deal with side effects from anti-HIV medicines or with symptoms of the illness.

**An important note about St. John's wort.** St. John's wort is an herbal medicine that is used by some people to treat depression. It interacts with the liver and can change how some drugs work in your body, including some anti-HIV drugs (for example, protease inhibitors and non-nucleoside reverse-transcriptase inhibitors (NNRTIs)). If you are taking antiviral drugs for your HIV, you should NOT take St. John's wort. Be sure you tell your provider if you are using St. John's wort. You should also not take St. John's wort if you are taking other antidepressants.

## *Before Giving Complementary Treatments a Try*

If you want to try complementary treatments to help you cope with HIV/AIDS, please remember these things:

- Always talk to your healthcare provider before you start any kind of treatment, even if you think it is safe.

- Just because something is "natural" (an herb, for example) doesn't mean that it is safe to take. Sometimes these products can interact with your HIV medicines or cause side effects on their own. St. John's wort, for example, decreases levels of some HIV medications in your blood.

574

- The federal government does not require that herbal remedies and dietary supplements be tested in the same way that standard medicines are tested before they are sold. Many of the treatments out there have not been studied as much as the HIV drugs you are taking. It is always a risk to take something or try something that hasn't been fully studied or researched.

- Be careful of treatments that claim to be "miracle cures"—ones that claim to cure HIV/ acquired immunodeficiency syndrome (AIDS). There are people out there who may try to trick you into buying an expensive product that doesn't work. Always do your research and ask your doctor for help.

- Complementary therapies are not substitutes for the treatment and drugs you receive from your doctor. Never stop taking your anti-HIV drugs just because you've started an alternative therapy.

- The federal government is funding studies of how well some alternative therapies work to treat disease, so keep your eyes open for news about these studies.

# Chapter 84

# *Irritable Bowel Syndrome and CAM*

Irritable bowel syndrome (IBS) is a chronic disorder that affects the large intestine and causes symptoms such as abdominal pain, cramping, constipation, and diarrhea. As many as one in five Americans have symptoms of IBS. The cause of IBS isn't well understood but stress, large meals, certain foods, and alcohol may trigger symptoms in people with this disorder.

## *What the Science Says about the Effectiveness of Complementary Health Approaches for Irritable Bowel Syndrome (IBS)*

Some evidence is emerging that a few complementary health approaches may be helpful for IBS. However, the research is limited so we don't know for sure.

### *Acupuncture*

For easing the severity of IBS, actual acupuncture wasn't better than simulated acupuncture, a 2012 systematic review reported. A clinical trial included in the review found that of the 230 participants

---

This chapter includes text excerpted from "Irritable Bowel Syndrome: In Depth," National Center for Complementary and Integrative Health (NCCIH), March 2015.

with IBS, those who received either actual or simulated acupuncture did better than those who received no acupuncture.

### Hypnotherapy (Hypnosis)

Researchers are studying gut-directed hypnotherapy (GDH), which focuses on improving bowel symptoms. Several IBS studies have found an association between hypnotherapy and long-term improvement in gastrointestinal symptoms, anxiety, depression, disability, and quality of life. The American College of Gastroenterology (ACG) stated in a 2014 paper that there is some evidence that hypnosis helps with IBS symptoms, but the research is very uncertain. Just more than half of the study participants who had 10 GDH sessions over 12 weeks felt better, compared with 25 percent of participants not assigned to undergo GDH, a 2013 study of 90 adults with IBS showed. The benefits lasted for at least 15 months. The non-GDH group had the same number of sessions of supportive talks with a physician who was trained in diseases related to stress and other factors. A research review suggested that children with IBS who underwent GDH had greater reductions in abdominal pain than children who received standard treatment. This was true whether the children underwent GDH with a therapist or listened to an audio recording. However, the result may not be reliable, as the researchers found only three small studies that met their standards. Many children and adolescents with mild IBS symptoms who get only reassurance from their healthcare provider improve over time.

### Mindfulness Meditation Training

Some studies suggest that mindfulness training helps people with IBS, but there's not enough evidence to draw firm conclusions. The ACG stated in a 2014 paper that the few studies that have looked at mindfulness meditation training for IBS found no significant effects. But the authors noted that given the limited number of studies, they can't be sure it doesn't help. A 2013 review that included these and other studies concluded that mindfulness training improved IBS-associated pain and quality of life but not depression or anxiety. The amount of improvement was small. A 2011 National Center for Complementary and Integrative Health (NCCIH) supported clinical trial (which was in the 2013 review) of 75 women with IBS showed that mindfulness training may decrease the severity of IBS symptoms, including psychological distress, compared to attending a support group. The benefits lasted for at least 3 months after the training ended.

## *Yoga*

In a small 2014 NCCIH-supported study, young adults (18–26 years old) reported generally feeling better and having less pain, constipation, and nausea after completing a series of yoga classes, compared with a waitlist control group. They were still feeling better at the study's 2-month follow-up. There's too little evidence to draw conclusions about the effectiveness of meditation, relaxation training, and reflexology for IBS.

## *About Dietary Supplements for IBS*

A variety of dietary supplements, many of which are Chinese herbs and herb combinations, have been investigated for IBS, but we can't draw any conclusions about them because of the poor quality of many of the studies.

- **Chinese herbs.** In a systematic review, a combination of Chinese herbs was associated with improved IBS symptoms, but extracts of three single herbs had no beneficial effects.

- **Peppermint oil.** Peppermint oil capsules may be modestly helpful in reducing several common symptoms of IBS, including abdominal pain and bloating. It's superior to placebo in improving IBS symptoms, the ACG stated in a 2014 paper.

- **Probiotics.** Generally, probiotics improve IBS symptoms, bloating, and flatulence, the ACG stated in a 2014 paper. However, it noted that the quality of existing studies is limited. It's not possible to draw firm conclusions about specific probiotics for IBS in part because studies have used different species, strains, preparations, and doses.

- IBS patients given probiotics did no better than those who got a placebo, a 2013 clinical trial of 131 patients found. The group received either the placebo or probiotics for 6 months.

- In a 2012 review, 34 of 42 studies of probiotics for IBS symptoms found greater improvement in people taking probiotics than a placebo. However, the difference in improvement between the probiotic and placebo groups varied a lot among the studies.

- A 2011 review of studies on a strain of probiotic bacteria showed associations between taking probiotics and a decrease in symptoms in children with IBS.

## *More to Consider*

If you are considering complementary health approaches for IBS then consider the following:

- Unproven products or practices should not be used to replace conventional treatments for IBS or as a reason to postpone seeing a healthcare provider about IBS symptoms or any other health problem

- If you're considering a practitioner-provided complementary practice such as hypnotherapy, or acupuncture, ask a trusted source (such as the healthcare provider who treats your IBS or a nearby hospital) to recommend a practitioner. Find out about the training and experience of any practitioner you're considering.

- Keep in mind that dietary supplements may interact with medications or other supplements and may contain ingredients not listed on the label. Your healthcare provider can advise you. If you're pregnant or nursing a child, or if you're considering giving a child a dietary supplement, it's especially important to consult your (or your child's) healthcare provider.

- Tell all of your healthcare providers about any complementary health approaches you use. Give them a full picture of what you do to manage your health. This will help ensure coordinated and safe care.

# Chapter 85

# *Low-Back Pain and Complementary Approaches*

Low-back pain is a very common condition, but often the cause is unknown. Most people have significant acute back pain at least once in their lives. Usually, it resolves on its own without specific treatment.

But for some people, the pain can become chronic or even debilitating, and difficult to treat. Spinal manipulation, acupuncture, massage, and yoga are complementary health approaches often used by people with low-back pain. They are all included in a longer list of treatment options recommended by the APS and the ACP for patients whose low-back pain does not improve with more conservative care. Other options include exercise, physical/occupational rehabilitation, cognitive-behavioral therapy (CBT), and progressive relaxation.

Here's what you need to know about what the science says for chronic low-back pain and some of these practices.

1.  Overall, studies have provided good evidence that spinal manipulation is moderately effective for chronic low-back

---

This chapter contains text excerpted from the following sources: Text in this chapter begins with excerpts from "5 Things to Know about Chronic Low-Back Pain and Complementary Health Practices," National Center for Complementary and Integrative Health (NCCIH), September 24, 2015; Text under the heading "Chronic Low-Back Pain and Complementary Health Approaches" is excerpted from "Chronic Low-Back Pain and Complementary Health Approaches," National Center for Complementary and Integrative Health (NCCIH), November 19, 2015.

pain. Spinal manipulation includes various interventions administered by osteopathic physicians, chiropractors, and physical therapists.

2.  There is fair evidence that acupuncture is helpful in relieving chronic back pain. Current evidence suggests that factors such as expectations and beliefs of the patient and the provider, rather than acupuncture-specific effects of needling, are primarily responsible for beneficial effects of acupuncture on pain.

3.  There is also fair evidence that massage is helpful in relieving chronic low-back pain. In general, however, these effects appear to be short term.

4.  Research, while limited in scope, suggests that a carefully adapted set of yoga poses may reduce low-back pain and improve function. The National Center for Complementary and Integrative Health (NCCIH) is also supporting research specifically associated with the safety of this widely-used self-care practice. People with back pain should work with an experienced teacher who can help modify or avoid some yoga poses to prevent adverse effects.

5.  Be sure to tell your healthcare provider about any complementary health practice you are considering. This will help ensure coordinated, safe care.

## *Chronic Low-Back Pain and Complementary Health Approaches*

The scientific evidence about spinal manipulation, acupuncture, massage, and yoga, the complementary approaches most often used by people for chronic low-back pain is discussed below.

*   Evidence-based clinical practice guidelines from the American College of Physicians (ACP) and the American Pain Society (APS) provide a useful algorithm for diagnosis and treatment of patients with chronic low-back pain. In general, the guidelines recommend a conservative approach to diagnosis and treatment, except when patients have progressive neurologic deficits or cauda equina syndrome (CES), or are suspected of having underlying conditions requiring urgent intervention (e.g., vertebral infection, or cancer with impending spinal cord compression).

- The systematic review supporting these recommendations found:

  - Good evidence that cognitive-behavioral therapy (CBT), exercise, spinal manipulation, and interdisciplinary rehabilitation are all moderately effective for chronic or subacute (>4 weeks' duration) low-back pain.

  - Fair evidence that acupuncture, massage, yoga (Viniyoga), and functional restoration are also effective for chronic low-back pain.

  - The guidelines recommend that practitioners consider these nonpharmacological interventions as appropriate options when treating patients whose low-back pain does not improve with more conservative self-care.

  - Interpreting and summarizing current evidence about diagnosis and treatment of chronic low-back pain is particularly challenging because of major differences in patient populations, eligibility criteria, diagnostic studies, treatments, and outcome measures across different studies, and the variety of healthcare professions involved in the care of patients.

# Chapter 86

# *Menopausal Symptoms and CAM*

## *Menopause*

Menopause is the time when a woman's menstrual periods stop permanently. It usually occurs naturally, at an average age of 51, but surgery or the use of certain medications can make it happen earlier. During the years around menopause (a time called perimenopause or menopausal transition), some women have hot flashes, night sweats, difficulty sleeping, or other troublesome symptoms.

## *Conventional Treatment for Menopause Symptoms*

Hormone therapy, using either estrogen alone or estrogen and progestin, is the most effective therapy for menopausal hot flashes. However, hormone therapy may increase the risk of breast cancer, blood clots, and other serious medical problems. Therefore, if it's used at all, it should be used at the lowest dose and for the shortest period that will control symptoms. Women with certain medical conditions (such as breast cancer, liver disease, or a history of blood clots) shouldn't use hormone therapy.

Nonhormonal medicines may also be used to treat menopause symptoms. In 2013, the U.S. Food and Drug Administration (FDA)

This chapter includes text excerpted from "Menopausal Symptoms: In Depth," National Center for Complementary and Integrative Health (NCCIH), May 2017.

approved a nonhormonal treatment for hot flashes and a treatment for vaginal symptoms associated with menopause.

## What the Science Says about Complementary Health Approaches for Menopause Symptoms

### Natural Products

Many natural products have been studied for menopause symptoms. However, none has clearly been shown to be helpful. There's little information on the long-term safety of natural products, and some can have harmful side effects or interact with drugs.

#### Phytoestrogens

Phytoestrogens are substances from plants that have chemical structures similar to those of the female hormone estrogen. The isoflavones found in soy and red clover are examples of phytoestrogens. Flaxseed is another phytoestrogen source. Studies that tested isoflavones from soy or red clover for their ability to relieve menopause symptoms have had inconsistent results. Studies of flaxseed products found them to be no more effective than a placebo (an inactive substance) in reducing hot flashes.

Phytoestrogens appear to be safe for short-term use, but their long-term safety hasn't been established. Because phytoestrogen supplements may have effects like those of the hormone estrogen, they may not be safe for women who shouldn't take estrogen.

#### Black Cohosh

Black cohosh is an herb native to North America. The roots and rhizomes (underground stems) of the plant are used in dietary supplements. Studies that tested black cohosh for menopause symptoms have had inconsistent results. A 2012 research review concluded that there's not enough evidence to support its use for menopause symptoms.

Black cohosh generally has only mild side effects, if any. However, rare cases of liver damage—some of them very serious—have been reported in people taking commercial black cohosh products. It's uncertain whether black cohosh was responsible for the liver damage. Nevertheless, people with liver disorders should consult a healthcare provider before taking black cohosh products. Anyone who develops symptoms of liver trouble, such as abdominal pain, dark urine, or jaundice, while taking black cohosh should stop using it and consult a healthcare provider.

### Dehydroepiandrosterone (DHEA)

Dehydroepiandrosterone (DHEA) is a substance that's naturally made in the body, where it's converted into the hormones testosterone and estrogen. DHEA production decreases as people grow older, but the significance of this change, including whether it affects aging and menopause symptoms, is unclear. It's uncertain whether DHEA is useful in treating menopause symptoms

The long-term safety of taking DHEA supplements is unknown. Some evidence suggests that even short-term use of these supplements may have harmful effects, including liver damage.

### Dong Quai

In traditional Chinese medicine (TCM), the herb dong quai is often used for women's health problems, including menopause. However, very little research has been done on dong quai for menopausal symptoms, so no conclusions can be reached about its effects. Dong quai may interact with the anticoagulant (blood-thinning) drug warfarin (Coumadin).

### Vitamin E

A few studies have suggested that vitamin E supplements might be helpful for menopause symptoms. However, the amount of research is small, and the effect is also small. For example, in one study, women taking vitamin E averaged one fewer hot flash per day.

Vitamin E, in the high doses found in supplements, may increase the risk of bleeding (including strokes due to bleeding in the brain) and interact with anticoagulant (blood-thinning) medications such as warfarin (Coumadin).

### Other Natural Products

Other natural products that have been studied for menopause symptoms include evening primrose oil, ginseng, kava, melatonin, and wild yam. However, very little research has been done on these products for menopausal symptoms, so no conclusions can be reached about their effectiveness. Kava supplements have been linked to a risk of severe liver disease.

## Mind and Body Practices

Only a small amount of research has been done on most mind and body practices for menopause symptoms. However, the limited evidence currently available suggests that some of these practices might help to relieve symptoms or make them less bothersome.

### Acupuncture

Acupuncture is a technique in which practitioners stimulate specific points on the body, most often by inserting thin needles through the skin. In studies that compared acupuncture to no treatment, acupuncture reduced the frequency and severity of hot flashes. However, studies that compared acupuncture with simulated acupuncture, including a 2016 study from Australia, showed no difference between the effects of the two treatments. Acupuncture appears to be less effective than hormone therapy in reducing the frequency of hot flashes.

Acupuncture is generally considered safe when performed by an experienced practitioner using sterile needles. Improperly performed acupuncture can cause potentially serious side effects.

### Hypnotherapy

Hypnotherapy is the use of hypnosis for health-related purposes. Hypnosis is a state in which a person's attention is concentrated and focused. In this hypnotic state, people have a heightened responsiveness to verbal messages (suggestions).

In a study funded by the National Center for Complementary and Integrative Health (NCCIH), hypnotherapy reduced the frequency of hot flashes in menopausal women who had hot flashes often. The women in the study also said that hot flashes didn't interfere with their lives as much and they slept better.

Hypnosis is generally safe when practiced by trained, licensed healthcare providers. Side effects are rare, but hypnosis might worsen some types of psychological problems.

### Mindfulness Meditation

Mindfulness meditation is a type of meditation that involves completely focusing on experiences on a moment-to-moment basis. In an NCCIH-funded study, mindfulness meditation training reduced the bothersomeness of hot flashes in menopausal women and led to improvements in anxiety, perceived stress, self-reported sleep quality, and quality of life. However, the intensity of hot flashes did not change.

Meditation is generally considered to be safe for healthy people. However, there have been reports that it might worsen symptoms in people with certain chronic physical or mental health problems. If you have an ongoing health issue, talk with your healthcare provider before starting meditation.

### Yoga

Yoga is a mind and body practice with historical origins in ancient Indian philosophy. Various styles of yoga typically combine physical postures and movement, breathing techniques, and meditation or relaxation. An evaluation of five studies concluded that yoga can provide short-term relief of some symptoms associated with menopause, but it doesn't decrease hot flashes.

Overall, people who practice yoga have a low rate of side effects. However, injuries—some of them serious—have been reported. People with health conditions may need to modify or avoid some yoga poses.

## Other Complementary Approaches

### Bioidentical Hormones

Bioidentical hormones are hormones from plant sources that are chemically similar or identical to hormones produced in the human body. Two kinds of bioidentical hormone products are used to treat menopause symptoms:

1. Those that have gone through the same FDA approval process as other types of hormone therapy

2. Custom-mixed preparations that compounding pharmacies prepare individually for patients.

This chapter discusses only the custom-mixed products. It's been claimed that custom-mixed bioidentical hormone preparations are more effective and safer than conventional hormone therapy, but scientific evidence to support this idea is lacking. Custom-mixed bioidentical hormones may actually be riskier than conventional treatment because less is known about their safety. Also, no regulatory agency oversees their preparation, and therefore, their content may vary from batch to batch.

## More to Consider

Keep in mind that although many dietary supplements come from natural sources, "natural" does not always mean "safe." Also, a manufacturer's use of the term "standardized" (or "verified" or "certified") does not necessarily guarantee product quality or consistency. Tell all your healthcare providers about any complementary or integrative health approaches you use. Give them a full picture of what you do to manage your health. This will help ensure coordinated and safe care.

# Chapter 87

# *Mental Healthcare and CAM*

## *Chapter Contents*

# Section 87.1

## *CAM Therapies for Behavioral Health*

This section contains text excerpted from the following sources: Text
in this section begins with excerpts from "Behavioral Health Trends
in the United States: Results from the 2014 National Survey on
Drug Use and Health," Substance Abuse and Mental Health Services
Administration (SAMHSA), September 2015; Text beginning with the
heading "What Is the Appeal of Complementary Health Approaches
for Behavioral Health Treatment?" is excerpted from "Advisory,"
Substance Abuse and Mental Health Services Administration
(SAMHSA), 2015; Text under the heading "What Can Complementary
and Alternative Medicine (CAM) Do for Anxiety?" is excerpted from
"Safe Use of Complementary Health Products and Practices for
Anxiety," MedlinePlus, National Institutes of Health (NIH), 2015.

Behavioral health disorders, which include substance use and mental health disorders, affect millions of adolescents and adults in the United States and contribute heavily to the burden of disease. The Substance Abuse and Mental Health Services Administration (SAMHSA) seeks to improve behavioral health in the United States through implementation of evidence-based approaches to prevent behavioral health problems and by promoting recovery support services for those with behavioral health conditions.

## What Is the Appeal of Complementary Health Approaches for Behavioral Health Treatment?

For a variety of reasons, complementary health approaches can be especially appealing to behavioral health clients. Individuals who have not been successful with a particular conventional treatment maybe curious about trying complementary therapies as adjuncts or treatment alternatives. Or, such individuals may hope that augmenting conventional treatment will enhance their recovery. Some clients may have a lifestyle preference for products and healing systems they perceive as natural, want to avoid medication side effects, or appreciate the hands-on care they receive from a complementary health practitioner. From the standpoint of the behavioral health treatment program, offering a complementary therapy that is culturally relevant or popular in the community may attract prospective clients to the program's conventional treatment offerings and support retention. Some practices, such as meditation or movement-based therapies, may help clients gain self-efficacy skills. Complementary practices offered to groups may also enhance clients' socialization skills and support systems.

## How Effective Are Complementary Health Approaches?

Complementary health approaches have been insufficiently studied compared with conventional treatments. Many of the studies that have been conducted lack one or more features of the randomized controlled trial (RCT), which is the gold standard for evaluating biomedical or behavioral interventions. An RCT compares a treatment with a different treatment or with a placebo and randomly assigns subjects to experimental and control (comparison) groups. RCTs are often blinded (that is, the subjects or the scientists administering the experiment, or both, do not know which treatment each subject is receiving) and, ideally, include sample sizes large enough for study results to achieve statistical significance. A well-designed RCT seeks to account for all possible variables that may influence the study results

These features of the RCT can present challenges when assessing complementary practices. For example, some complementary practices involve multiple components (e.g., movement combined with meditation and deep breathing); teasing apart the effects of each component adds to the already considerable amount of time, funds, and labor required to conduct an RCT. Also, when studying interventions such as yoga or acupuncture, it is often not feasible to blind study participants and those administering the intervention. Yet another challenge is that complementary health practitioners typically customize the treatment to the individual. For purposes of an RCT, however, the intervention must be standardized, which can make a study's results less relevant to real-world application. The challenges of evaluating complementary health approaches through well-designed RCTs are prompting health researchers to explore alternative trial designs. Another challenge in evaluating the efficacy of complementary health approaches is the ongoing debate over the value of the placebo effect. Evidence on a variety of complementary practices indicates that positive effects that occur may be attributable not to the treatment itself, but rather to the interaction between the complementary health practitioner and the patient, the patient's beliefs and expectations about the treatment, and the setting and cultural context in which it is provided. Evidence that the placebo effect may play a potentially significant role in some complementary therapies has led some researchers to label complementary health approaches as "placebos." However, some researchers claim that the placebo effect is a powerful force that can be effectively harnessed through complementary health approaches to facilitate the body's ability to heal itself. The task of helping clients make informed, evidence-based decisions about complementary health approaches is complicated by—as just described—the lack of convincing data, questions about the most appropriate means of evaluating these practices, and the unresolved controversy over the role of placebo in treatment.

Presented below are summaries of the existing evidence on selected complementary health approaches for mental or substance use disorders, as provided by systematic reviews and meta-analyses.

## *Acupuncture*

Acupuncture is a low-risk, low-cost therapy that, based on anecdotal evidence, can relieve physical withdrawal symptoms, help with relaxation, and suppress cravings for drugs and alcohol. A small percentage of substance abuse treatment programs—4.4 percent—offer acupuncture as an adjunct therapy. Some systematic reviews have focused specifically on acupuncture for treatment of disorders involving opioids, alcohol, and cocaine. These reviews did not find evidence of efficacy, and the authors have concluded that more research is needed. A 2009 review of clinical trials found some evidence for acupuncture's effectiveness with opioid withdrawal but not for treatment of other conditions such as alcohol withdrawal, nicotine relapse prevention, or cocaine dependence. A 2013 review of 48 RCTs testing acupuncture for use with patients who had alcohol, cocaine, nicotine, or opioid dependence concluded that nearly half of the clinical trials reviewed had at least one positive result (e.g., on craving), indicating that different types of acupuncture may have beneficial effects at different points in the withdrawal and recovery process. A substantial number of studies have been done on acupuncture as a treatment for mental disorders. A review published by the American Psychiatric Association's Task Force on Complementary and Alternative Medicine concluded that the data do not suggest that acupuncture is effective in treating major depressive disorder.

## Mindfulness Meditation

An increasing amount of research has focused on mindfulness meditation, with 477 articles published in academic journals in 2012 alone. In a systematic review of 14 randomized and 10 nonrandomized controlled trials, the authors found evidence that mindfulness-based interventions can reduce consumption of substances of abuse when compared with various controls, and they found preliminary evidence that the interventions can reduce cravings.

## Movement Therapies

For the treatment of mental or substance use disorders, exercise is theorized to provide social and psychological benefits by increasing socialization, improving emotional regulation, decreasing sensitivity to anxiety, and improving stress management. It is also postulated that because exercise triggers neurological effects similar to those produced by opioid drugs, exercise may serve as a substitute for substance use.

Exercise to promote physical, mental, emotional, or spiritual health is called movement therapy. Some studies have investigated movement therapies in relation to specific mental or substance use disorders. A 2013 meta-analysis of 37 RCTs found that exercise is moderately more effective than no therapy or a control intervention for reducing symptoms of depression. A 2011 meta-analysis of 10 RCTs found that yoga-based interventions have a statistically significant effect when used as an adjunct for treating severe mental illness, especially when current treatment modalities are inadequate or have adverse effects (e.g., weight gain, cardiovascular disease). A 2014 review of eight studies on yoga for treatment of addictions reported that seven of those studies showed positive effects; the article authors concluded that the results are "encouraging but inconclusive" because of methodological limitations.

Although evidence of exercise's effect on mental and substance use disorders is inconclusive, the benefits of routine physical exercise for overall health, wellness, and quality of life are well documented. At the least, exercise can be a helpful adjunct therapy to behavioral health treatment, and clients may benefit from participation in a movement-based complementary practice such as yoga, Pilates, or tai chi. A doctor's guidance on appropriate types of exercise or movement therapy is advised for clients who are pregnant, have a specific medical condition (e.g., multiple sclerosis (MS), back injury, osteoporosis), or have not exercised in a long time.

*Natural Products*

Of the many dietary supplements marketed to consumers as having mental health benefits, two of the most popular are omega-3 supplements and SAMe (S-adenosyl-L-methionine). Some omega-3 fatty acids are essential nutrients obtained from food sources such as fatty fish and certain plants such as flax. SAMe is a chemical that is naturally found in almost all tissues in the body. Table 87.1 provides evidence of effectiveness and cautions for both of these products. Many herbal products are also marketed to consumers for treatment of mental disorders. Table 87.1 lists two examples, kava and St. John's wort. Among the many other botanicals marketed as treatments for mental health conditions are brook mint for anxiety or insomnia, chamomile for insomnia, lavender for anxiety or insomnia, linden for insomnia and nervous tension, passionflower for insomnia and anxiety, and valerian for anxiety. RCTs and systematic reviews provide little evidence that homeopathic medicines are effective for any specific condition. The key ingredient can be extremely diluted, so the principle of action does not appear to be science-based. Even when the main ingredient is highly diluted, there may be other active ingredients in the mixture, including alcohol and metals, that can cause side effects and drug interactions.

## What Can Complementary and Alternative Medicine (CAM) Do for Anxiety?

Anxiety has now surpassed depression as the most common mental health diagnosis among college students," even though depression is also increasing among young people. In fact, "more than half of students visiting campus clinics cite anxiety as a health concern," according to a recent study of more than 100,000 students nationwide by the Center for Collegiate Mental Health (CCMH) at Penn State.

A yearly survey conducted by the American College Health Association found that "nearly one in six college students has been diagnosed with or treated for anxiety within the last 12 months." Unlike the relatively mild, brief anxiety caused by a specific event (such as speaking in public or a first date), severe anxiety that lasts at least six months is generally considered to be a problem that might benefit from evaluation and treatment, according to the National Institutes of Health's (NIH) National Institute for Mental Health (NIMH).

Each anxiety disorder has different symptoms, but all the symptoms cluster around excessive, irrational fear and dread. Anxiety disorders commonly occur along with other mental or physical illnesses,

**Table 87.1.** Examples of Natural Products Marketed to Consumers for Treatment of Mental Disorders

| Product | Example of Use | Evidence of Effectiveness | Cautions |
|---|---|---|---|
| Omega-3 fatty acids (found in fatty fish, flax, and other dietary sources) | Depression | May have benefit as an adjunct to standard pharmacologic therapy for depression | May interact with anticoagulants |
| SAMe (chemical found naturally in the body) | Depression | May have benefit as an adjunct to standard pharmacologic therapy for depression | Close medical supervision is advised for patients with bipolar disorder or on tricyclic antidepressants. |
| Kava (*Piper methysticum*, plant) | Anxiety | May have anxiolytic effect | Safety risks outweigh benefits. Adversely interacts with several classes of drugs, including some sedatives, benzodiazepines, and monoamine oxidase inhibitors (MAOIs). Has been linked to severe liver damage. Should not be taken with alcohol because of risk of excessive sedation and harm to the liver. |
| St. John's wort (Hypericum perforatum, herb) | Depression | Some evidence exists to support use for treating mild to moderate depression in adults | Active compounds in St. John's wort interact with other medications to render them less effective and potentially cause serious side effects. Such herb–drug interactions have been documented for MAOIs and selective serotonin reuptake inhibitors, used to treat depression. Interactions have also been documented for medications to treat other conditions, including HIV/AIDS, Parkinson disease (PD), and cancer. St. John's wort can also interfere with the efficacy of oral contraceptives, anticonvulsants, immunosuppressants used with transplantation, anticoagulants, and other types of medications. Products made from St. John's wort vary considerably in the quantity and quality of their active compounds, leading to variability in interactive and other side effects. |

including alcohol or substance abuse, which may mask anxiety symptoms or make them worse.

Research studies funded by the NIH's National Center for Complementary and Integrative Health (NCCIH) have investigated several natural products and mind and body practices for anxiety. As with any treatment, it is important to consider safety before using complementary health products and practices. Safety depends on the specific therapy, and each complementary product or practice should be considered on its own.

Mind and body practices such as meditation and yoga, for example, are generally considered to be safe in healthy people when practiced appropriately. Natural products such as herbal medicines or botanicals are often sold as dietary supplements and are readily available to consumers; however, there is a lot we don't know about the safety of many of these products, in part because a manufacturer does not have to prove the safety and effectiveness of a dietary supplement before it is available to the public.

Two of the main safety concerns for dietary supplements are:

1.  The possibilities of drug interactions—for example, research has shown that St. John's wort interacts with drugs, such as antidepressants, in ways that can interfere with their intended effects.

2.  The possibilities of product contamination—supplements have been found to contain hidden prescription drugs or other compounds, particularly in dietary supplements marketed for weight loss, sexual health, including erectile dysfunction, and athletic performance or body-building.

# Section 87.2

# *Attention Deficit Hyperactivity Disorder (ADHD) and CAM*

This section includes text excerpted from "Attention-Deficit Hyperactivity Disorder at a Glance," National Center for Complementary and Integrative Health (NCCIH), September 24, 2017.

People with attention deficit hyperactivity disorder (ADHD) may have trouble paying attention or controlling impulsive behavior, and they may be overly active. Difficulty paying attention is the main problem for some people, hyperactivity and impulsiveness for others. Surveys estimate that as many as 9 percent of American children and 4 percent of adults have ADHD. Conventional treatment for ADHD includes medication, behavior therapy, or a combination of both. Stimulant medication (the most commonly used type of medication) has been shown to be helpful for at least 70 percent of children with ADHD.

## *What the Science Says*

Although conventional treatment has been proven helpful for ADHD symptoms in children and adults, complementary approaches have not. Complementary health approaches studied for ADHD include the following:

- **Dietary supplements.** The possibility that omega-3 fatty acids could be helpful for ADHD is being investigated, but the evidence is inconclusive.

- Correcting deficiencies in the minerals zinc, iron, or magnesium may improve ADHD symptoms, but this does not mean that supplements of these minerals would be helpful for people with ADHD who are not deficient, and all three minerals can be toxic if taken in excessive amounts.

- Melatonin has not been shown to relieve ADHD symptoms, but it may help children with ADHD who have sleep problems to fall asleep sooner.

- Research on L-carnitine/acetyl-L-carnitine and various herbs, such as St. John's wort, French maritime pine bark extract (also known as Pycnogenol), and Ginkgo biloba, has not demonstrated that these supplements are helpful for ADHD.

- **Special diets.** Despite much research, the role of foods and food ingredients (such as color additives) in ADHD remains controversial. Some evidence suggests that only a small number of people with ADHD are affected by substances in food, and that different individuals may react to different foods or food components.

- **Neurofeedback.** Some research has suggested that neurofeedback, a technique in which people are trained to alter their brain wave patterns, may improve ADHD symptoms, but several small studies that compared neurofeedback with a simulated (sham) version of the procedure did not find differences between the two treatments.

- **Other complementary health approaches.** An assessment of research on homeopathy concluded that there is no evidence that it is helpful for ADHD symptoms. Several mind and body practices, including acupuncture, chiropractic care, massage therapy, meditation, and yoga, have been studied for ADHD. However, the amount of evidence on each of these practices is small, and no conclusions can be reached about whether they are helpful.

## Side Effects and Risks

Dietary supplements may have side effects and may interact with drugs. In particular, St. John's wort can speed up the process by which the body breaks down many drugs, thus making the drugs less effective. Zinc, iron, and magnesium can all be toxic in high doses.

If you're interested in trying a special diet, consult your healthcare provider and consider getting guidance from a registered dietitian. Planning, evaluating, and following special diets can be challenging, and it is important to ensure that the diet meets nutritional needs. If you're considering using any of the approaches discussed here for ADHD, discuss this decision with your (or your child's) healthcare provider.

## Section 87.3

# Posttraumatic Stress Disorder (PTSD) and Acupuncture

This section contains text excerpted from the following sources:
Text in this section begins excerpts from "What Is PTSD?" U.S.
Department of Veterans Affairs (VA), September 15, 2017; Text
beginning with the heading "Complementary and Alternative
Medicine (CAM) Therapies" is excerpted from "Complementary and
Alternative Medicine (CAM) for PTSD," National Center
for Posttraumatic Stress Disorder (NCPTSD), U.S. Department
of Veterans Affairs (VA), March 30, 2017.

Posttraumatic stress disorder (PTSD) is a mental health problem that some people develop after experiencing or witnessing a life-threatening event, like combat, a natural disaster, a car accident, or sexual assault.

It's normal to have upsetting memories, feel on edge, or have trouble sleeping after this type of event. At first, it may be hard to do normal daily activities, like go to work, go to school, or spend time with people you care about. But most people start to feel better after a few weeks or months.

If it's been longer than a few months and you're still having symptoms, one may have PTSD. For some people, PTSD symptoms may start later on, or they may come and go over time.

## Complementary and Alternative Medicine (CAM) Therapies

The use of complementary and alternative medicine (CAM) is widespread for the management of mental health problems, including posttraumatic stress disorder (PTSD). There is only limited evidence about the effectiveness of CAM as a treatment for PTSD; however, the evidence suggests that some CAM approaches have modest beneficial effects as a treatment for PTSD.

Broadly conceptualized, CAM refers to treatments not considered to be standard in the current practice of Western medicine.

601

Complementary refers to the use of these techniques in combination with conventional approaches and alternative refers to their use in lieu of conventional practices.

Many treatments and techniques that are considered CAM within the U.S. are part of conventional medicinal practices in other parts of the world. As Western practitioners and consumers increasingly adopt these approaches, the boundaries between conventional medicine and CAM continue to shift.

## Conventional Posttraumatic Stress Disorder (PTSD) Treatment and CAM

Some conventional therapies for PTSD (e.g., cognitive behavioral therapies (CBT)) include elements that are consistent with CAM approaches. They are not considered to be CAM herein because CBT has a separate and well-developed basis in cognitive and behavioral theories. The CAM techniques that are used in CBT (e.g., relaxation, mindfulness) are conceptualized as supporting cognitive-behavioral mechanisms as opposed to operating on their own to create change. For example, relaxation may be used during exposure-based treatment for PTSD to manage arousal, thereby helping the patient to tolerate the exposure, which is believed to be the major change agent.

Psychotherapies such as Acceptance and Commitment Therapy (ACT), Dialectical Behavior Therapy (DBT), and Mindfulness-Based Cognitive Therapy (MBCT) include mindfulness, which has been defined as "paying attention in a particular way: on purpose, in the present moment, and nonjudgmentally." Mindfulness is seen as an important agent of change in these approaches because it shifts the individual's perspective in a way that counteracts psychopathological processes. Within these approaches, mindfulness is coupled with cognitive and behavioral principles and techniques to affect change. For this reason, such interventions are not considered to be CAM.

## Widespread Use of CAM for PTSD in Veteran and Civilian Populations

In general, reported rates of CAM use are similar in veteran and civilian samples, ranging from approximately one-quarter to one-half of respondents, depending on the type of CAM and health conditions assessed. Active military personnel are not captured in nationally representative or veteran samples, but research suggests rates of CAM use in the military are similar, if not higher than rates of CAM use among veterans and civilians.

The use of CAM therapies specifically for management and treatment of mental health problems is common and increasing. Among a nationally representative sample, rates of CAM increased for managing anxiety (20.2–27.9%) and depression (40.9–42.7%). In another nationally representative sample, survey results showed that CAM therapies were used more commonly than conventional therapies to treat self-defined anxiety attacks (51.9 versus 40.8%) and severe depression (63.9 versus 36.4%).

Research on use of CAM specific to individuals with PTSD is emerging and suggests extensive utilization.

- A study in veterans found that those with PTSD were 25 percent more likely than veterans without PTSD to report CAM use, in particular, biofeedback and relaxation.

- In a sample of older veterans, some diagnoses, including PTSD, were more common among CAM users.

- Results from the National Comorbidity Survey Replication (NCS-R) study indicated that 12.6 percent of individuals with PTSD accessed provider administered CAM in the past year (e.g., chiropractor, acupuncture, self-help group). This is likely an underestimate, as measurement of CAM excluded self-administered therapies, such as herbal therapy, relaxation techniques, or homeopathy.

- One study looked at use of CAM specifically for the management of PTSD symptoms. In a nationally representative sample, 39 percent of those with PTSD indicated that they had used CAM in the previous year to address self-reported emotional and mental health problems.

## Limited Evidence for the Effectiveness of CAM in PTSD

Despite the widespread use of CAM among individuals with PTSD, evidence to support the efficacy of CAM for treating PTSD is limited. The current empirical evidence for different CAM modalities in PTSD is described below. This is not an exhaustive list of potential applications of CAM in PTSD. It is limited to those CAM modalities that have been tested in controlled studies in patients with PTSD. For each modality, treatment effects on PTSD symptoms and key limitations are summarized.

## Acupuncture

There has been one published randomized clinical trial of acupuncture as a treatment for PTSD. In that study, acupuncture was superior to waitlist and comparable to group CBT for PTSD in a nonveteran sample. Although the effect size was large, the sample was small and there was no control for the nonspecific features of acupuncture (i.e., sham acupuncture). A systematic review described the evidence for the effectiveness of acupuncture for PTSD as encouraging, but concluded that further trials are needed. Of note, five of the six studies examined in that review were conducted in China, where acupuncture is a mainstream treatment. Therefore, findings may not generalize to the use of acupuncture as a CAM modality in Western medicine.

## Meditation

Several studies have evaluated different meditative practices. A randomized controlled trial found that a six-week group intervention that provided training in mantram repetition (silent repetition of a spiritually meaningful word) in conjunction with treatment as usual (medication and case management) had a small to moderate effect on PTSD symptoms among veterans with chronic PTSD as compared to treatment as usual alone. It is difficult to interpret the observed benefits in the mantram repetition group as due only to the intervention because there was no control for the nonspecific treatment effects, such as additional clinical contact, of the group-based mantram repetition intervention.

Niles et al. found that an eight-week mindfulness intervention was superior to psychoeducation, both delivered by telehealth. Those in the mindfulness condition showed greater improvement in PTSD symptoms, but these improvements were not sustained after treatment ended. It is not clear if the brief nature of the intervention or the modality of delivery (telehealth versus face-to-face) affected the results. A randomized controlled pilot study compared Mindfulness Based Stress Reduction (MBSR) plus usual care to usual care alone. Both groups had improved PTSD symptoms at posttreatment, but between-group differences were not observed in intent-to-treat analyses, although the observed within-group effect were larger in the group that received MBSR in addition to usual care. As with the trial of mantram repetition described above, the nonspecific treatment effects of MBSR, such as additional clinical contact and group support, were not controlled for in this pilot study, which leaves the possibility that the few differences that were observed could be attributable to these other factors.

### Relaxation

Results are somewhat variable regarding the impact of relaxation on PTSD symptoms. Some studies have found no benefit associated with relaxation as compared to other PTSD treatments. Other trials have shown that relaxation is associated with clinically meaningful, albeit modest, changes in PTSD symptoms.

### Yoga

One small randomized controlled trial (RCT) compared an adjunctive, 12-session yoga intervention to an assessment control in a sample of veteran and civilian women. Although there were significant decreases in PTSD symptoms (specifically re-experiencing and hyperarousal symptoms) in both groups, there were no between-group differences. Both treatment arms required weekly, structured group interactions and general behavioral activation, which may have partially contributed to the similar levels of clinical change (small to moderate effect sizes) observed in both study arms.

### Other CAM Mind-Body Practices

Research is emerging with preliminary evidence for other CAM mind-body therapies, such as energy therapy for PTSD. An initial study of Emotional Freedom Techniques (EFT), in which the patient taps acupuncture points to stimulate energy meridians, compared the approach to Eye Movement Desensitization and Reprocessing ((EMDR); n = 46, 19 of whom withdrew before posttreatment). EFT and EMDR did not differ statistically, and the effect size observed in both groups was small. In another study EFT plus standard care was compared to standard care alone in a sample of veterans (n = 59), and EFT was associated with improved PTSD symptoms. Because of methodological limitations of these trials, strong conclusions about EFT cannot be drawn from these findings. Another study compared treatment as usual plus adjunctive healing touch and guided imagery to treatment as usual alone in an active duty sample who had returned from deployment and screened positive for PTSD symptoms (although PTSD diagnosis was not established). There were statistically significant decreases in PTSD symptoms for the group who received adjunctive healing touch plus guided imagery, but not for the treatment as usual control group. Here again, controls for the effects of usual treatment were not clearly specified, and adherence to between-session use of guided imagery was not assessed. These initial studies begin to demonstrate acceptability and feasibility of adjunctive CAM mind-body approaches, but do not provide conclusive information about efficacy.

## *Clinical Implications*

Based on the available evidence, it is difficult to draw firm conclusions about the efficacy of any type of CAM for PTSD. Acupuncture appears to have benefit but needs to be evaluated relative to sham acupuncture in order to control for the nonspecific benefits of treatment. Mindfulness-based meditation and relaxation appear to have modest benefit; little is known about the effect of other meditative practices and other CAM modalities.

Overall, the current evidence base does not support the use of CAM interventions as an alternative to current empirically-established approaches for PTSD, or as first-line interventions recommended within evidence-based clinical guidelines. CAM may be best applied as an adjunct to other PTSD treatments or as a gateway to additional services for patients who initially refuse other approaches.

# Chapter 88

# *Osteoarthritis and CAM*

Osteoarthritis (OA) is the most common type of arthritis. It occurs most often in the hands, knees, hips, and spine. OA affects cartilage — the slippery tissue that covers the ends of bones in a joint. Cartilage allows bones to glide over each other and absorbs the shock of movement. In OA, the top layer of cartilage breaks down and wears away, allowing the bones under it to rub against each other. This can cause pain, swelling, and difficulty in moving the joint.

OA is most common in older people, but younger people can have it too, especially in joints that have been injured.

## What the Science Says about Complementary Health Approaches for Osteoarthritis (OA)

A variety of complementary approaches have been studied for OA, including natural products, mind and body practices, and others. The following chapter summarizes the evidence on the effectiveness and safety of specific approaches.

### *Natural Products*

*Glucosamine and Chondroitin Sulfate*

Glucosamine and chondroitin are substances found in cartilage. Both are produced naturally in the body. They are also available as

---

This chapter includes text excerpted from "Osteoarthritis: In Depth," National Center for Complementary and Integrative Health (NCCIH), September 2016.

dietary supplements. Researchers have studied their effects, individually or in combination, in people with OA.

Studies of glucosamine for pain in knee OA have had conflicting results. Some, including a major National Institutes of Health (NIH)-sponsored study, found little or no evidence that glucosamine can relieve pain, but several other studies indicated that it can. Studies of chondroitin for pain from OA of the knee have had inconsistent results, but in general, the largest, highest quality studies have not shown an effect. There isn't enough evidence to show whether glucosamine or chondroitin lessens pain from OA in other joints.

A few studies have looked at whether glucosamine or chondroitin or the combination can have beneficial effects on the joint structure in people with OA. Some but not all of these studies found evidence that chondroitin or a glucosamine/chondroitin combination might help, but the improvements seen in most studies may be too small to make a difference to patients. There's little evidence that glucosamine alone has beneficial effects on the joint structure.

Glucosamine and chondroitin supplements may interact with the anticoagulant (blood-thinning) drug warfarin (Coumadin). Overall, studies have not shown any other serious side effects.

*Dimethyl Sulfoxide (DMSO) and Methylsulfonylmethane (MSM)*

Dimethyl sulfoxide (DMSO) and methylsulfonylmethane (MSM) are two chemically related substances that have been studied for OA. DMSO is applied to the skin. MSM is used as a dietary supplement. Very little research has been done on DMSO and MSM, so it's uncertain whether they're helpful for OA symptoms.

Both DMSO and MSM can have side effects. DMSO can cause digestive upset, skin irritation, and a garlic-like taste, breath, and body odor. MSM can cause allergic reactions, digestive upsets, and skin rashes.

*S-Adenosyl-L-Methionine (SAMe)*

S-Adenosyl-L-methionine (SAMe) is a molecule that is naturally produced in the body. It's also sold in the United States as a dietary supplement. Studies of SAMe for OA have had inconsistent results. In some studies, SAMe appeared to be as effective as nonsteroidal anti-inflammatory drugs (NSAIDs) in relieving symptoms associated with OA, but in others, it was no more helpful than a placebo (an inactive substance).

Side effects of SAMe are uncommon and usually mild. However, little is known about the long-term safety of SAMe because most studies have been brief. SAMe may have special risks for people with bipolar disorder and those who are human immunodeficiency virus (HIV) positive. It also may interact with drugs, including some antidepressants and levodopa, a drug used for Parkinson disease (PD).

## Oral Herbal Remedies

A variety of herbal products that are taken orally (by mouth) have been studied for OA. A 2014 evaluation of oral herbal remedies for OA found enough evidence to conclude that avocado-soybean unsaponifiables (ASU) and Boswellia serrata, an herb used in Ayurvedic medicine, may produce slight improvements in pain and function; however, the improvements were so small that patients might not consider them meaningful. For all other herbal products, the amount of research is too small to allow any conclusions to be reached.

Little information is available on the safety of most herbal products used for OA, including ASUs and Boswellia serrata. Herbs and other dietary supplements may cause health problems if not used correctly, and some may interact with prescription or nonprescription medications or other dietary supplements.

## Topical Herbal Remedies

Some herbal products have been used topically (applied to the skin) for OA. A 2013 evaluation of the evidence on topical herbal products concluded that arnica gel and comfrey extract gel might be helpful, and capsicum extract gel probably is not. The evidence on other products was insufficient to allow conclusions to be reached.

There's not much information on the safety of topical herbal therapies for OA, but it's been reported that some products, such as capsicum extract gel, can cause skin irritation or other side effects.

## Mind and Body Practices

### Acupuncture

A 2012 combined analysis of data from several studies indicated that acupuncture can be helpful and a reasonable option to consider for OA pain. A 2013 analysis using different statistical methods also concluded that acupuncture may help relieve knee OA pain. After these analyses were completed, a 2014 Australian study showed that

609

both needle and laser acupuncture were modestly better at relieving knee pain from OA than no treatment but not better than simulated (sham) laser acupuncture. These results are generally consistent with previous studies, which showed that acupuncture is consistently better than no treatment but not necessarily better than simulated acupuncture at relieving OA pain. A 2016 review of U.S. studies found evidence that acupuncture, as practiced in the United States, may help some patients with knee OA manage their pain.

How acupuncture works to relieve pain is unclear. Evidence available suggests that many factors—like expectation and belief—that are unrelated to acupuncture needling may play important roles in the beneficial effects of acupuncture on pain. Acupuncture is generally considered safe when performed by an experienced practitioner using sterile needles. Improperly performed acupuncture can cause potentially serious side effects.

### *Cupping and Moxibustion*

In addition to acupuncture, other traditional Asian practices that have been used for OA include cupping (applying a cup to the skin and creating suction either mechanically or by using heat) and moxibustion (burning an herb above the skin to apply heat to acupuncture points). Only a small amount of research has been done on the use of these practices for OA. A single study evaluated cupping for OA; its results were promising, but it's a very preliminary study. Several studies evaluated moxibustion for OA symptoms and found that it might be helpful; however, because the amount of research was small and the studies may have been biased, definite conclusions cannot be reached.

Both cupping and moxibustion can leave marks on the skin, which are usually temporary. Because cupping may draw blood, it could expose people to disease-causing microorganisms if the same device is used on more than one person without being sterilized after each use. Moxibustion has been linked to allergic reactions, burns, and infections.

### *Massage Therapy*

Very few studies have evaluated massage therapy for OA. The small amount of available evidence suggests that massage may help to reduce symptoms in people with knee OA. Massage therapy appears to have few risks when performed by a trained practitioner. However, arthritis-stressed joints are sensitive, so massage therapists who treat people with OA need to be familiar with the special needs of people with this condition.

### Tai Chi and Qi Gong

Tai chi and qi gong are traditional mind and body practices of Chinese origin. They combine certain postures and gentle, dance-like body movements with mental focus, breathing, and relaxation.

Several studies have evaluated the effects of tai chi on knee OA. In general, they showed short-term improvements in pain, stiffness, and physical function. Some studies also showed other desirable changes, such as improved balance or reduced depression. In a 2016 study in which tai chi was compared with physical therapy for knee OA and patients were encouraged to continue their exercises after the 12-week study period ended, patients in both the tai chi and physical therapy groups showed improvement in pain for a full year. Much less research has been done on qi gong, but the few studies that have been completed showed improvements in some OA symptoms.

Tai chi and qi gong are generally considered to be safe practices. However, side effects, such as temporarily increased knee pain, have been reported in some people with OA.

### Yoga

Yoga incorporates several elements of exercise that may be beneficial for arthritis, including activities that may help improve strength and flexibility. However, very little research has been done on yoga for OA, so it's uncertain whether it's helpful. Before starting to do yoga, people with OA should discuss their special needs with their healthcare provider and the yoga instructor. Props and modifications may be necessary to make yoga safe and comfortable for people with OA.

## Other Complementary Health Approaches for OA

### Balneotherapy

Balneotherapy is the technique of bathing in mineral water for health purposes; it also includes related practices such as mud packs. Although some studies have reported that balneotherapy can reduce pain in OA, the amount of high-quality research is too small for definite conclusions to be reached.

Balneotherapy has a good safety record.

*Homeopathy*

There's little evidence to support homeopathy as an effective approach for OA symptoms, particularly pain. There's been no research on the effects of homeopathy on OA. Although most homeopathic products are highly dilute and, therefore, considered to be safe, some contain ingredients in amounts large enough that they could cause harmful effects. There have also been instances when potentially harmful contaminants have been found in homeopathic products.

*Magnets*

The available scientific evidence does not support using static magnets for pain relief. Static magnets are magnets often sold in shoe insoles, wrist wraps, headbands, and similar products. A small amount of evidence suggests that electromagnetic field therapy, which involves the use of small machines or mats to deliver an electromagnetic field to a joint or to the whole body, may provide some pain relief in OA, but it's unclear whether it has a meaningful effect on physical function or quality of life for OA patients.

Static magnets are generally considered safe. Information about the safety of electromagnetic field therapy is limited, but few adverse effects have been reported in studies of this technique. Magnetic devices of any kind may be hazardous for people with certain types of implanted medical devices, such as pacemakers.

# Chapter 89

# *Seasonal Allergies and CAM*

If you have an allergy, your immune system reacts to something that doesn't bother most other people. People with seasonal allergies (also called hay fever or allergic rhinitis) react to pollen from plants. Symptoms may include sneezing, coughing, a runny or stuffy nose, and itching in the eyes, nose, mouth, and throat.

This chapter discusses complementary health approaches for allergic rhinitis.

## What the Science Says

Many complementary health approaches have been studied for allergic rhinitis. There's some evidence that a few may be helpful.

### *Mind and Body Practices*

A 2015 evaluation of 13 studies of acupuncture for allergic rhinitis, involving a total of 2,365 participants, found evidence that this approach may be helpful. Rinsing the sinuses with a neti pot (a device that comes from the Ayurvedic tradition) or with other devices, such as nebulizers or spray, pump, or squirt bottles, may be a useful addition to conventional treatment for allergic rhinitis.

---

This chapter includes text excerpted from "Seasonal Allergies at a Glance," National Center for Complementary and Integrative Health (NCCIH), September 24, 2017.

### Natural Products

**Butterbur.** An evaluation of six studies of the herb butterbur for allergic rhinitis, involving a total of 720 participants, indicated that butterbur may be helpful.

**Probiotics.** Researchers have been investigating probiotics (live microorganisms that may have health benefits) for diseases of the immune system, including allergies. Although some studies have had promising results, the overall evidence on probiotics and allergic rhinitis is inconsistent. It's possible that some types of probiotics might be helpful but that others are not.

**Honey.** It's been thought that eating honey might help to relieve pollen allergies because honey contains small amounts of pollen and might help people build up a tolerance to it. Another possibility is that honey could act as an antihistamine or anti-inflammatory agent. Only a few studies have examined the effects of honey in people with seasonal allergies, and their results have been inconsistent.

**Other natural products.** Many other natural products have been studied for allergic rhinitis, including astragalus, capsaicin, grape seed extract, omega-3 fatty acids, Pycnogenol (French maritime pine bark extract), quercetin, spirulina, stinging nettle, and an herb used in Ayurvedic medicine called tinospora, or guduchi. In all instances, the evidence is either inconsistent or too limited to show whether these products are helpful.

## *Side Effects and Risks*

- People can get infections if they use neti pots or other nasal rinsing devices improperly. Following steps will help you in rinsing your sinuses safely:

  - Most important is the source of water that is used with nasal rinsing devices. According to the U.S. Food and Drug Administration (FDA), tap water that is not filtered, treated, or processed in specific ways is not safe for use as a nasal rinse. Sterile water is safe; over-the-counter (OTC) nasal rinsing products that contain sterile saline (salt water) are available.

  - Some tap water contains low levels of organisms, such as bacteria and protozoa, including amoebas, which may be safe to swallow because stomach acid kills them. But these organisms can stay alive in nasal passages and cause potentially serious infections. Improper use of neti pots may have caused two deaths in 2011 in Louisiana from a rare brain infection that the state health department linked to tap water contaminated with an amoeba called Naegleria fowleri.

- Acupuncture is generally considered safe when performed by an experienced practitioner using sterile needles. Improperly performed acupuncture can cause potentially serious side effects.

- Raw butterbur extracts contain pyrrolizidine alkaloids, which can cause liver damage and cancer. Extracts of butterbur that are almost completely free from these alkaloids are available. However, no studies have proven that the long-term use of butterbur products, including the reduced-alkaloid products, is safe.

- In healthy people, probiotics usually have only minor side effects, if any. However, in people with underlying health problems (for example, weakened immune systems), serious complications such as infections have occasionally been reported.

- Be cautious about using herbs or bee products for any purpose. Some herbs, such as chamomile and echinacea, may cause allergic reactions in people who are allergic to related plants. Also, people with pollen allergies may have allergic reactions to bee products, such as bee pollen, honey, royal jelly, and propolis (a hive sealant made by bees from plant resins). Children under 1 year of age should not eat honey.

- Talk to your healthcare provider about the best way to manage your seasonal allergies, especially if you're considering or using a dietary supplement. Be aware that some supplements may interact with medications or other supplements or have side effects of their own. Keep in mind that most dietary supplements have not been tested in pregnant women, nursing mothers, or children.

# Chapter 90

# *Sleep Disorders and CAM*

There are more than 80 different sleep disorders. This chapter focuses on insomnia—difficulty falling asleep or difficulty staying asleep. Insomnia is one of the most common sleep disorders. Chronic, long-term sleep disorders affect millions of Americans each year. These disorders and the sleep deprivation they cause can interfere with work, driving, social activities, and overall quality of life, and can have serious health implications. Sleep disorders account for an estimated $16 billion in medical costs each year, plus indirect costs due to missed days of work, decreased productivity, and other factors.

## What the Science Says about Complementary Health Approaches and Insomnia

Research has produced promising results for some complementary health approaches for insomnia, such as relaxation techniques. However, evidence of effectiveness is still limited for most products and practices, and safety concerns have been raised about a few.

### *Mind and Body Practices*

* There is evidence that relaxation techniques can be effective in treating chronic insomnia.

---

This chapter includes text excerpted from "Sleep Disorders: In Depth," National Center for Complementary and Integrative Health (NCCIH), October 2015.

- Progressive relaxation may help people with insomnia and nighttime anxiety.

- Music-assisted relaxation may be moderately beneficial in improving sleep quality in people with sleep problems, but the number of studies has been small.

- Various forms of relaxation are sometimes combined with components of cognitive-behavioral therapy (CBT) (such as sleep restriction and stimulus control), with good results.

- Using relaxation techniques before bedtime can be part of a strategy to improve sleep habits that also includes other steps, such as maintaining a consistent sleep schedule; avoiding caffeine, alcohol, heavy meals, and strenuous exercise too close to bedtime; and sleeping in a quiet, cool, dark room.

- Relaxation techniques are generally safe. However, rare side effects have been reported in people with serious physical or mental health conditions. If you have a serious underlying health problem, it would be a good idea to consult your healthcare provider before using relaxation techniques.

- In a preliminary study, mindfulness-based stress reduction, a type of meditation, was as effective as a prescription drug in a small group of people with insomnia.

- Preliminary studies in postmenopausal women and women with osteoarthritis (OA) suggest that yoga may be helpful for insomnia.

- Some practitioners who treat insomnia have reported that hypnotherapy enhanced the effectiveness of CBT and relaxation techniques in their patients, but very little rigorous research has been conducted on the use of hypnotherapy for insomnia.

- A small 2012 study on massage therapy showed promising results for insomnia in postmenopausal women. However, conclusions cannot be reached on the basis of a single study.

- Most of the studies that have evaluated acupuncture for insomnia have been of poor scientific quality. The evidence available so far is not rigorous enough to show whether acupuncture is helpful for insomnia.

### Dietary Supplements

*Melatonin and Related Supplements*

- Melatonin may help with jet lag and sleep problems related to shift work.

- A 2013 evaluation of the results of 19 studies concluded that melatonin may help people with insomnia fall asleep faster, sleep longer, and sleep better, but the effect of melatonin is small compared to that of other treatments for insomnia.

- Studies of melatonin in children with sleep problems suggest that it may be helpful, both in generally healthy children and in those with conditions such as autism or attention deficit hyperactivity disorder (ADHD). However, both the number of studies and the number of children who participated in the studies are small, and all of the studies tested melatonin only for short periods of time.

- Melatonin supplements appear to be relatively safe for short-term use, although the use of melatonin was linked to bad moods in elderly people (most of whom had dementia) in one study.

- The long-term safety of melatonin supplements has not been established.

- Dietary supplements containing substances that can be changed into melatonin in the body—L-tryptophan and 5-hydroxytryptophan (5-HTP)—have been researched as sleep aids.

- Studies of L-tryptophan supplements as an insomnia treatment have had inconsistent results, and the effects of 5-HTP supplements on insomnia have not been established.

- The use of L-tryptophan supplements may be linked to eosinophilia-myalgia syndrome (EMS), a complex, potentially fatal disorder with multiple symptoms including severe muscle pain. It is uncertain whether the risk of EMS associated with L-tryptophan supplements is due to impurities in L-tryptophan preparations or to L-tryptophan itself.

*Herbs*

- Although chamomile has traditionally been used for insomnia, often in the form of a tea, there is no conclusive evidence from clinical trials showing whether it is helpful. Some people, especially those who are allergic to ragweed or related plants, may have allergic reactions to chamomile.

- Although kava is said to have sedative properties, very little research has been conducted on whether this herb is helpful for insomnia. More importantly, kava supplements have been linked to a risk of severe liver damage.

- Clinical trials of valerian (another herb said to have sedative properties) have had inconsistent results, and its value for insomnia has not been demonstrated. Although few people have reported negative side effects from valerian, it is uncertain whether this herb is safe for long-term use.

- Some "sleep formula" dietary supplements combine valerian with other herbs such as hops, lemon balm, passionflower, and kava or other ingredients such as melatonin and 5-HTP. There is little evidence on these preparations from studies in people.

### *Other Complementary Health Approaches*

Aromatherapy is the therapeutic use of essential oils from plants. It is uncertain whether aromatherapy is helpful for treating insomnia because little rigorous research has been done on this topic. A systematic review concluded that current evidence does not demonstrate significant effects of homeopathic medicines for insomnia.

## Considering Complementary Health Approaches for Sleep Problems

If you're considering complementary health approaches for sleep problems:

- Talk to your healthcare providers. Tell them about the complementary health approach you are considering and ask any questions you may have. Because trouble sleeping can be an indication of a more serious condition, and because some prescription and over-the-counter (OTC) drugs can contribute to sleep problems, it is important to discuss your sleep-related symptoms with your healthcare providers before trying any complementary health product or practice.

- Be cautious about using any sleep product—prescription medications, OTC medications, dietary supplements, or homeopathic remedies. Find out about potential side effects and any risks from long-term use or combining products.

- Keep in mind that "natural" does not always mean safe. For example, kava products can cause serious harm to the liver. Also, a manufacturer's use of the term "standardized" (or "verified" or "certified") does not necessarily guarantee product quality or consistency. Natural products can cause health problems if not used correctly. The healthcare providers you see about your sleep problems can advise you.

- If you are pregnant, nursing a child, or considering giving a child a dietary supplement or other natural health product, it is especially important to consult your (or your child's) healthcare provider.

If you are considering a practitioner-provided complementary health practice, check with your insurer to see if the services will be covered, and ask a trusted source (such as your healthcare provider or a nearby hospital or medical school) to recommend a practitioner.

Tell all your healthcare providers about any complementary health approaches you use. Give them a full picture of what you do to manage your health. This will help ensure coordinated and safe care.

# Part Nine


# Additional Help and Information

# Chapter 91

# *Glossary of Terms Related to Complementary and Alternative Medicine*

**acupuncture:** A family of procedures that originated in traditional Chinese medicine. Acupuncture is the stimulation of specific points on the body by a variety of techniques, including the insertion of thin metal needles through the skin. It is intended to remove blockages in the flow of qi and restore and maintain health.

**Alexander technique:** A movement therapy that uses guidance and education on ways to improve posture and movement. The intent is to teach a person how to use muscles more efficiently in order to improve the overall functioning of the body. Examples of the Alexander technique as complementary and alternative medicine (CAM) are using it to treat low-back pain and the symptoms of Parkinson disease (PD).

**aromatherapy:** The use of essential oils from plants to support and balance the mind, body, and spirit. Aromatherapy may be combined with other complementary treatments like massage therapy and acupuncture, as well as with standard treatments.

**Ayurvedic medicine:** One of the world's oldest medical systems. It originated in India and has evolved there over thousands of years. In

This glossary contains terms excerpted from documents produced by several sources deemed reliable.

625

the United States, Ayurvedic medicine is considered CAM. The aim of Ayurvedic medicine is to integrate and balance the body, mind, and spirit. This is believed to help prevent illness and promote wellness.

**biofeedback:** A method of learning to voluntarily control certain body functions such as heartbeat, blood pressure, and muscle tension with the help of a special machine. This method can help control pain.

**botanical:** A plant or plant part valued for its medicinal or therapeutic properties, flavor, and/or scent. Herbs are a subset of botanicals. Products made from botanicals that are used to maintain or improve health may be called herbal products, botanical products, or phytomedicines.

**Chelation therapy:** An investigational therapy using a artificial amino acid, called ethylenediaminetetraacetic acid (EDTA). It is added to the blood through a vein. Disodium EDTA has been in widespread use since the 1970s for disease of the heart and arteries.

**chiropractic:** A whole medical system that focuses on the relationship between the body's structure—mainly the spine—and function. Practitioners perform adjustments (also called manipulation) with the goal of correcting structural alignment problems to assist the body in healing.

**chiropractic care:** This care involves the adjustment of the spine and joints to influence the body's nervous system and natural defense mechanisms to alleviate pain and improve general health. It is primarily used to treat back problems, headaches, nerve inflammation, muscle spasms, and other injuries and traumas.

**cholesterol:** A fat-like substance that is made by your body and found naturally in animal foods such as dairy products, eggs, meat, poultry, and seafood. Foods high in cholesterol include dairy fats, egg yolks, and organ meats such as liver. Cholesterol is needed to carry out functions such as hormone and vitamin production. It is carried through the blood by [lipoproteins].

**clinical trial:** A type of research study that uses volunteers to test the safety and efficacy (the ability to produce a beneficial effect) of new methods of screening (checking for disease when there are no symptoms), prevention, diagnosis, or treatment of a disease. Also called a clinical study.

**complementary and alternative medicine (CAM):** A group of diverse medical and healthcare systems, practices, and products that are not presently considered to be part of conventional medicine. Complementary medicine is used together with conventional medicine, and alternative medicine is used in place of conventional medicine.

**conventional medicine:** Medicine as practiced by holders of MD (medical doctor) or DO (doctor of osteopathy) degrees and by their allied health professionals such as physical therapists, psychologists, and registered nurses.

**Daily Value (DV):** A term used on a food or dietary supplement product label to describe the recommended levels of intake of a nutrient. The percent Daily Value (% DV) represents how much of a nutrient is provided in one serving of the food or dietary supplement. For example, the DV for calcium is 1,000 mg (milligrams); a food that has 200 mg of calcium per serving would state on the label that the % DV for calcium is 20 percent.

**dietary supplement:** A product that is intended to supplement the diet; contains one or more dietary ingredients (including vitamins, minerals, herbs or other botanicals, amino acids, and certain other substances) or their constituents; and is intended to be taken by mouth, in forms such as tablet, capsule, powder, softgel, gelcap, or liquid.

**Feldenkrais:** A movement therapy that uses a method of education in physical coordination and movement. Practitioners use verbal guidance and light touch to teach the method through one-on-one lessons and group classes. The intent is to help the person become more aware of how the body moves through space and to improve physical functioning.

**guided imagery:** A type of CAM that encourages imagining a pleasant scene to take your mind off your pain or anxiety.

**herbal supplements:** One type of dietary supplement. An herb is a plant or plant part (such as leaves, flowers, or seeds) that is used for its flavor, scent, and/or therapeutic properties. Botanical is often used as a synonym for herb. An herbal supplement may contain a single herb or mixtures of herbs.

**homeopathy:** A whole medical system that originated in Europe. Homeopathy seeks to stimulate the body's ability to heal itself by giving very small doses of highly diluted substances that in larger doses would produce illness or symptoms (an approach called "like cures like").

**hypnosis:** A trance-like state in which a person becomes more aware and focused and is more open to suggestion.

**magnet therapy:** A magnet produces a measurable force called a magnetic field. Magnets are used for many different types of pain, including foot pain and back pain from conditions such as arthritis and fibromyalgia. Magnets in products such as magnetic patches and disks, shoe insoles, bracelets, and mattress pads are used for pain in the foot, wrist, back, and other parts of the body.

**manipulation:** The application of controlled force to a joint, moving it beyond the normal range of motion in an effort to aid in restoring health. Manipulation may be performed as a part of other therapies or whole medical systems, including chiropractic medicine, massage, and naturopathy.

**massage:** Pressing, rubbing, and moving muscles and other soft tissues of the body, primarily by using the hands and fingers. The aim is to increase the flow of blood and oxygen to the massaged area.

**meditation:** Refers to a variety of techniques or practices intended to focus or control attention. Most of them are rooted in Eastern religious or spiritual traditions. These techniques have been used by many different cultures throughout the world for thousands of years.

**mind-body medicine:** Medicine that focuses on the interactions among the brain, mind, body, and behavior, and the powerful ways in which emotional, mental, social, spiritual, and behavioral factors can directly affect health. It regards as fundamental an approach that respects and enhances each person's capacity for self-knowledge and self-care, and it emphasizes techniques that are grounded in this approach.

**mineral:** In nutrition, an inorganic substance found in the earth that is required to maintain health.

**naturopathy:** A whole medical system that originated in Europe. Naturopathy aims to support the body's ability to heal itself through the use of dietary and lifestyle changes together with CAM therapies such as herbs, massage, and joint manipulation.

**omega-3 fatty acids:** Polyunsaturated fatty acids that come from foods such as fish, fish oil, vegetable oil (primarily canola and soybean), walnuts, and wheat germ. Omega-3s are important in a number of bodily functions, including the movement of calcium and other substances in and out of cells, the relaxation and contraction of muscles, blood clotting, digestion, fertility, cell division, and growth. In addition, omega-3s are thought to protect against heart disease, reduce inflammation, and lower triglyceride levels.

**osteopathic manipulation:** A full-body system of hands-on techniques to alleviate pain, restore function, and promote health and well-being.

**pilates:** A movement therapy that uses a method of physical exercise to strengthen and build control of muscles, especially those used for posture. Awareness of breathing and precise control of movements are integral components of Pilates. Special equipment, if available, is often used.

**polyunsaturated fat:** This type of fat is liquid at room temperature. There are two types of polyunsaturated fatty acids (PUFAs): omega-6 and omega-3. Omega-6 fatty acids are found in liquid vegetable oils, such as corn oil, safflower oil, and soybean oil. Omega-3 fatty acids come from plant sources—including canola oil, flaxseed, soybean oil, and walnuts—and from fish and shellfish.

**probiotics:** Live microorganisms (in most cases, bacteria) that are similar to beneficial microorganisms found in the human gut. They are also called friendly bacteria or good bacteria. Probiotics are available to consumers mainly in the form of dietary supplements and foods.

**progressive relaxation:** Is used to relieve tension and stress by systematically tensing and relaxing successive muscle groups.

**qi:** In traditional Chinese medicine, the vital energy or life force proposed to regulate a person's spiritual, emotional, mental, and physical health and to be influenced by the opposing forces of yin and yang.

**qi gong:** An ancient Chinese discipline combining the use of gentle physical movements, mental focus, and deep breathing directed toward specific parts of the body. Performed in repetitions, the exercises are normally performed two or more times a week for 30 minutes at a time.

**reflexology:** A type of massage, which applies pressure to the feet (or sometimes the hands or ears), to promote relaxation or healing in other parts of the body.

**Reiki:** A healing practice that originated in Japan. Its practitioners place their hands lightly on or just above the person receiving treatment, with the goal of facilitating the person's own healing response.

**saturated fat:** Fat that consists of triglycerides containing only saturated fatty acid radicals (i.e., they have no double bonds between the carbon atoms of the fatty acid chain and are fully saturated with hydrogen atoms). Dairy products, animal fats, coconut oil, cottonseed oil, palm kernel oil, and chocolate can contain high amounts of saturated fats.

**spirituality:** Defined as an individual's sense of peace, purpose, and connection to others, and beliefs about the meaning of life. Spirituality may be found and expressed through an organized religion or in other ways.

**tai chi:** A martial art originated in China, is a mind-body practice in CAM. It is sometimes referred to as moving meditation — practitioners move their bodies slowly, gently, and with awareness, while breathing deeply.

**traditional Chinese medicine:** A whole medical system that originated in China. It is based on the concept that disease results from disruption in the flow of qi and imbalance in the forces of yin and yang. Practices such as herbs, meditation, massage, and acupuncture seek to aid healing by restoring the yin-yang balance and the flow of qi.

**vegan:** A person who does not eat any foods that come from animals, including meat, eggs, and dairy products.

**vegetarian:** A person who eats a diet free of meat. Lacto-vegetarians consume milk and milk products along with plant-based foods. They do not eat eggs. Lacto-ovo vegetarians eat eggs and milk and milk products, in addition to plant-based foods.

**vitamin:** A nutrient that the body needs in small amounts to function and maintain health. Examples are vitamins A, C, and E.

**whole medical system:** A complete system of theory and practice that has evolved over time in different cultures and apart from conventional medicine. Examples of whole medical systems include traditional Chinese medicine, Ayurvedic medicine, homeopathy, and naturopathy.

**X-ray:** A type of high-energy radiation. In low doses, X-rays are used to diagnose diseases by making pictures of the inside of the body.

**yin and yang:** The concept of two opposing yet complementary forces described in traditional Chinese medicine. Yin represents cold, slow, or passive aspects of the person, while yang represents hot, excited, or active aspects. A major theory is that health is achieved through balancing yin and yang and disease is caused by an imbalance leading to a blockage in the flow of qi.

**yoga:** A mind-body practice in CAM with origins in ancient Indian philosophy. The various styles of yoga that people use for health purposes typically combine physical postures, breathing techniques, and meditation or relaxation.

Chapter 92

# Directory of Organizations That Provide Information about Complementary and Alternative Medicine

## Government Agencies That Provide Information about Complementary and Alternative Medicine

*Agency for Healthcare Research and Quality (AHRQ)*
5600 Fishers Ln.
Rockville, MD 20857
Phone: 301-427-1364
Website: www.ahrq.gov

*Centers for Disease Control and Prevention (CDC)*
1600 Clifton Rd.
Atlanta, GA 30329-4027
Toll-Free: 800-CDC-4636
(800-232-4636)
Toll-Free TTY: 888-232-6348
Website: www.cdc.gov
E-mail: cdcinfo@cdc.gov

Resources in this chapter were compiled from several sources deemed reliable; all contact information was verified and updated in May 2018.

### Healthcare.gov
Centers for Medicare and
Medicaid Services (CMS)
7500 Security Blvd.
Baltimore, MD 21244
Toll-Free: 800-318-2596
Toll-Free TTY: 855-889-4325
Website: www.healthcare.gov

### Healthfinder®
National Health Information
Center (NHIC)
1101 Wootton Pkwy
Rockville, MD 20852
Website: www.healthfinder.gov
E-mail: healthfinder@hhs.gov

### National Cancer Institute (NCI)
9609 Medical Center Dr.
BG 9609 MSC 9760
Bethesda, MD 20892-9760
Toll-Free: 800-4-CANCER
(800-422-6237)
Website: www.cancer.gov

### National Institute of Arthritis and Musculoskeletal and Skin Diseases (NIAMS)
NIAMS Information
Clearinghouse
National Institutes of Health
(NIH)
Bethesda, MD 20892-3675
Toll-Free: 877-22-NIAMS
(877-226-4267)
Phone: 301-495-4484
TTY: 301-565-2966
Fax: 301-718-6366
Website: www.niams.nih.gov
E-mail: NIAMSinfo@mail.nih.gov

### National Institute of Diabetes, Digestive and Kidney Diseases (NIDDK)
Health Information Center
Toll-Free: 800-860-8747
Toll-Free TTY: 866-569-1162
Website: www.niddk.nih.gov
E-mail: healthinfo@niddk.nih.gov

### National Institute of Neurological Disorders and Stroke (NINDS)
NIH Neurological Institute
P.O. Box 5801
Bethesda, MD 20824
Toll-Free: 800-352-9424
Phone: 301-496-5751
Website: www.ninds.nih.gov

### National Institute on Aging (NIA)
31 Center Dr. MSC 2292
Bldg. 31 Rm. 5C27
Bethesda, MD 20892
Toll-Free: 800-222-2225
Toll-Free TTY: 800-222-4225
Website: www.nia.nih.gov
E-mail: niaic@nia.nih.gov

### National Institutes of Health (NIH)
9000 Rockville Pike
Bethesda, MD 20892
Phone: 301-496-4000
TTY: 301-402-9612
Website: www.nih.gov
E-mail: NIHinfo@od.nih.gov

*Substance Abuse and*
*Mental Health Services*
*Administration (SAMHSA)*
5600 Fishers Ln.
Rockville, MD 20857
Toll-Free: 877-SAMHSA-7
(877-726-4727)
Toll-Free TTY: 800-487-4889
Fax: 240-221-4292
Website: www.samhsa.gov

*U.S. Department of Health*
*and Human Services (HHS)*
200 Independence Ave. S.W.
Washington, DC 20201
Toll-Free: 877-696-6775
Website: www.hhs.gov

*U.S. Food and Drug*
*Administration (FDA)*
10903 New Hampshire Ave.
Silver Spring, MD 20993
Toll-Free: 888-INFO-FDA
(888-463-6332)
Website: www.fda.gov

*U.S. National Library of*
*Medicine (NLM)*
8600 Rockville Pike
Bethesda, MD 20894
Toll-Free: 888-FIND-NLM
(888-346-3656)
Phone: 301-594-5983
Website: www.nlm.nih.gov
E-mail: publicinfo@nlm.nih.gov

## Private Agencies That Provide Information about Complementary and Alternative Medicine

*Academy of Integrative*
*Health & Medicine (AIHM)*
6919 La Jolla Blvd.
San Diego, CA 92037
Phone: 858-240-9033
Website: www.aihm.org
E-mail: info@aihm.org

*Acupressure*
Website: www.acupressure.com
E-mail: info@acupressure.com

*Alexander Technique*
*International (ATI)*
1692 Massachusetts Ave.
Cambridge, MA 02138
Toll-Free: 888-668-8996 (toll-free
from Canada and USA)
Phone: 617-497-5151
Fax: 617-497-2615
Website: www.
alexandertechniqueinternational.
com

*Alliance of International
Aromatherapists (AIA)*
3000 S. Jamaica Ct.
Ste. 145
Aurora, CO 80014
Toll-Free: 877-531-6377
Phone: 303-531-6377
Website: aia.memberclicks.net
E-mail: info@alliance-
aromatherapists.org

*Alternative Medicine
Foundation Inc.*
Website: www.amfoundation.org

*American Academy of Anti-
Aging Medicine (A4M)*
1801 N. Military Trail
Ste. 200
Boca Raton, FL 33431
Toll-Free: 888-997-0112
Phone: 561-997-0112
Fax: 561-997-0287
Website: www.a4m.com
E-mail: info@a4m.com

*American Academy of Family
Physicians (AAFP)*
11400 Tomahawk Creek Pkwy
Leawood, KS 66211-2680
Toll-Free: 800-274-2237
Phone: 913-906-6000
Fax: 913-906-6075
Website: www.nf.aafp.org
E-mail: aafp@aafp.org

*American Academy of
Medical Acupuncture
(AAMA)*
2512 Artesia Blvd.
Ste. 200
Redondo Beach, CA 90278
Phone: 310-379-8261
Website: www.
medicalacupuncture.org
E-mail: info@
medicalacupuncture.org

*American Apitherapy Society*
500 Arthur St.
Centerport, NY 11721
Phone: 631-470-9446
Fax: 631-693-2528
Website: www.apitherapy.org
E-mail: aasoffice@apitherapy.org

*American Association of
Acupuncture and Oriental
Medicine (AAAOM)*
P.O. Box 96503
#44114
Washington, DC 20090-6503
Website: www.aaaomonline.org
E-mail: admin@aaaomonline.org

*American Association of
Colleges of Osteopathic
Medicine (AACOM)*
7700 Old Georgetown Rd.
Ste. 250
Bethesda, MD 20814
Phone: 301-968-4100
Fax: 301-968-4101
Website: www.aacom.org
E-mail: webmaster@aacom.org

**American Association of Naturopathic Physicians (AANP)**
818 18th St. N.W., Ste. 250
Washington, DC 20006
Toll-Free: 866-538-2267
Phone: 202-237-8150
Fax: 202-237-8152
Website: www.naturopathic.org
E-mail: member.services@naturopathic.org

**American Botanical Council (ABC)**
6200 Manor Rd.
Austin, TX 78723
Toll-Free: 800-373-7105
Phone: 512-926-4900
Fax: 512-926-2345
Website: abc.herbalgram.org
E-mail: abc@herbalgram.org

**American Chiropractic Association (ACA)**
1701 Clarendon Blvd.
Ste. 200
Arlington, VA 22209
Phone: 703-276-8800
Fax: 703-243-2593
Website: www.acatoday.org
E-mail: memberinfo@acatoday.org

**American Dance Therapy Association (ADTA)**
10632 Little Patuxent Pkwy
Ste. 108
Columbia, MD 21044
Phone: 410-997-4040
Fax: 410-997-4048
Website: www.adta.org
E-mail: info@adta.org

**American Feng Shui Institute (AFSI)**
7220 N. Rosemead Blvd.
Ste. 204
San Gabriel, CA 91775
Phone: 626-571-2757
Website: www.amfengshui.com
E-mail: fsinfo@amfengshui.com

**American Herbalists Guild (AHG)**
P.O. Box 3076
Asheville, NC 28802-3076
Phone: 617-520-4372
Website: www.americanherbalistsguild.com
E-mail: office@americanherbalistsguild.com

**American Holistic Health Association (AHHA)**
P.O. Box 17400
Anaheim, CA 92817-7400
Phone: 714-779-6152
Website: www.ahha.org
E-mail: mail@ahha.org

**American Massage Therapy Association (AMTA)**
500 Davis St.
Ste. 900
Evanston, IL 60201-4695
Toll-Free: 877-905-2700
Phone: 847-864-0123
Fax: 847-864-5196
Website: www.amtamassage.org
E-mail: info@amtamassage.org

### American Music Therapy Association (AMTA)
8455 Colesville Rd.
Ste 1000
Silver Spring, MD 20910
Phone: 301-589-3300
Fax: 301-589-5175
Website: www.musictherapy.org
E-mail: info@musictherapy.org

### American Naturopathic Medical Association (ANMA)
P.O. Box 96273
Las Vegas, NV 89193
Phone: 702-450-3477
Website: www.anma.org
E-mail: admin@anma.org

### American Organization for Bodywork Therapies of Asia (AOBTA)
P.O. Box 343
West Berlin, NJ 08091
Phone: 856-809-2953
Fax: 856-809-2958
Website: www.aobta.org
E-mail: office@aobta.org

### American Polarity Therapy Association (APTA)
P.O. Box 10942
Parkville, MD 21234
Phone: 336-574-1121
Fax: 336-574-1151
Website: polaritytherapy.org
E-mail: aptaoffices@
polaritytherapy.org

### American Psychological Association (APA)
750 First St. N.E.
Washington, DC 20002-4242
Toll-Free: 800-374-2721
Phone: 202-336-5500
Website: www.apa.org

### American Reflexology Certification Board (ARCB)
2586 Knightsbridge Rd. S.E.
Grand Rapids, MI 49546
Phone: 303-933-6921
Fax: 303-904-0460
Website: www.arcb.net
E-mail: info@arcb.net

### American Society of Clinical Hypnosis (ASCH)
140 N. Bloomingdale Rd.
Bloomingdale, IL 60108
Phone: 630-980-4740
Fax: 630-351-8490
Website: www.asch.net
E-mail: info@asch.net

### American Tai Chi and Qigong Association (ATCQA)
2465 J-17 Centreville Rd.
Ste. 150
Herndon, VA 20171
Website: www.americantaichi.org
E-mail: TC@AmericanTaiChi.net

### Anthroposophical Society in America
1923 Geddes Ave.
Ann Arbor, MI 48104-1797
Phone: 734-662-9355
Fax: 734-662-1727
Website: www.rudolfsteiner.org
E-mail: info@anthroposophy.org

*Associated Bodywork and Massage Professionals (ABMP)*
25188 Genesee Trail Rd.
Ste.200
Golden, CO 80401
Toll-Free: 800-458-2267
Phone: 303-674-8478
Toll-Free Fax: 800-667-8260
Website: www.abmp.com
E-mail: expectmore@abmp.com

*Association for Applied Psychophysiology and Biofeedback (AAPB)*
10200 W. 44th Ave.
Ste. 304
Wheat Ridge, CO 80033
Toll-Free: 800-477-8892
Phone: 303-422-8436
Website: www.aapb.org
E-mail: info@aapb.org

*Atlantic Institute of Aromatherapy*
16018 Saddlestring Dr.
Tampa, FL 33618
Phone: 813-265-2222
Website: www.atlanticinstitute.com

*The Ayurvedic Institute*
11311 Menaul Blvd. N.E.
Albuquerque, NM 87112
Phone: 505-291-9698
Fax: 505-294-7572
Website: www.ayurveda.com
E-mail: office@ayurveda.com

*Bastyr Center for Natural Health*
3670 Stone Way N.
Seattle, WA 98103
Phone: 206-834-4100
Fax: 206-834-4131
Website: www.bastyrcenter.org

*Benson-Henry Institute (BHI) for Mind Body Medicine*
151 Merrimac St.
Fourth Fl.
Boston, MA 02114
Phone: 617-643-6090
Fax: 617-643-6077
Website: www.
bensonhenryinstitute.org
E-mail: mindbody@partners.org

*Biodynamic Craniosacral Therapy Association of North America (BCTA/NA)*
Phone: 734-904-0546
Website: www.
craniosacraltherapy.org/
contact-us

*Biofeedback Certification Institute of America (BCIA)*
5310 Ward Rd.
Ste. 201
Arvada, CO 80002
Phone: 720-502-5829
Website: www.bcia.org
E-mail: info@bcia.org

*Center for Mindfulness in Medicine, Health Care, and Society*
University of Massachusetts
Medical School (UMMS)
55 Lake Ave. N.
Worcester, MA 01655
Phone: 508-856-2656
Fax: 508-856-1977
Website: www.umassmed.edu
E-mail: mindfulness@umassmed.edu

*DrWeil.com*
Website: www.drweil.com

*Feldenkrais Educational Foundation of North America (FEFNA)*
401 Edgewater Place
Ste. 600
Wakefield, MA 01880
Phone: 781-876-8935
Fax: 781-645-1322
Website: www.feldenkrais.com

*Feldenkrais Resources*
3680 Sixth Ave.
San Diego, CA 92103
Toll-Free: 800-765-1907
Phone: 619-220-8776
Fax: 619-330-4993
Website: www.feldenkraisresources.com

*Hellerwork International*
300 Avenida Adobe
San Clemente, CA 92672
Phone: 714-873-6131
Website: www.hellerwork.com
E-mail: admin@hellerwork.com

*Holistic Network International*
Website: www.holisticnetworkofflorida.com
E-mail: info@HolisticNetworkInternational.com

*Homeopathic Educational Services*
812C Camelia St.
Berkeley, CA 94710
Toll-Free: 800-359-9051
Phone: 510-649-0294
Fax: 510-649-1955
Website: www.homeopathic.com
E-mail: email@homeopathic.com

*Institute of Traditional Medicine (ITM)*
553 Queen St. W.
Second Fl.
Toronto, ON M5V2B6
Phone: 416-537-0928
Website: www.itmworld.org
E-mail: info@itmworld.org

*International Association of Reiki Professionals (IARP)*
Website: www.iarp.org

*International Association of Yoga Therapists (IAYT)*
P.O. Box 251563
Little Rock, AR 72225
Phone: 928-541-0004
Website: iayt.site-ym.com/general/?type=CONTACT

# Directory of Organizations

**The International Center for Reiki Training (ICRT)**
21421 Hilltop St.
Unit #28
Southfield, MI 48033
Toll-Free: 800-332-8112
Phone: 248-948-8112
Fax: 248-948-9534
Website: www.reiki.org
E-mail: center@reiki.org

**International Chiropractors Association (ICA)**
6400 Arlington Blvd.
Ste. 800
Falls Church, VA 22042
Toll-Free: 800-423-4690
Phone: 703-528-5000
Fax: 703-528-5023
Website: www.chiropractic.org
E-mail: info@chiropractic.org

**International College of Applied Kinesiology (ICAK)**
Website: www.icak.com

**International Feng Shui Guild (IFSG)**
705 B S.E. Melody Ln., Ste. 166
Lees Summit, MO 64063
Phone: 816-246-1898
Website: www.ifsguild.org
E-mail: office@ifsguild.org

**International Institute of Reflexology**
P.O. Box 12642
St Petersburg, FL 33733-2642
Phone: 727-343-4811
Website: www.reflexology-usa.net
E-mail: info@reflexology-usa.net

**International Medical & Dental Hypnotherapy Association (IMDHA)**
8852 SR 3001
Laceyville, PA 18623
Phone: 570-869-1021
Fax: 570-869-1249
Website: www.hypnosisalliance.com
E-mail: info@imdha.com

**National Association for Holistic Aromatherapy (NAHA)**
P.O. Box 27871
Raleigh, NC 27611-7871
Phone: 919-894-0298
Fax: 919-894-0271
Website: naha.org/contact
E-mail: info@naha.org

**National Association of Cognitive-Behavioral Therapists (NACBT)**
P.O. Box 2195
Weirton, WV 26062
Toll-Free: 800-253-0167
Phone: 304-224-2534
Fax: 304-224-2584
Website: www.nacbt.org/contact-us

**National Association of Nutrition Professionals (NANP)**
P.O. Box 348028
Sacramento, CA 95834
Toll-Free: 800-342-8037
Fax: 510-580-9429
Website: www.nanp.org
E-mail: info@nanp.org

### National Ayurvedic Medical Association (NAMA)
8605 Santa Monica Blvd.
#46789
Los Angeles, CA 90069-4109
Toll-Free: 800-669-8914
Website: www.ayurvedanama.
org
E-mail: nama@ayurvedaNAMA.
org

### National Center for Homeopathy (NCH)
1120 Route 73
Ste. 200
Mount Laurel, NJ 08054
Phone: 856-437-4752
Fax: 856-439-0525
Website: www.
homeopathycenter.org

### National Center on Health, Physical Activity and Disability (NCHPAD)
4000 Ridgeway Dr.
Birmingham, AL 35209
Toll-Free: 800-900-8086
Fax: 205-313-7475
Website: www.nchpad.org
E-mail: email@nchpad.org

### National Certification Commission for Acupuncture and Oriental Medicine (NCCAOM)
2025 M St. N.W.
Ste. 800
Washington DC, 20036
Toll-Free: 888-381-1140
Phone: 202-381-1140
Fax: 202-381-1141
Website: www.nccaom.org

### National Headache Foundation
820 N. Orleans
Ste. 217
Chicago, IL 60610-3131
Phone: 312-274-2650
Website: www.headaches.org
E-mail: info@headaches.org

### National Qigong Association (NQA)
P.O. Box 270065
St. Paul, MN 55127
Toll-Free: 888-815-1893
Website: www.nqa.org
E-mail: info@NQA.org

### Reflexology Association of America (RAA)
P.O. Box 44324
Madison, WI 53744-4324
Phone: 980-234-0159
Website: www.reflexology-usa.
org
E-mail: infoRAA@reflexology-
usa.org

### Rolf Institute of Structural Integration (RISI)
5055 Chaparral Ct.
Ste. 103
Boulder, CO 80301
Phone: 303-449-5903
Fax: 303-449-5978
Website: www.rolf.org

### The Thai Yoga Center (TYC)
5401 Saving Grace Ln.
Brooksville, FL 34602
Phone: 706-358-8646
Website: www.thaiyogacenter.
com

**Therapeutic Touch International Association (TTIA)**
P.O. Box 130
Delmar, NY 12054
Phone: 518-325-1185
Fax: 509-693-3537
Website: therapeutictouch.org
E-mail: info@therapeutictouch.org

**The University of Arizona Center for Integrative Medicine (UACIM)**
P.O. Box 245153
Tucson, AZ 85724-5153
Phone: 520-626-6489
Website: integrativemedicine.arizona.edu

**University of Minnesota Center for Spirituality and Healing (CSH)**
420 Delaware St. S.E.
MMC 505
Minneapolis, MN 55455
Phone: 612-624-9459
Fax: 612-626-5280
Website: www.csh.umn.edu
E-mail: csh@umn.edu

**The Vegetarian Resource Group (VRG)**
P.O. Box 1463
Baltimore, MD 21203
Phone: 410-366-8343
Website: www.vrg.org
E-mail: vrg@vrg.org

**Zero Balancing Health Association (ZBHA)**
8640 Guilford Rd.
Ste. 224
Columbia, MD 21046
Phone: 410-381-8956
Fax: 410-381-9634
Website: www.zerobalancing.com

# Index

# *Index*

647

digestive tract
  calcium 265
  detoxification 354
  echinacea 279
  probiotics 295
digoxin, St. John's wort 291
Dilantin®, vitamin D 202
dimethylamylamine (DMAA), banned
  dietary supplements 310
diuretics
  calcium 268
  detoxification 355
  magnesium 239
  zinc 285
DMAA *see* dimethylamylamine
DNA *see* deoxyribonucleic acid
docosahexaenoic acid (DHA)
  dietary supplements regulation 324
  omega-3 fatty acids 247
dong quai
  astragalus 276
  menopausal symptoms 587
dosha, Ayurvedic medicine 75
DRIs *see* Dietary Reference Intakes
drug interactions
  dietary supplements 108
  homeopathy 82
  mental healthcare and CAM 596
  older adults 21
"Drugs—Health Information on the
  Web" (FDA) 51n
DrWeil.com, website address 638
dry mouth (Xerostomia)
  acupuncture 71
  St. John's wort 291
DSHEA *see* Dietary Supplement
  Health and Education Act
DV *see* Daily Value

## E

echinacea
  CAM use and children 14
  dietary supplements 105, 322
  flu and cold 554
  overview 278–9
  seasonal allergies 615
  *see also Echinacea angustifolia;
    Echinacea purpurea*

"Echinacea" (NCCIH) 278n
*Echinacea angustifolia*, immune
  system support supplements 278
*Echinacea purpurea*, immune system
  support supplements 278
eczema
  apitherapy 342
  probiotics 294
  *see also* atopic dermatitis
EGCG *see* epigallocatechin gallate
Elderberry, immune system support
  supplements 280
electrocardiograph (ECG), biofeedback
  therapies 376
electrodermograph (EDG),
  biofeedback therapies 376
electroencephalograph (EEG),
  biofeedback therapies 376
electromagnets
  acupuncture 58
  magnet therapy 493
  osteoarthritis (OA) 612
electromyography (EMG), biofeedback
  376
*Eleutherococcus senticosus*, sports and
  energy supplements 306
EMS *see* eosinophilia-myalgia
  syndrome
endometriosis, chronic pain 530
enemas, Gerson therapy 358
energy drinks
  overview 314–6
  sports and energy supplements 305
"Energy Drinks" (NCCIH) 314n
enzymes
  apitherapy 342
  bogus dietary supplements 48
  calcium 262
  coenzyme $Q_{10}$ ($CoQ_{10}$) 147
  dietary supplements 104, 120
  Gerson therapy 356
  vitamin $B_6$ 185
eosinophilia-myalgia syndrome
  (EMS), sleep disorders 619
ephedra
  sports and energy supplements 311
  traditional Chinese medicine
    (TCM) 97
ephedrine, sports and energy
  supplements 311